Illustrated Handbook of Medical Physiology

Illustrated Handbook of Medical Physiology

C.T. Kirkpatrick BSc MB BCh BAO MD

Medical Director, Pfizer Clinical Research Unit, Kent and Canterbury Hospital, Canterbury, UK

and formerly

Clinical Research Director, BIOS Ltd, Surrey, UK
Medical Officer (Research), Institute of Aviation Medicine, Farnborough, UK
Lecturer in Physiology, Queen's University of Belfast, Northern Ireland

A Wiley Phoenix Publication

JOHN WILEY & SONS
Chichester • New York • Brisbane • Toronto • Singapore

Copyright © 1992 by John Wiley & Sons Ltd.
Baffins Lane, Chichester
West Sussex PO19 1UD, England

Other Wiley Editorial Offices

John Wiley & Sons, Inc., 605 Third Avenue,
New York, NY 10158-0012, USA

Jacaranda Wiley Ltd, G.P.O. Box 859, Brisbane,
Queensland 4001, Australia

John Wiley & Sons (Canada) Ltd, 22 Worcester Road,
Rexdale, Ontario M9W 1L1, Canada

John Wiley & Sons (SEA) Pte Ltd, 37 Jalan Pemimpin #05-04,
Block B, Union Industrial Building, Singapore 2057

Library of Congress Cataloging-in-Publication Data

Kirkpatrick, C. T.
    Illustrated handbook of medical physiology / C. T. Kirkpatrick.
      p.   cm.
    "A Wiley Phoenix Publication."
    Includes index.
    ISBN 0 471 91455 X
    1. Human physiology — Handbooks, manuals, etc. I. Title.
    [DNLM: 1. Physiology — handbooks. QT 39 K59i]
  QP34.5.K565   1991
  612—dc20
DNLM/DLC
for Library of Congress   91-8312
                                                CIP

British Library Cataloguing in Publication Data

A catalogue record of this book is available from the British Library

ISBN 0 471 91455 X

Phototypset by MHL Typesetting Ltd, Coventry
Printed and bound in Great Britain by Courier International Ltd, East Kilbride

Contents

Preface

Physiology, the study of the mechanisms of the body, is essentially a dynamic subject, dealing with active processes and concentrating on explanation rather than description. When I was asked to write a textbook which was to be extensively illustrated, my first response was to wonder just how an illustrator could produce suitable pictures to explain mechanisms rather than describe structures. However, I submitted my first chapter of text, and when I saw the diagrams which were produced, I became very happy with the concept, and satisfied that pictures could, indeed, illuminate the explanation of mechanism.

Inevitably there were mistakes and misunderstandings — for instance, in the description of the autonomic nervous system, an early draft attempted to illustrate the concept of 'fight or flight' with a picture of a jumbo-jet! After many discussions, re-drafts and corrections, we have arrived at a set of illustrations which I feel helps in the understanding of the fundamental mechanisms of the body, and I hope acts as an aid to the retention of the information for the student faced with undergraduate or postgraduate examinations.

The text is based on lecture material evolved during my period in the Physiology Department at Queen's University, but has undergone considerable refinement, digestion and re-synthesis in the light of experience gained in my subsequent appointments. I must thank my colleagues for many helpful discussions during the gestation of the book, but accept full responsibility for the content.

I must also thank my wife, Melanie, for her support during the writing process; she has put up with late nights and early mornings, telephone calls from editor and publishers, piles of paper and floppy disks all over the house, and periods of gloom and despondency. She has encouraged me throughout the project, and given invaluable help.

C.T. KIRKPATRICK
Farnborough, December 1991

Introduction

Physiology is the study of **mechanisms**, of how things work. If we were to consider a motor car, **anatomy** would describe the number and size of the cylinders, the position of the carburettor and the layout of the controls, the capacity of the fuel tank and radiator, and the upholstery of the seats.

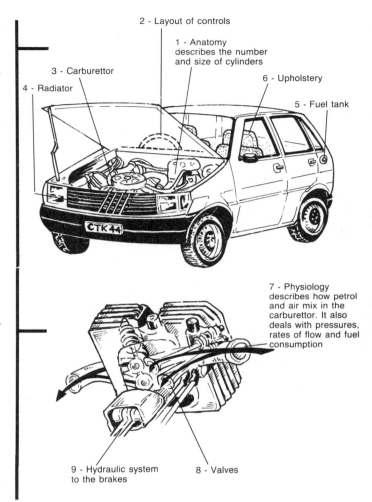

2 - Layout of controls

1 - Anatomy describes the number and size of cylinders

3 - Carburettor

4 - Radiator

6 - Upholstery

5 - Fuel tank

Physiology would describe how petrol and air were mixed in the carburettor, the way in which the combustion of the mixture resulted in expansion of gases, the sequence of opening of the valves, the mechanism of generation of the spark, the transfer of pressure down the hydraulic system to the brakes, and the forces producing acceleration and deceleration. Anatomy would deal with sizes and cubic capacities; physiology would deal with pressures, rates of flow and fuel consumption, revolutions per minute and miles per hour.

7 - Physiology describes how petrol and air mix in the carburettor. It also deals with pressures, rates of flow and fuel consumption

9 - Hydraulic system to the brakes

8 - Valves

Similarly, for the human or animal body anatomy describes the structure, position and size of the various organs; it describes the minute structure of the cells and organelles, and clearly defines the locations of structures relative to their neighbours.

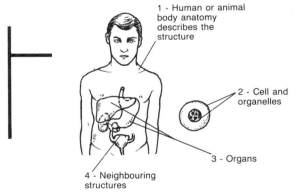

1 - Human or animal body anatomy describes the structure

2 - Cell and organelles

3 - Organs

4 - Neighbouring structures

Physiology gives a function to these structures; it describes the way in which they work; it describes **how** and attempts to discover **why**. Where the anatomist describes the structure, position and size of an organ like the **heart** with its chambers, valves and great vessels, the physiologist describes pressures, rates of flow, the sequence of opening and closing of valves, the migration of waves of electrical excitation and the concentration of oxygen in the blood.

The disciplines of anatomy and physiology are interlinked and inseparable; a knowledge of structure is essential to any discussion of function, and a knowledge of function illuminates what might otherwise be a tedious catalogue of structural data.

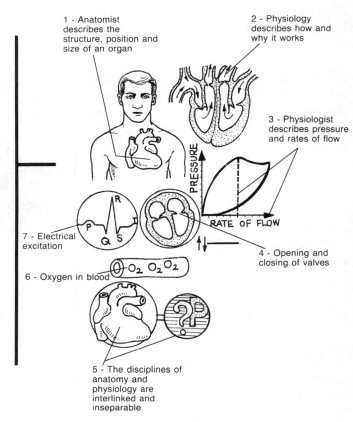

Physiology describes mechanisms at the level of the **cell**, and then how the cells interact in **tissues**. It considers how tissues combine to form **organs**, and how organs function together as **systems**. Finally it shows how several organ systems can be **integrated** to produce an efficiently functioning **body**. The functions of groups of individual bodies and even nations then become the province of the sociologist or the politician.

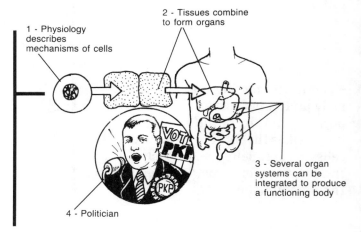

The **cell** is the fundamental building block of the body; many cells can function, at least briefly, in a more or less independent way, but others are so specialized that they can only function as part of a larger group.

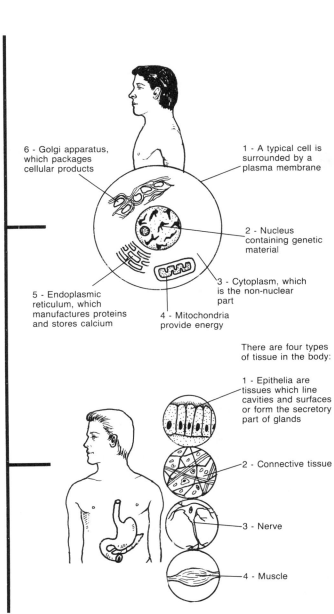

1 - The cell is the fundamental building block of the body

A typical cell is surrounded by a **plasma membrane**, which acts as a boundary and a barrier between that cell and its neighbours or the environment. It usually has a **nucleus** containing the genetic material which programs the manufacture of proteins and other substances within the cell, and it is composed largely of **cytoplasm**, which is the non-nuclear part where most of the cell's functions are performed. Among the **organelles** found in the cytoplasm are the **mitochondria** which provide energy for cellular reactions, **endoplasmic reticulum** where proteins are manufactured or substances like calcium are stored, the **Golgi apparatus** where cellular products are packaged for export, and various vesicles and contractile mechanisms according to the function of the cell.

Groups of cells, sometimes exclusively of one kind, but more often of various related kinds, are linked together to form **tissues** which serve a common function.

There are four types of tissue in the body: epithelia, connective tissue, nerves and muscles. **Epithelia** are tissues which line cavities and surfaces or form the secretory part of glands, and consist of sheets or layers of contiguous cells that form a more or less impermeable barrier.

6 - Golgi apparatus, which packages cellular products

1 - A typical cell is surrounded by a plasma membrane

2 - Nucleus containing genetic material

3 - Cytoplasm, which is the non-nuclear part

5 - Endoplasmic reticulum, which manufactures proteins and stores calcium

4 - Mitochondria provide energy

There are four types of tissue in the body:

1 - Epithelia are tissues which line cavities and surfaces or form the secretory part of glands

2 - Connective tissue

3 - Nerve

4 - Muscle

Connective tissues consist of collections of cells together with non-cellular material which they produce, such as fibres or bone; they act as structural, supporting or packing components of the body.

Muscular tissues have cells which can contract to produce movement, beating of the heart or control of fluid flow in internal organs. **Nervous** tissue contains cells with the specialized property of conducting electrical impulses and transmitting information around the body. All the tissues of the body can be placed in one of these four categories.

Organs are the functional units of the body, such as the heart, brain, kidney and spleen, and can be seen as separate entities when one looks inside the body or at the body surface. An organ may consist predominantly of one type of cell or tissue, or may contain a very large variety of tissues and cells; an organ may have a single specialized function, such as the heart, or it may have very many functions, like the liver.

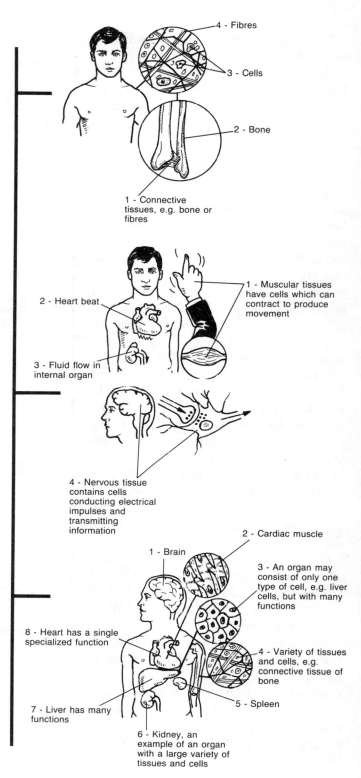

4 - Fibres

3 - Cells

2 - Bone

1 - Connective tissues, e.g. bone or fibres

1 - Muscular tissues have cells which can contract to produce movement

2 - Heart beat

3 - Fluid flow in internal organ

4 - Nervous tissue contains cells conducting electrical impulses and transmitting information

1 - Brain

2 - Cardiac muscle

3 - An organ may consist of only one type of cell, e.g. liver cells, but with many functions

8 - Heart has a single specialized function

4 - Variety of tissues and cells, e.g. connective tissue of bone

5 - Spleen

7 - Liver has many functions

6 - Kidney, an example of an organ with a large variety of tissues and cells

While several organs have a more or less independent function, the majority of organs are parts of more complex **organ systems**, in which groups of related organs function together.

For instance, the digestive system consists of the stomach and intestine together with a number of accessory glands.

The circulatory system consists of the heart and all the blood vessels.

The nervous system consists of the brain and spinal cord, as well as all the nerves which supply individual organs. Many of the organ systems are interconnected and interdependent; for example, almost all the body's organs receive branches of the circulatory and nervous systems.

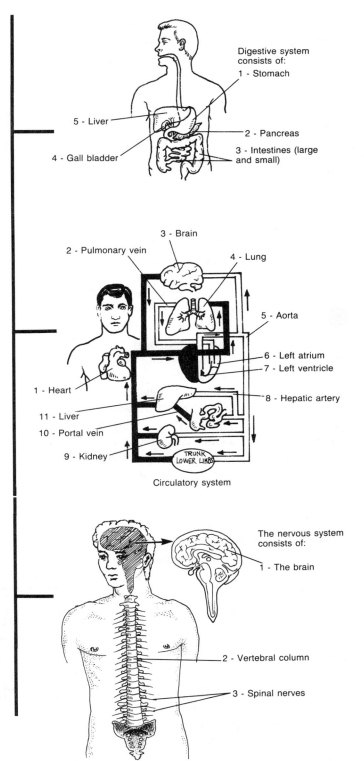

Digestive system consists of:
1 - Stomach
2 - Pancreas
3 - Intestines (large and small)
4 - Gall bladder
5 - Liver

3 - Brain
2 - Pulmonary vein
4 - Lung
5 - Aorta
6 - Left atrium
7 - Left ventricle
8 - Hepatic artery
1 - Heart
11 - Liver
10 - Portal vein
9 - Kidney
TRUNK LOWER LIMBS

Circulatory system

The nervous system consists of:
1 - The brain
2 - Vertebral column
3 - Spinal nerves

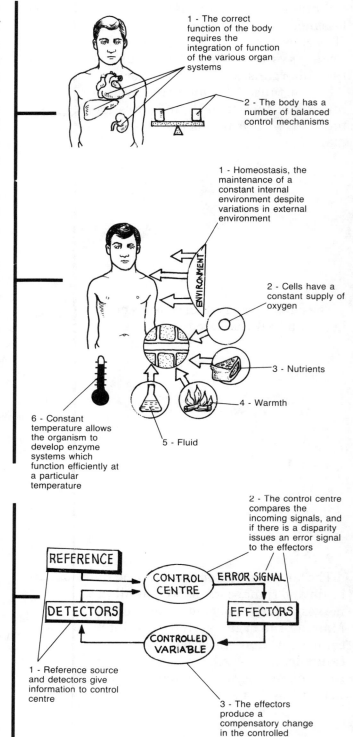

The correct function of the body requires the **integration** of function of the various organ systems, and much of this book will describe the way in which this integration is achieved. The body has a number of very delicately balanced control mechanisms, whose function is to ensure the **constancy of the internal environment**; such mechanisms are known as **homeostatic** mechanisms.

Homeostasis, the maintenance of a constant internal environment despite variations in external conditions, is a prerequisite for independent existence. If cells can expect to have a constant supply of oxygen, nutrients, warmth and fluid they can become specialized in their tasks, as they no longer have to expend energy in foraging for food or eliminating waste; a constant temperature allows the organism to develop enzyme systems which function efficiently at one particular temperature. It is, of course, necessary to allocate some cells and organs to the specialized tasks of keeping the internal environment constant for all the other cells.

All homeostatic mechanisms have a number of common components. These include one or more **detectors** to give information to the control mechanism about the variable being controlled; a **source of reference** which informs the system about what is the expected or preferred value of the variable; a **control centre** which compares the incoming information from the detectors with the reference information, and responds to any errors with an appropriate signal to one or more **effectors** which produce changes in the value of the variable being controlled.

1 - The correct function of the body requires the integration of function of the various organ systems

2 - The body has a number of balanced control mechanisms

1 - Homeostasis, the maintenance of a constant internal environment despite variations in external environment

2 - Cells have a constant supply of oxygen

3 - Nutrients

4 - Warmth

5 - Fluid

6 - Constant temperature allows the organism to develop enzyme systems which function efficiently at a particular temperature

REFERENCE

CONTROL CENTRE

ERROR SIGNAL

DETECTORS

EFFECTORS

CONTROLLED VARIABLE

2 - The control centre compares the incoming signals, and if there is a disparity issues an error signal to the effectors

1 - Reference source and detectors give information to control centre

3 - The effectors produce a compensatory change in the controlled variable

Detectors may be of two types: those which inform about the absolute value of a variable, and those which inform about the rate of change in the variable.

An important feature of most homeostatic mechanisms is **redundancy**; there may be several different types of detectors conveying information to the control centre by different pathways, and there may be a number of parallel effector mechanisms responding to the signals generated by the controller. The control system may be able to operate with only one input and one output, but more normally the controller evaluates data from a number of sources and uses more than one pathway for corrective action. If the controller has information arriving along diverse detector pathways, it is better able to decide on the necessary action; the more alternative effector pathways that are open to the controller, the more precise and flexible will be the control afforded by the system.

Most homeostatic mechanisms make use of **negative feedback**; that is, the signal sent to the effectors produces a change opposite in direction to the change sensed by the detectors. For example, if the arterial blood pressure **falls** due to blood loss or postural change, the regulatory centre sends signals to the heart and blood vessels which accelerate the heart and constrict the vessels, causing a **rise** in pressure.

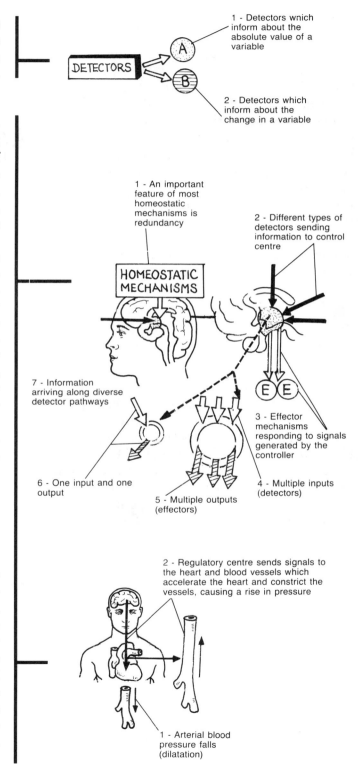

1 - Detectors which inform about the absolute value of a variable

2 - Detectors which inform about the change in a variable

1 - An important feature of most homeostatic mechanisms is redundancy

2 - Different types of detectors sending information to control centre

7 - Information arriving along diverse detector pathways

3 - Effector mechanisms responding to signals generated by the controller

6 - One input and one output

5 - Multiple outputs (effectors)

4 - Multiple inputs (detectors)

2 - Regulatory centre sends signals to the heart and blood vessels which accelerate the heart and constrict the vessels, causing a rise in pressure

1 - Arterial blood pressure falls (dilatation)

The control of body temperature illustrates many of these features. If the body temperature is altered from its 'normal' value of 37 °C (98.6 °F) a **control centre** in the brain receives sensory information from **temperature receptors**, both in the skin and more centrally, and issues commands to **effector organs** such as the circulatory system (to modify the blood flow through the skin and eliminate or conserve heat) and the sweating or shivering apparatus (to eliminate or generate heat).

Other important homeostatic mechanisms include those which regulate the volume and composition of the blood and tissue cells, the pH of the tissue fluids, the supply of oxygen to the tissues and the posture of the body. These will form much of the content of the remaining chapters of this book.

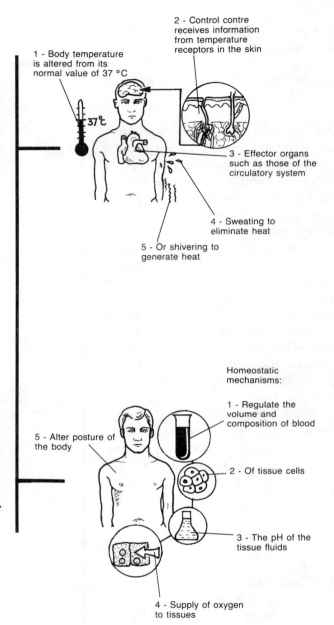

1 - Body temperature is altered from its normal value of 37 °C

2 - Control contre receives information from temperature receptors in the skin

3 - Effector organs such as those of the circulatory system

4 - Sweating to eliminate heat

5 - Or shivering to generate heat

Homeostatic mechanisms:

1 - Regulate the volume and composition of blood

2 - Of tissue cells

3 - The pH of the tissue fluids

4 - Supply of oxygen to tissues

5 - Alter posture of the body

The Nervous System

Introduction to the Nervous System

The next few chapters will describe various aspects of the nervous system, including the function of the neurones and synapses (its component building blocks); the sensory system with its receptors and complex pathways for information flow; the motor system with the mucles and the nervous pathways for their control; and the autonomic nervous system for the control of visceral function and temperature.

This chapter presents a broad outline of the functions and structure of the nervous system. The most important functions are the acquisition of **information**, the **communication** of this information to the correct destination, and the **control** of the body's function, with execution of actions appropriate to the incoming information. The human brain is also capable of **abstract thinking**, an activity about which physiologists still have very little information.

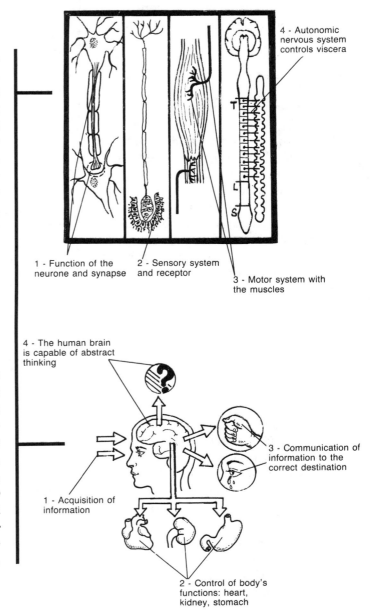

4 - Autonomic nervous system controls viscera

1 - Function of the neurone and synapse

2 - Sensory system and receptor

3 - Motor system with the muscles

4 - The human brain is capable of abstract thinking

3 - Communication of information to the correct destination

1 - Acquisition of information

2 - Control of body's functions: heart, kidney, stomach

The nervous system receives signals from sense organs, registers them in the brain, and makes muscles move, glands secrete and blood vessels constrict or dilate. It is the initiator and coordinator of the body's actions; even when some body systems seem to be largely under non-nervous, hormonal (chemical) control, there is almost always a step involving the nervous system somewhere in the process.

The direction of signals in the nervous system is conventionally defined in relation to the centre, and relative to the 'highest' parts or those nearest to the head. Signals coming from the periphery towards the spinal cord and brain are known as **afferent** (or 'coming towards') signals, while those going from the brain or spine out along the nerves to the muscles or glands are known as **efferent** (or 'going away') signals. The terms afferent and efferent look and sound so similar that they can be confusing; as far as possible this nomenclature will not be used in this book. The more explicit terms 'sensory' for incoming information and 'motor' for outgoing information will be used where appropriate, but the reader should be familiar with the other terms in case of encountering them in other textbooks of physiology or medicine.

There are two main parts: the **central nervous system**, comprising the brain and the spinal cord, and the **peripheral nervous system**, comprising the sensory receptors, the connections to muscles and glands, and the nerves which join these structures to the central nervous system.

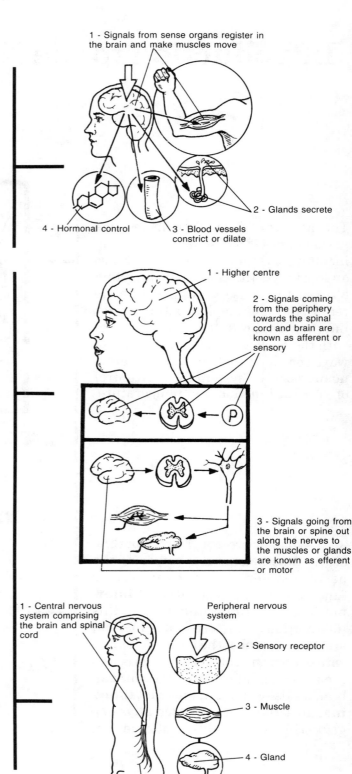

1 - Signals from sense organs register in the brain and make muscles move

2 - Glands secrete

3 - Blood vessels constrict or dilate

4 - Hormonal control

1 - Higher centre

2 - Signals coming from the periphery towards the spinal cord and brain are known as afferent or sensory

3 - Signals going from the brain or spine out along the nerves to the muscles or glands are known as efferent or motor

1 - Central nervous system comprising the brain and spinal cord

Peripheral nervous system

2 - Sensory receptor

3 - Muscle

4 - Gland

5 - Nerves

The central nervous system consists of the spinal cord and the brain, as mentioned earlier. The organization of the spinal cord is simpler and will be described first. In the centre of the spinal cord is the **grey matter**, so called because it appears slightly greyish on cross-section. It is composed largely of the cell bodies of **neurones** or nerve cells, and the surrounding **white matter** is composed of the long processes or nerve fibres (**axons**) which arise from these cell bodies. White matter is white because most of the axons are covered with **myelin**, a fatty insulating material.

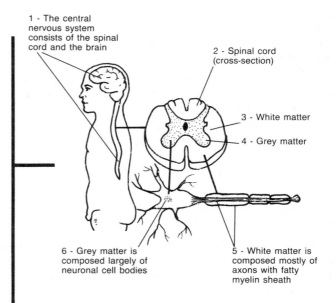

1 - The central nervous system consists of the spinal cord and the brain

2 - Spinal cord (cross-section)

3 - White matter

4 - Grey matter

6 - Grey matter is composed largely of neuronal cell bodies

5 - White matter is composed mostly of axons with fatty myelin sheath

The spinal cord is **segmented**, in that the structure and organization are based on a series of similar segments which are repeated along the cord. In each segment there are spinal nerves entering and leaving, and the input and output side of each segment have certain connections to produce simple reflexes. This segmentation is also reflected in the structure of the backbone with its separate vertebrae, and the segmental spinal nerves leave the spinal canal in the gaps between the vertebrae. In the thoracic region the segmentation is further seen in the repetitive structure of the ribs, with their intercostal muscles, blood vessels and nerves.

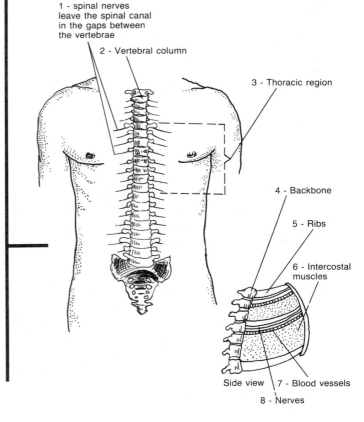

1 - spinal nerves leave the spinal canal in the gaps between the vertebrae

2 - Vertebral column

3 - Thoracic region

4 - Backbone

5 - Ribs

6 - Intercostal muscles

Side view

7 - Blood vessels

8 - Nerves

At the upper end of the nervous system the segmentation is lost in favour of **cephalization**, the specialization of structure and function at the head end of the system. There is an increased concentration of sensory organs around the brain, and in particular the organs of special sense (the eyes, ears and chemical sensors of the nose and mouth) are located in the head.

The lowest part of the brain, the **brain stem**, is really the upward continuation of the spinal cord, with the main nerve fibre tracts running longitudinally through it. However, it also contains a number of integrative centres for some of the major body systems, notably the cardiovascular and respiratory centres, as well as the sensory nuclei for most of the cranial nerves. The brain stem is divided into the **medulla oblongata** (lowest), the **pons** (or bridge, since there is a very large transversely running tract of nerve fibres here) and the **midbrain**.

1 - Sensory organs around the brain, in particular the organs of special sense for eyes, ears, nose and mouth

6 - Centres for the cardiovascular and respiratory systems

5 - Midbrain or uppermost part of brain stem

4 - Pons with transverse tract of nerve fibres

3 - Medulla oblongata or lowest part of brain stem

2 - Sensory nuclei

1 - Spinal cord

The same distinction between grey matter (predominantly cell bodies) and white matter (predominantly nerve fibre tracts) is found in the brain, but the arrangement is not so simple. In the lower parts of the brain the long fibre tracts can still be recognized as the white matter, but the grey matter is much more broken up than in the spinal cord, and is organized as a very large number of separate nuclei or clumps of cells, with extremely complicated interconnections.

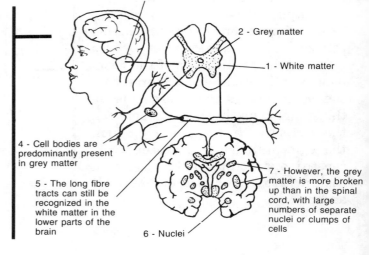

3 - In the lower parts of the brain the long fibre tracts can be recognized as white matter

2 - Grey matter

1 - White matter

4 - Cell bodies are predominantly present in grey matter

5 - The long fibre tracts can still be recognized in the white matter in the lower parts of the brain

6 - Nuclei

7 - However, the grey matter is more broken up than in the spinal cord, with large numbers of separate nuclei or clumps of cells

In the highest parts of the brain, the cerebrum and cerebellum, there are central areas where large clumps of grey matter are found ('nuclei' or 'basal ganglia'); these are surrounded by extensive tracts of white matter, and then on the surface is found another layer of grey matter, the cerebral or cerebellar **cortex**. The outermost layer of the brain is thus composed largely of nerve cell bodies with their attached processes.

1 - Cerebrum

2 - Cerebellum

3 - Large clumps of grey matter: 'nuclei' or 'basal ganglia'

4 - Extensive tracts of white matter

5 - Cerebral and cerebellar cortex of grey matter is composed of nerve cell bodies and is the outermost layer of the brain

When the brain is viewed from the top we see the **cerebrum**, which is split by a deep fissure into two hemispheres; each hemisphere when viewed from the side is split into lobes. The surface of the cerebrum is extensively folded, resulting in an enormous surface area and allowing for the presence of a very complex cerebral cortex with a consequently huge capacity for higher brain functions. The folds are known as **gyri**, and the crevices between them are known as **sulci**.

1 - Cerebrum is split by a deep fissure into two hemispheres

2 - Folds are known as gyri

5 - The folds and gyri allow a large surface area of the cerebral cortex with a huge capacity for higher brain functions

3 - Sulci

4 - Cerebral hemisphere (seen in cross-section)

The cerebellum, which is found under the cerebrum and behind the brain stem, is also extensively folded, with much finer gyri and sulci than in the cerebral cortex. Each part of the brain stem is connected to the cerebellum, through the superior, middle and inferior cerebellar **peduncles**.

1 - Cerebrum

7 - Posterior view of brain stem with cerebellum removed

2 - Brain stem

3 - Cerebellum has finer gyri and sulci and is extensively folded

6 - Superior

5 - Middle

4 - Inferior

Cerebellar peduncles which are connected to the brain stem

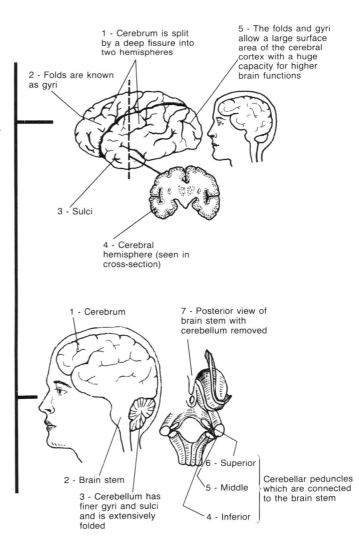

When the brain is split in half sagitt-ally and viewed from the midline, the inner surfaces of the cerebral hemi-spheres are seen, as well as the large **commissures** or fibre tracts which join the two hemispheres. Another impor-tant structure seen in the midline is the **hypothalamus**, an area where most of the body's visceral functions are regulated. We can also see two of the main cavities of the brain, the third and fourth ventricles (the first two are buried deep within the cerebral hemispheres).

The peripheral nervous system con-sists of the spinal nerves, the cranial nerves and the associated sensory and motor structures. The spinal nerves leave the spinal cord in pairs, one from each segment of the cord. Each spinal nerve has two roots, a dorsal root which consists almost entirely of sensory nerve fibres bringing information into the central nervous system, and a ventral root which consists almost entirely of motor fibres carrying infor-mation out from the nervous system to the muscles and glands. The roots fuse within the spinal canal (inside the bones of the vertebral column or back-bone) and leave the spine (as mixed spinal nerves) in the gaps between vertebrae.

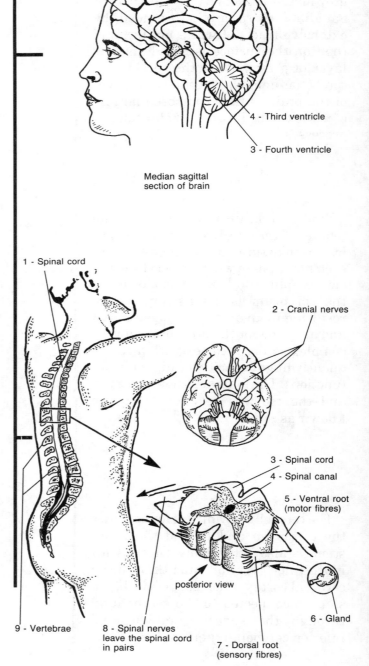

2 - Hypothalamus

1 - Commissures or fibre tracts which join the two hemispheres

4 - Third ventricle

3 - Fourth ventricle

Median sagittal section of brain

1 - Spinal cord

2 - Cranial nerves

3 - Spinal cord

4 - Spinal canal

5 - Ventral root (motor fibres)

6 - Gland

posterior view

7 - Dorsal root (sensory fibres)

8 - Spinal nerves leave the spinal cord in pairs

9 - Vertebrae

The cranial nerves, i.e. the nerves attached to various parts of the brain, are functionally very similar to the spinal nerves but are not arranged in such a stereotyped manner, and they often carry complex information relating to the organs of special sense, which are found in the head near to the brain.

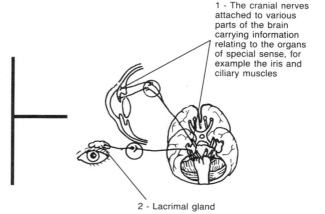

1 - The cranial nerves attached to various parts of the brain carrying information relating to the organs of special sense, for example the iris and ciliary muscles

2 - Lacrimal gland

CELL TYPES IN THE NERVOUS SYSTEM

The **neurones** are the main functional cell type in the nervous system; they are the cells which carry the signals around the body. Almost as important are the supporting and nutritive cells. Within the central nervous system these are called **glia**, and there are several types, including the oligodendrocytes which make myelin, the insulating material for nerve axons. In the peripheral nerves the nutritive, supporting and myelinating functions are provided by the **Schwann cells**.

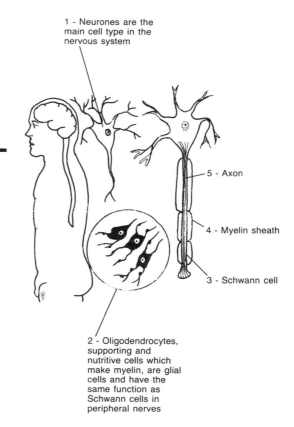

1 - Neurones are the main cell type in the nervous system

5 - Axon

4 - Myelin sheath

3 - Schwann cell

2 - Oligodendrocytes, supporting and nutritive cells which make myelin, are glial cells and have the same function as Schwann cells in peripheral nerves

COVERINGS OF THE CENTRAL NERVOUS SYSTEM

The brain and spinal cord are covered by a series of protective layers, the **meninges**. The layer closest to the brain surface is the **pia mater**, a fine epithelial layer under which the major blood vessels run before they split into their finer branches supplying the brain tissue. Surrounding the pia mater is a fluid-filled cavity, on the outside of which is another layer, the **arachnoid mater**. This has numerous fibrous vascular connections which run between the arachnoid and pia, bridging the pia—arachnoid space and looking like a spider's web, which is why the arachnoid (web-like) is so called. Around the arachnoid, and lining the inner surfaces of the skull and vertebral bones, is the **dura mater** (dura = hard), which is continuous with the periosteum.

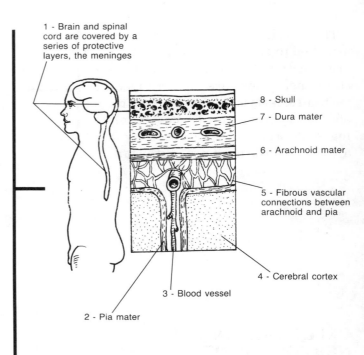

1 - Brain and spinal cord are covered by a series of protective layers, the meninges

8 - Skull

7 - Dura mater

6 - Arachnoid mater

5 - Fibrous vascular connections between arachnoid and pia

4 - Cerebral cortex

3 - Blood vessel

2 - Pia mater

THE VENTRICULAR SYSTEM

The pia—arachnoid space, or subarachnoid space, is continuous with a series of cavities inside the brain, called **ventricles**. There is one **lateral** ventricle inside the centre of each cerebral hemisphere, and these communicate with the **third** ventricle through narrow canals, the **foramina of Munro**. The third ventricle communicates with the **fourth** ventricle, located between the cerebellum and the back of the brain stem, through the **aqueduct of Sylvius**. The fourth ventricle opens into the subarachnoid space through two laterally placed **foramina of Magendie** and a medial **foramen of Luschka**.

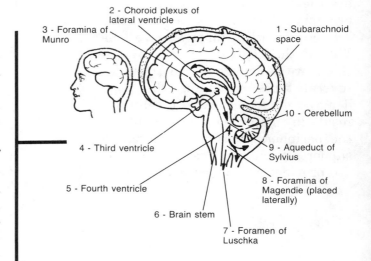

2 - Choroid plexus of lateral ventricle

3 - Foramina of Munro

1 - Subarachnoid space

4 - Third ventricle

10 - Cerebellum

9 - Aqueduct of Sylvius

8 - Foramina of Magendie (placed laterally)

5 - Fourth ventricle

6 - Brain stem

7 - Foramen of Luschka

THE CEREBROSPINAL FLUID

The ventricles are lined with a fine epithelial layer, the **ependyma**, which is continuous with the lining of the central canal of the spinal cord. Each ventricle contains a highly vascular meshwork of tissue, the **choroid plexus**, which secretes the fluid filling the ventricles and the subarachnoid space, the **cerebrospinal fluid (CSF)**. This watery fluid is slightly different in composition from plasma, and is thus not a simple ultrafiltrate; there is a potential difference of about +5 mV between the CSF and the blood, suggesting that there may be active transport mechanisms operating, and the pH remains at an almost constant level of 7.33 despite wide variations in the pH of plasma. There is considerably less protein in the CSF than in plasma, rather less glucose and potassium but rather more sodium and chloride.

The CSF is continuously produced in the choroid plexuses, at a rate of about 700–800 ml per day, sufficient to exchange the whole CSF volume every 4 hours. It flows from ventricle to ventricle through the various foramina and aqueducts and then into the subarachnoid space around the brain and spinal cord. It becomes reabsorbed into the blood again in **arachnoid villi**, which are invaginations of the subarachnoid space into the walls of large blood vessels in the skull, such as the **superior sagittal sinus**. If any of the channels for the flow of CSF become blocked, the pressure within the subarachnoid space or the ventricle system increases, and **hydrocephalus** ('water on the brain') results. Such blockage may be congenital, or may result from infections of the meninges or brain tumours.

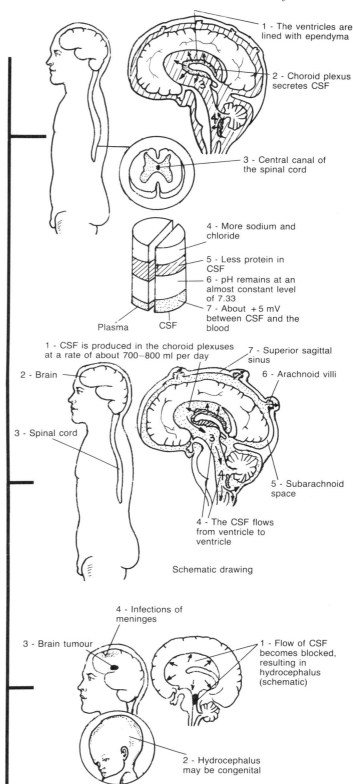

1 - The ventricles are lined with ependyma

2 - Choroid plexus secretes CSF

3 - Central canal of the spinal cord

4 - More sodium and chloride

5 - Less protein in CSF

6 - pH remains at an almost constant level of 7.33

7 - About +5 mV between CSF and the blood

Plasma   CSF

1 - CSF is produced in the choroid plexuses at a rate of about 700–800 ml per day

2 - Brain

3 - Spinal cord

7 - Superior sagittal sinus

6 - Arachnoid villi

5 - Subarachnoid space

4 - The CSF flows from ventricle to ventricle

Schematic drawing

4 - Infections of meninges

3 - Brain tumour

1 - Flow of CSF becomes blocked, resulting in hydrocephalus (schematic)

2 - Hydrocephalus may be congenital

Samples of CSF may be obtained in patients by the procedure known as **lumbar puncture**. The spinal cord is rather shorter than the length of the spinal canal within the vertebrae, and the spinal subarachnoid space extends for some distance distal to the end of the cord, so it can be punctured safely at about the level of the space between the 3rd and 4th or 4th and 5th lumbar vertebrae. The puncture must be performed with full aseptic precautions; it is usual to measure the CSF pressure with a simple water manometer, and to observe whether it rises and falls with respiration (reflecting changes in venous pressure in the cerebral sinuses).

If the neck veins are manually compressed, there is normally an increase in CSF pressure as reabsorption is temporarily halted; failure of the pressure to rise indicates blockage in the system (Queckenstedt's test). The normal pressure of CSF is about 10 cm of water (100 mm water, almost 1 kPa).

Following the measurement of pressure, some of the fluid is withdrawn for laboratory analysis and microscopic examination.

4 - Spinal cord

3 - Vertebrae

2 - Water manometer to measure pressure of CSF. It rises and falls with respiration. Normal pressure of CSF is 10 cm of water

5 - Spinal subarachnoid space

1 - CSF may be obtained in patients by lumbar puncture at the level of the space between 3rd and 4th or 4th and 5th lumbar vertebrae

1 - Neck veins are manually compressed; CSF pressure failing to rise indicates blockage in the system

2 - Fluid is withdrawn for microscopic examination

The **functions** of the CSF include support and protection against damage (the brain is of a very soft and fragile consistency, and 'floats' in the CSF); the removal of excess metabolites, rather like the function of lymphatic vessels elsewhere; and the buffering of the brain against large changes in the concentration of substances in the plasma.

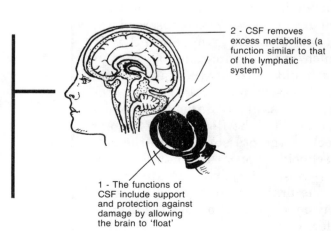

2 - CSF removes excess metabolites (a function similar to that of the lymphatic system)

1 - The functions of CSF include support and protection against damage by allowing the brain to 'float'

The blood supply to the brain comes from branches of the carotid arteries and from the vertebral arteries which arise from the subclavians. The various arteries form a rather complex network at the base of the brain (the 'circle of Willis') from which the anterior, middle and posterior cerebral arteries arise to supply blood to the substance of the brain. If one of the major arteries becomes blocked, it is often still possible for the brain to obtain all of the blood which it needs from the other arteries in the network.

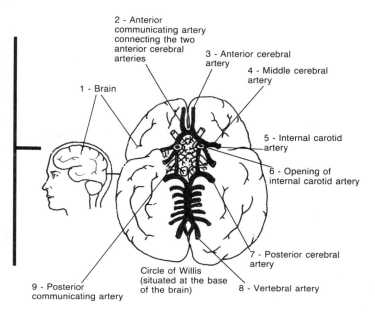

2 - Anterior communicating artery connecting the two anterior cerebral arteries

1 - Brain

3 - Anterior cerebral artery

4 - Middle cerebral artery

5 - Internal carotid artery

6 - Opening of internal carotid artery

7 - Posterior cerebral artery

Circle of Willis (situated at the base of the brain)

9 - Posterior communicating artery

8 - Vertebral artery

The brain requires a very high rate of blood flow (about 15% of the cardiac output), as its metabolic rate is very high (largely as a result of the operation of ion pumps — see next chapter) and it cannot store glucose or use anaerobic metabolism.

The rate of cerebral blood flow is very sensitive to changes in arterial oxygen and carbon dioxide levels; both hypoxia and hypercapnia cause dilatation of cerebral vessels, which can produce cerebral oedema in patients with head injury.

It is thus very important that brain-injured patients be artificially ventilated to prevent a catastrophic rise in intracranial pressure; this attention to the respiratory functions has an even higher priority than any specific neurosurgical treatment.

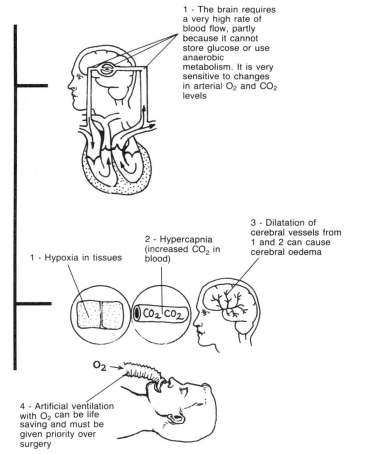

1 - The brain requires a very high rate of blood flow, partly because it cannot store glucose or use anaerobic metabolism. It is very sensitive to changes in arterial O_2 and CO_2 levels

3 - Dilatation of cerebral vessels from 1 and 2 can cause cerebral oedema

2 - Hypercapnia (increased CO_2 in blood)

1 - Hypoxia in tissues

CO_2 CO_2

O_2 →

4 - Artificial ventilation with O_2 can be life saving and must be given priority over surgery

The cerebral capillaries are much less permeable to many of the constituents of plasma than are capillaries elsewhere in the body. The endothelial cells have a continuous band of tight junctions, and most substances which gain access to the interstitial fluid of the brain must pass through the cells lining the capillaries, rather than through gaps between the cells. It is thus easier for lipid-soluble substances and drugs to get access to the interstitial spaces than for ions and polar molecules; the same is true of the blood vessels of the choroid plexus, and these barriers to free diffusion are known as the **blood–brain barrier** and the **blood–CSF barrier**.

There is one region of the brain where the blood–brain barrier is incomplete: this is the hypothalamus, where the plasma constituents can permeate freely into the interstitial space, and where there are numerous receptors which sample the plasma and measure its osmolality and the concentrations of constituents such as glucose and hormones.

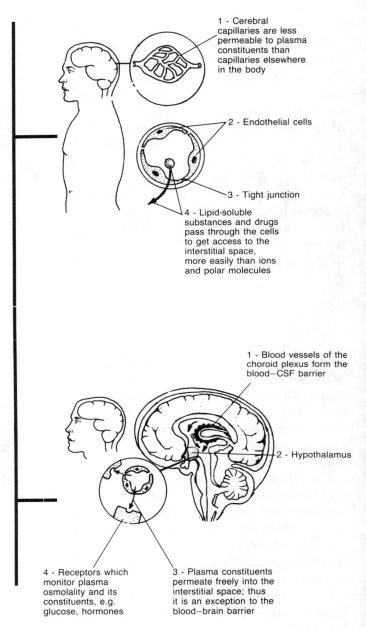

1 - Cerebral capillaries are less permeable to plasma constituents than capillaries elsewhere in the body

2 - Endothelial cells

3 - Tight junction

4 - Lipid-soluble substances and drugs pass through the cells to get access to the interstitial space, more easily than ions and polar molecules

1 - Blood vessels of the choroid plexus form the blood–CSF barrier

2 - Hypothalamus

4 - Receptors which monitor plasma osmolality and its constituents, e.g. glucose, hormones

3 - Plasma constituents permeate freely into the interstitial space; thus it is an exception to the blood–brain barrier

Principles of Excitable Membranes

An excitable membrane is one which is capable of producing an electrical change in response to an external or internal stimulus, which can be conducted or propagated along the membrane, resulting in contraction of the cell or the release of some chemical by the cell.

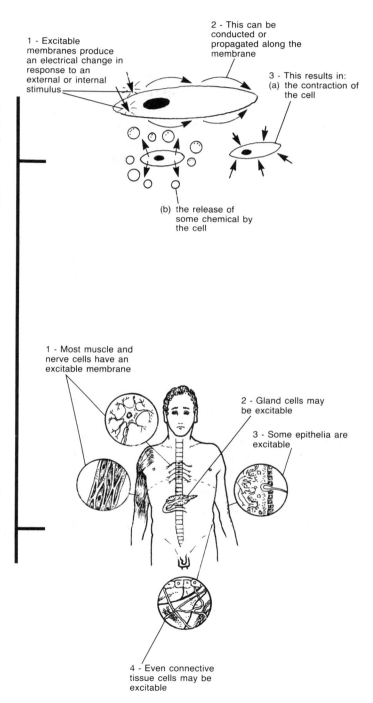

1 - Excitable membranes produce an electrical change in response to an external or internal stimulus

2 - This can be conducted or propagated along the membrane

3 - This results in:
(a) the contraction of the cell

(b) the release of some chemical by the cell

1 - Most muscle and nerve cells have an excitable membrane

2 - Gland cells may be excitable

3 - Some epithelia are excitable

4 - Even connective tissue cells may be excitable

Most muscle and nerve cells have excitable membranes, but excitability is also a feature of many gland cells, some epithelia and even some of the cells found in connective tissue.

An example of a chain of excitable cells is provided by a **simple reflex arc** such as the familiar knee-jerk response. A sharp tap to the patellar tendon of the flexed knee produces a brisk contraction of the quadriceps muscle which straightens the knee.

The tap on the tendon stretches the muscle, activating stretch **receptors** (muscle spindles) in the muscle. This provokes the membrane of the sensory nerve (connected to the receptors) to generate an **action potential**, a large rapid change in the potential difference across the membrane. This action potential is conducted along the nerve until it reaches the spinal cord, where it causes the release of chemicals (neurotransmitters) from the end of the nerve.

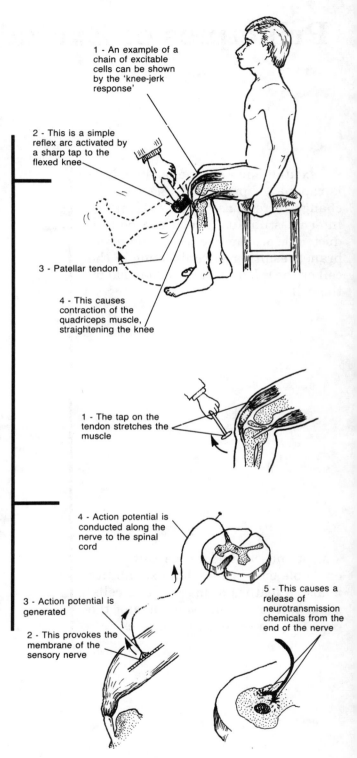

1 - An example of a chain of excitable cells can be shown by the 'knee-jerk response'

2 - This is a simple reflex arc activated by a sharp tap to the flexed knee

3 - Patellar tendon

4 - This causes contraction of the quadriceps muscle, straightening the knee

1 - The tap on the tendon stretches the muscle

4 - Action potential is conducted along the nerve to the spinal cord

3 - Action potential is generated

2 - This provokes the membrane of the sensory nerve

5 - This causes a release of neurotransmission chemicals from the end of the nerve

The chemicals diffuse across a very narrow gap (**synapse**) between nerve cells and initiate excitation in another nerve cell.

This second nerve cell propagates an action potential out along its peripheral fibre (axon) until it reaches the muscle; there it causes release of another chemical transmitter close to the surface of a muscle cell, and this chemical causes excitation of the muscle cell membrane.

An action potential is propagated all along the muscle membrane and causes the contraction of the muscle fibres, producing movement of the knee.

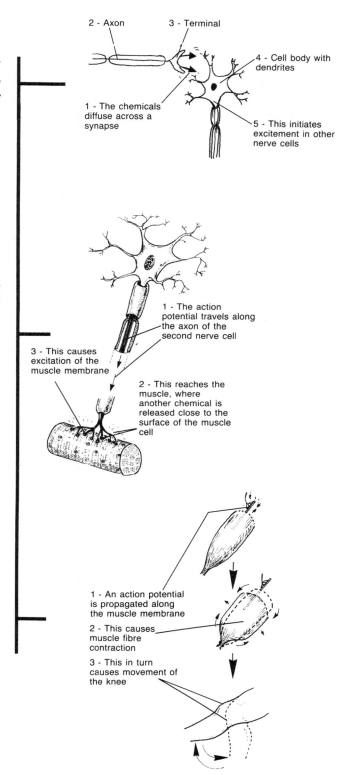

2 - Axon   3 - Terminal

4 - Cell body with dendrites

1 - The chemicals diffuse across a synapse

5 - This initiates excitement in other nerve cells

1 - The action potential travels along the axon of the second nerve cell

3 - This causes excitation of the muscle membrane

2 - This reaches the muscle, where another chemical is released close to the surface of the muscle cell

1 - An action potential is propagated along the muscle membrane

2 - This causes muscle fibre contraction

3 - This in turn causes movement of the knee

STRUCTURE OF NERVE CELLS

A typical nerve cell has a **cell body** or **soma** which lies in the central nervous system or in a ganglion, and one or more long processes which connect the neurone with other elements of the nervous system.

Most nerve cells or **neurones** have one very long process or **axon**, which may be a few millimetres long or up to a metre in the case of the nerves supplying the toes, and a series of short processes known as **dendrites** because they are arranged like the branches of a tree.

The cell body or soma contains the nucleus, which has a prominent nucleolus.

In the cytoplasm there are numerous mitochondria to supply energy for cellular metabolism, and a prominent Golgi apparatus and numerous **Nissl** granules, which are concerned with the synthesis of substances which are to be transported to remote parts of the cell.

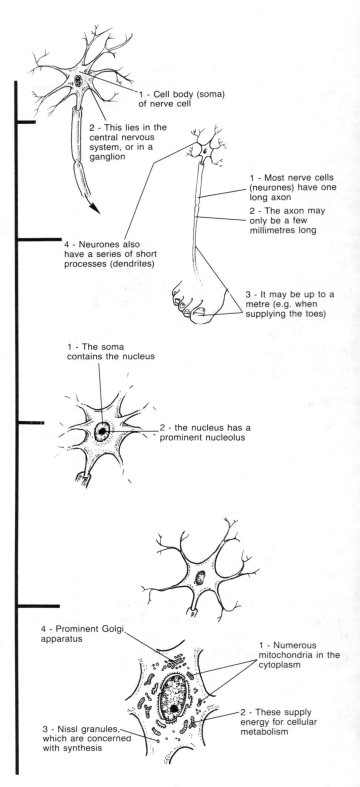

1 - Cell body (soma) of nerve cell

2 - This lies in the central nervous system, or in a ganglion

1 - Most nerve cells (neurones) have one long axon

2 - The axon may only be a few millimetres long

4 - Neurones also have a series of short processes (dendrites)

3 - It may be up to a metre (e.g. when supplying the toes)

1 - The soma contains the nucleus

2 - the nucleus has a prominent nucleolus

4 - Prominent Golgi apparatus

1 - Numerous mitochondria in the cytoplasm

3 - Nissl granules, which are concerned with synthesis

2 - These supply energy for cellular metabolism

The axon has a central core of cytoplasm (often called axoplasm) surrounded by the cell membrane. In the axoplasm there are fine filaments, the **neurofilaments**, whose function is still obscure, and a collection of fine tubules which run axially along the axon, carrying neurotransmitters and other chemicals which are synthesized in the soma, out to the more peripheral parts of the cell.

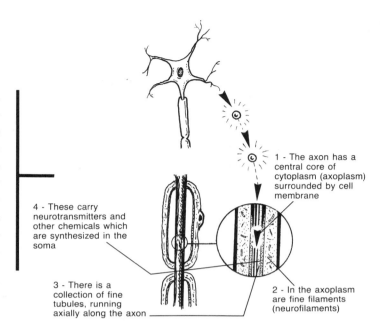

1 - The axon has a central core of cytoplasm (axoplasm) surrounded by cell membrane

2 - In the axoplasm are fine filaments (neurofilaments)

3 - There is a collection of fine tubules, running axially along the axon

4 - These carry neurotransmitters and other chemicals which are synthesized in the soma

Around the outside of the axon are found various supportive and nutritive cells, which are called **Schwann** cells in the peripheral nerves, but are called **glial** cells in the central nervous system.

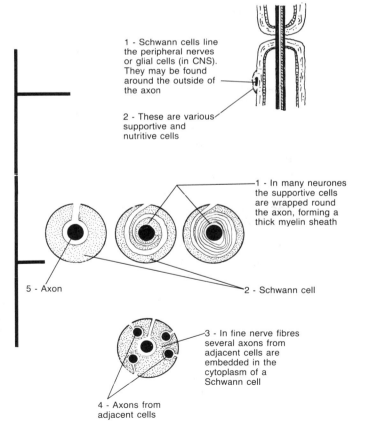

1 - Schwann cells line the peripheral nerves or glial cells (in CNS). They may be found around the outside of the axon

2 - These are various supportive and nutritive cells

In many neurones the supportive cells are wrapped round and round the axon like a Swiss roll, to form a thick **myelin sheath**, but in the finer nerve fibres several axons from adjacent cells are embedded in the cytoplasm of a single Schwann cell, which has a simpler structure than in myelinated nerves.

1 - In many neurones the supportive cells are wrapped round the axon, forming a thick myelin sheath

2 - Schwann cell

5 - Axon

3 - In fine nerve fibres several axons from adjacent cells are embedded in the cytoplasm of a Schwann cell

4 - Axons from adjacent cells

The dendrites are usually finer than the axon process, and branch extensively; they are usually unmyelinated, and are found exclusively within the central nervous system or the substance of the peripheral ganglion in which the soma lies.

The dendrites are the site of most of the synaptic contacts with a given neurone; in other words, the dendrites represent the input side of the neurone, while the axon represents the output side.

The peripheral sensory nerves are an exception to this basic dendrite—soma—axon structure; these neurones have their cell bodies in the **dorsal root ganglia** of the spinal nerves, and have one long axon process carrying impulses in from the peripheral receptor organs and another (usually shorter) axon running into the spinal cord and forming synapses within the central nervous system. The input and output axons are more or less continuous with one another, and are connected with the soma by a short stalk.

The structure of synaptic connections and other relevant features of the neurone will be described later.

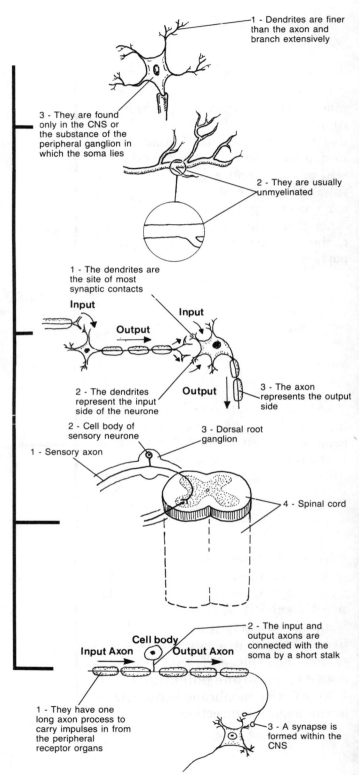

1 - Dendrites are finer than the axon and branch extensively

3 - They are found only in the CNS or the substance of the peripheral ganglion in which the soma lies

2 - They are usually unmyelinated

1 - The dendrites are the site of most synaptic contacts

Input

Input

Output

2 - The dendrites represent the input side of the neurone

Output

3 - The axon represents the output side

2 - Cell body of sensory neurone

1 - Sensory axon

3 - Dorsal root ganglion

4 - Spinal cord

Cell body

Input Axon

Output Axon

2 - The input and output axons are connected with the soma by a short stalk

1 - They have one long axon process to carry impulses in from the peripheral receptor organs

3 - A synapse is formed within the CNS

THE MEMBRANE POTENTIAL

All cells in the body have a potential difference between the inside of the membrane (in the cytoplasm) and the outside (in the interstitial fluid surrounding the cell).

The presence of the membrane seems to be essential for the generation of this potential difference, which is known as the **membrane potential**. The membrane potential can be measured by inserting a very fine glass micropipette (containing a conducting electrolyte such as concentrated KCl) through the cell membrane and recording the potential difference between this microelectrode and another electrode placed in the interstitial fluid.

In a typical nerve or muscle cell the inside of the cell is at a potential some 50–90 mV negative with respect to the outside, and the cell is said to have a **resting membrane potential** of (say) −70 mV; the membrane is **polarized** in the negative direction.

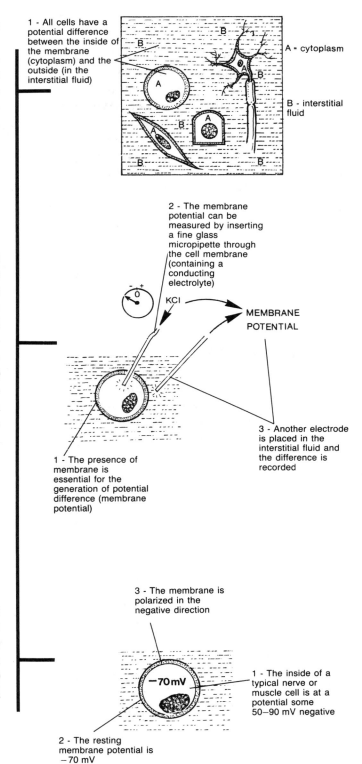

1 - All cells have a potential difference between the inside of the membrane (cytoplasm) and the outside (in the interstitial fluid)

A - cytoplasm

B - interstitial fluid

2 - The membrane potential can be measured by inserting a fine glass micropipette through the cell membrane (containing a conducting electrolyte)

KCl

MEMBRANE POTENTIAL

3 - Another electrode is placed in the interstitial fluid and the difference is recorded

1 - The presence of membrane is essential for the generation of potential difference (membrane potential)

3 - The membrane is polarized in the negative direction

−70 mV

1 - The inside of a typical nerve or muscle cell is at a potential some 50–90 mV negative

2 - The resting membrane potential is −70 mV

During excitation of the cell the membrane potential as recorded by an intracellular microelectrode changes very rapidly, becoming less negative (**depolarized**) and eventually becoming positive for a short time. The mechanism of this voltage change will be described later, but first we shall examine the basis for the resting membrane potential.

The membrane of the cell is polarized because of differences in concentrations of various ions between the inside and outside of the cell. These concentration gradients arise mainly because of differences in the permeability of the membrane to different ions.

For instance, there are large proteins and other organic molecules within cells which carry electric charge, but which cannot cross the cell membrane and are therefore trapped within the cell.

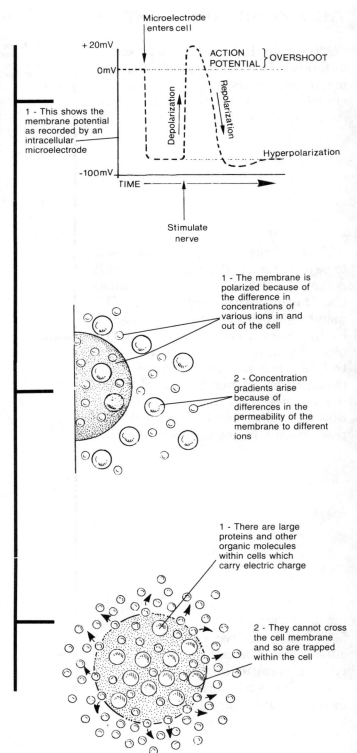

Microelectrode enters cell

+20mV

0mV

ACTION POTENTIAL } OVERSHOOT

Depolarization

Repolarization

Hyperpolarization

-100mV

TIME

Stimulate nerve

1 - This shows the membrane potential as recorded by an intracellular microelectrode

1 - The membrane is polarized because of the difference in concentrations of various ions in and out of the cell

2 - Concentration gradients arise because of differences in the permeability of the membrane to different ions

1 - There are large proteins and other organic molecules within cells which carry electric charge

2 - They cannot cross the cell membrane and so are trapped within the cell

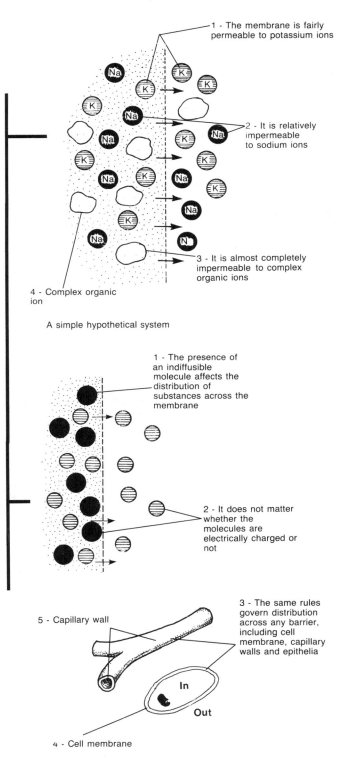

Some inorganic ions cross the membrane more easily than others; the membrane is considerably more permeable to potassium ions than to sodium ions, but the permeabilities to both of these ions are enormously greater than to complex organic ions.

1 - The membrane is fairly permeable to potassium ions

2 - It is relatively impermeable to sodium ions

3 - It is almost completely impermeable to complex organic ions

4 - Complex organic ion

A simple hypothetical system

Let us consider a simplified system, in order to see how the presence of an indiffusible molecule affects the distribution of substances across the membrane. For this part of the discussion it does not matter whether the various molecules are electrically charged, and the arguments apply equally to cell membranes, capillary walls and epithelia: in other words to any barrier between two phases or compartments.

1 - The presence of an indiffusible molecule affects the distribution of substances across the membrane

2 - It does not matter whether the molecules are electrically charged or not

5 - Capillary wall

3 - The same rules govern distribution across any barrier, including cell membrane, capillary walls and epithelia

In

Out

4 - Cell membrane

Suppose initially we have equal concentrations of molecule 'A' (diffusible) on both sides of the membrane; now if a quantity of molecule 'B' (indiffusible) is introduced on to the left side, the total concentration of molecules on the left will be larger than on the right, and some of the diffusible molecules will move from left to right (or some water may move from right to left: this will have the same effect) in response to an osmotic gradient.

This will lead to an increase in the concentration of 'A' on the right, but as molecules of each substance tend to move down their own concentration gradient, the molecules of 'A' will now tend to move back from right to left.

Eventually an equilibrium will be reached where a concentration gradient is formed which just balances an osmotic gradient in the opposite direction. Such a state is called a **Gibbs–Donnan** equilibrium, and partly explains how quite large concentration gradients can exist, even for freely diffusible molecules.

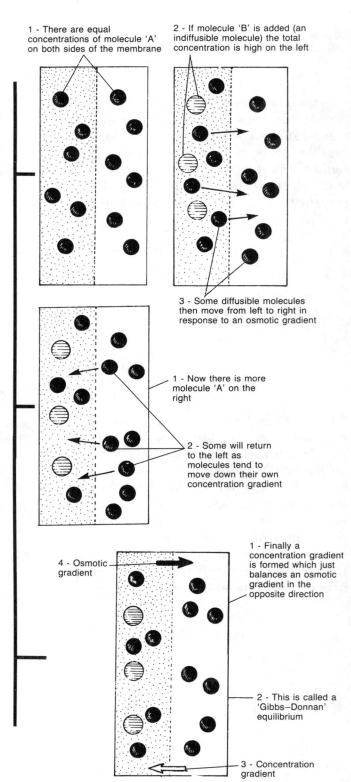

1 - There are equal concentrations of molecule 'A' on both sides of the membrane

2 - If molecule 'B' is added (an indiffusible molecule) the total concentration is high on the left

3 - Some diffusible molecules then move from left to right in response to an osmotic gradient

1 - Now there is more molecule 'A' on the right

2 - Some will return to the left as molecules tend to move down their own concentration gradient

4 - Osmotic gradient

1 - Finally a concentration gradient is formed which just balances an osmotic gradient in the opposite direction

2 - This is called a 'Gibbs–Donnan' equilibrium

3 - Concentration gradient

Let us now examine the situation where a concentration gradient already exists for an **electrically charged** ion; this gradient will have been established by the presence of indiffusible molecules, whose identity need not immediately concern us. Suppose we have different concentrations of a diffusible cation X^+ on the left and right of our membrane; the anion Y^- is indiffusible.

The presence of a concentration gradient will make X^+ tend to migrate from left to right, but this will transfer positive charge from left to right, making the right-hand compartment positive with respect to the left, and opposing the tendency of further positive ions to cross from left to right. It also makes the left compartment more negative, which exerts an attractive force on the positive ions which have crossed to the right.

Eventually an equilibrium is reached where the electrical force or potential difference produced by ion movement is just balanced by the concentration gradient for the diffusible ions, and a **Nernst** equilibrium is set up.

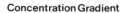

Concentration Gradient

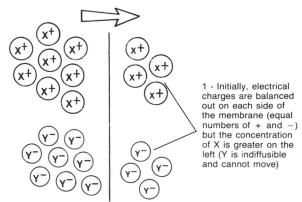

1 - Initially, electrical charges are balanced out on each side of the membrane (equal numbers of + and −) but the concentration of X is greater on the left (Y is indiffusible and cannot move)

Potential Gradient

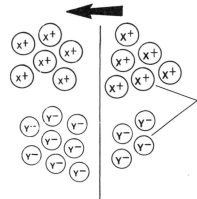

2 - Some X molecules have moved to make concentrations equal, but now there are more + than − on the right, and more − than + on the left. There is a potential difference across the membrane tending to move X^+ back from right to left

Concentration Gradient

Potential Gradient

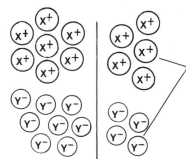

3 - Some X molecules move back, leaving a smaller potential gradient but re-establishing a concentration gradient. At equilibrium the potential gradient just balances the concentration gradient

The magnitude of the potential difference due to an imbalance in concentration of a single type of ion is found by the Nernst equation:

$$E = \frac{RT}{F} \log_e \frac{[A]_o}{[A]_i}$$

where E is the potential, R is the gas constant, T is the absolute temperature, F is Faraday's number and subscripts 'o' and 'i' refer to outside and inside the cell. The important feature of the Nernst equation is that the potential is proportional to the **logarithm** of the concentration ratio.

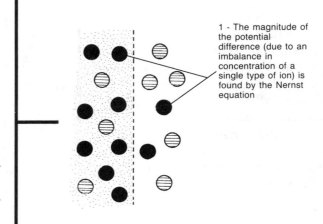

1 - The magnitude of the potential difference (due to an imbalance in concentration of a single type of ion) is found by the Nernst equation

So far we have considered purely imaginary membranes, which are freely permeable to some molecules and absolutely impermeable to others. In reality the cell membrane is permeable by different amounts to different ions, and a large number of different ionic types is involved. In a typical nerve cell there is a large intracellular concentration of protein and K^+ ions, with a large extracellular concentration of Na^+ ions; the membrane is only slightly permeable to Na^+, but much more permeable to K^+ and Cl^-.

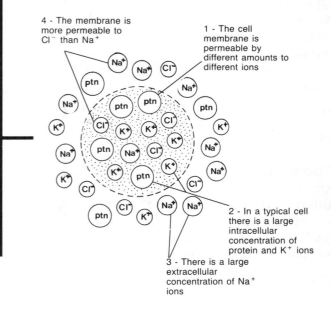

4 - The membrane is more permeable to Cl^- than Na^+

1 - The cell membrane is permeable by different amounts to different ions

2 - In a typical cell there is a large intracellular concentration of protein and K^+ ions

3 - There is a large extracellular concentration of Na^+ ions

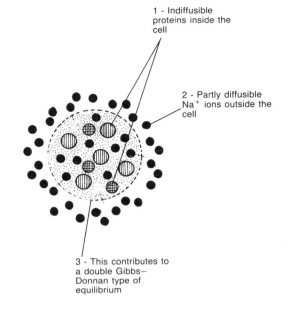

1 - Indiffusible proteins inside the cell

2 - Partly diffusible Na$^+$ ions outside the cell

3 - This contributes to a double Gibbs–Donnan type of equilibrium

The indiffusible proteins inside the cell and the partly diffusible sodium ions outside contribute to a double Gibbs–Donnan type of equilibrium.

The Nernst equation can be modified to take account of the different permeabilities and concentrations in the Goldman–Hodgkin–Katz equation:

$$E_\mathrm{m} = \frac{RT}{F} \log_e \frac{P_\mathrm{Na}[\mathrm{Na}]_o + P_\mathrm{K}[\mathrm{K}]_o + P_\mathrm{Cl}[\mathrm{Cl}]_i}{P_\mathrm{Na}[\mathrm{Na}]_i + P_\mathrm{K}[\mathrm{K}]_i + P_\mathrm{Cl}[\mathrm{Cl}]_o}$$

Note how the structure of the equation resembles the Nernst equation, but each ionic concentration is multiplied by the appropriate permeability coefficient (P); note also that the positions of intracellular and extracellular chloride concentrations are reversed, as chloride ions are negatively charged.

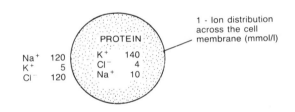

PROTEIN

Na$^+$	120	
K$^+$	5	
Cl$^-$	120	

K$^+$ 140
Cl$^-$ 4
Na$^+$ 10

1 - Ion distribution across the cell membrane (mmol/l)

THE NATURE AND STRUCTURE OF MEMBRANES

Many of the permeability properties of the cell membrane may be understood by reference to the structure of the membrane. Most of the membrane consists of a bilayer of phospholipid molecules with their hydrophilic heads facing towards the aqueous extracellular or intracellular fluids, and with their hydrophobic tails facing away from the aqueous phase but towards each other within the centre of the membrane.

Such a membrane is almost totally impermeable to water and to water-soluble molecules and ions; however, within the membrane are embedded protein molecules, some of which penetrate right through both layers of the membrane, and some of which are found in the inner or outer layer.

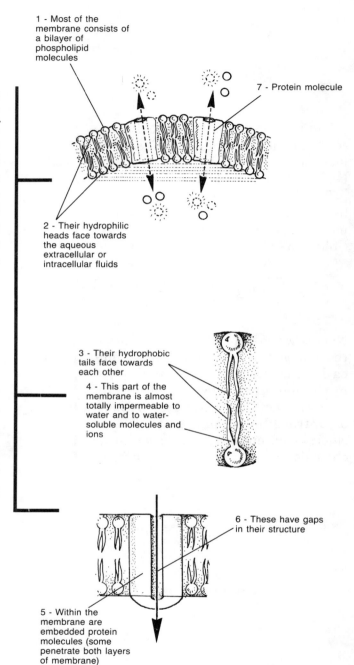

1 - Most of the membrane consists of a bilayer of phospholipid molecules

7 - Protein molecule

2 - Their hydrophilic heads face towards the aqueous extracellular or intracellular fluids

3 - Their hydrophobic tails face towards each other

4 - This part of the membrane is almost totally impermeable to water and to water-soluble molecules and ions

6 - These have gaps in their structure

5 - Within the membrane are embedded protein molecules (some penetrate both layers of membrane)

Many of these proteins have gaps in their structure which allow water and small molecules to penetrate through the membrane; others have such a structure that a very tiny gap can be made much larger by the binding of specific chemicals to the molecule (such molecules are known as **receptors**) or by a change in the potential difference across the membrane (these are the ionic channels which are involved in the action potential).

Others can bind specific substances and act as **carriers**, facilitating the transport of these substances across the membrane.

Still others are enzymatic in nature, using cellular chemical energy for the **active transport** of specific ions or other substances across the cell membrane (the sodium–potassium pump, which is an ATPase enzyme, is an example of such a molecule).

The density of such specialized molecules in the membrane is actually extremely low, and most of the membrane consists of uniform, impermeable phospholipid molecules.

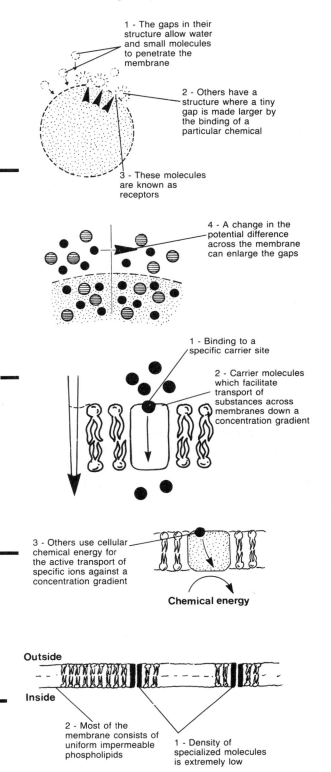

1 - The gaps in their structure allow water and small molecules to penetrate the membrane

2 - Others have a structure where a tiny gap is made larger by the binding of a particular chemical

3 - These molecules are known as receptors

4 - A change in the potential difference across the membrane can enlarge the gaps

1 - Binding to a specific carrier site

2 - Carrier molecules which facilitate transport of substances across membranes down a concentration gradient

3 - Others use cellular chemical energy for the active transport of specific ions against a concentration gradient

Chemical energy

Outside

Inside

2 - Most of the membrane consists of uniform impermeable phospholipids

1 - Density of specialized molecules is extremely low

THE ACTION POTENTIAL

When an electric shock or other suitable stimulus is applied to a nerve or muscle cell whose membrane potential is being recorded with an intracellular microelectrode, there is an initial slow depolarization due to current flow from the site of stimulus, then the membrane potential very rapidly decreases (depolarizes) and becomes positive inside, and then almost as rapidly becomes negative again and reverts towards the resting potential. The whole process takes a very few milliseconds, and is known as the **action potential**.

The action potential is the fundamental unit of information signalling in the nervous system; in any given cell it is a stereotyped event, the automatic response to an adequate stimulus.

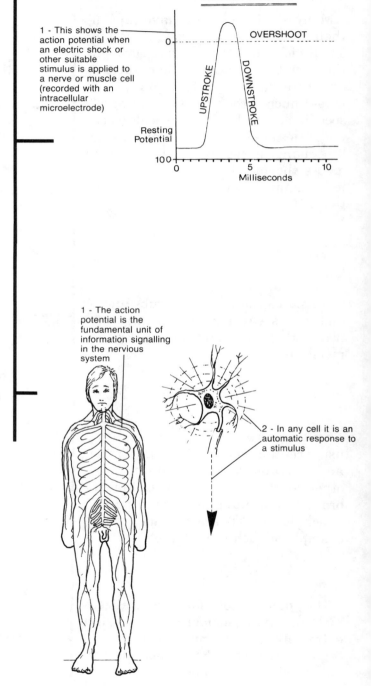

ACTION POTENTIAL

1 - This shows the action potential when an electric shock or other suitable stimulus is applied to a nerve or muscle cell (recorded with an intracellular microelectrode)

OVERSHOOT

UPSTROKE

DOWNSTROKE

Resting Potential

0

100

0   5   10

Milliseconds

1 - The action potential is the fundamental unit of information signalling in the nervous system

2 - In any cell it is an automatic response to a stimulus

If a small stimulus is applied to the cell, it may be insufficient to initiate an action potential; if it is a little larger, it may just succeed in exciting the cell. If the size of the stimulus is further increased, the resulting action potential is no greater than before; no matter how great the stimulus, the size of the action potential remains the same. It is either present or it is not: this is known as the 'all-or-none' law. Once a stimulus is adequate to excite the cell (a 'threshold' stimulus) it produces a stereotyped response.

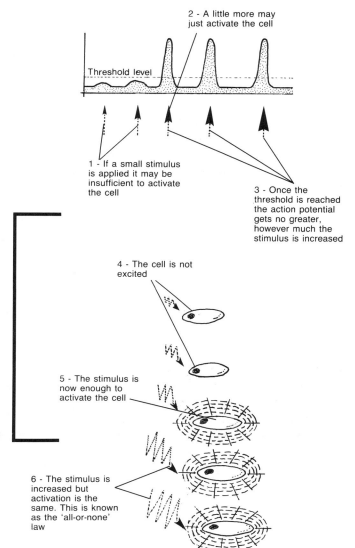

2 - A little more may just activate the cell

Threshold level

1 - If a small stimulus is applied it may be insufficient to activate the cell

3 - Once the threshold is reached the action potential gets no greater, however much the stimulus is increased

4 - The cell is not excited

5 - The stimulus is now enough to activate the cell

6 - The stimulus is increased but activation is the same. This is known as the 'all-or-none' law

If the size of an action potential is always the same, then how can the brain get information about the size of sensory stimuli being applied to the body?

An increase in light intensity does not produce bigger action potentials in the optic nerve, but it does produce more frequent impulses. In other words, the nervous system uses frequency of impulses to code for intensity.

In a similar way, the brain can make a muscle contract more forcefully, not by sending out bigger action potentials, but by sending action potentials of the same size more frequently.

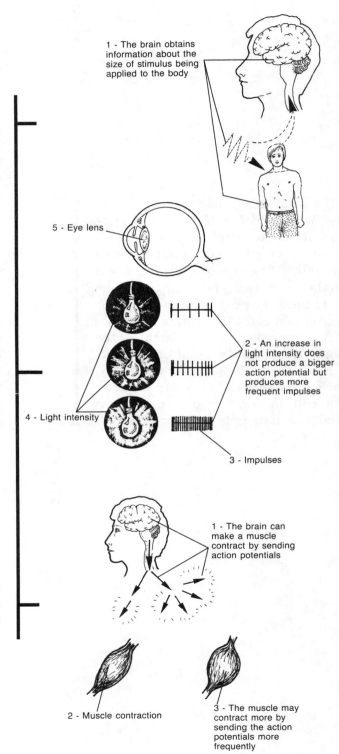

1 - The brain obtains information about the size of stimulus being applied to the body

5 - Eye lens

2 - An increase in light intensity does not produce a bigger action potential but produces more frequent impulses

4 - Light intensity

3 - Impulses

1 - The brain can make a muscle contract by sending action potentials

2 - Muscle contraction

3 - The muscle may contract more by sending the action potentials more frequently

There is a limit to the frequency at which a nerve can discharge action potentials; if we attempt to initiate a second action potential while one action potential is already proceeding, we find that the membrane is **refractory** to the stimulus, and another action potential cannot be started.

The **absolute refractory period** is defined as the period after the beginning of an action potential when another impulse cannot be started, no matter how strong the stimulus; this is followed by a **relative refractory period**, during which the membrane becomes excitable again, but requires a larger stimulus than usual to provoke the second impulse.

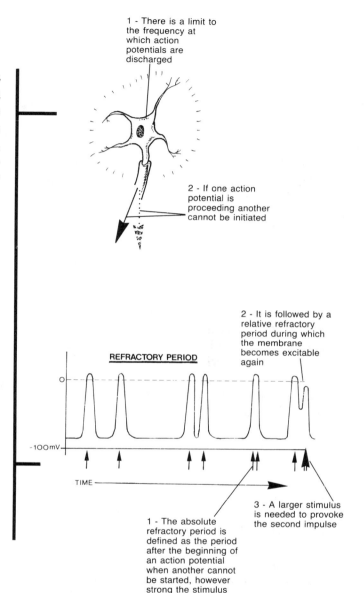

1 - There is a limit to the frequency at which action potentials are discharged

2 - If one action potential is proceeding another cannot be initiated

REFRACTORY PERIOD

2 - It is followed by a relative refractory period during which the membrane becomes excitable again

3 - A larger stimulus is needed to provoke the second impulse

1 - The absolute refractory period is defined as the period after the beginning of an action potential when another cannot be started, however strong the stimulus

TIME

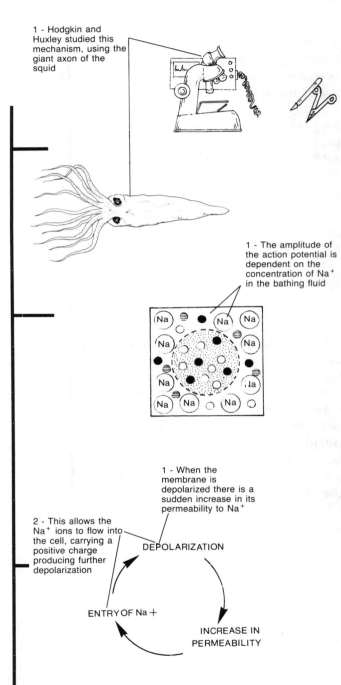

1 - Hodgkin and Huxley studied this mechanism, using the giant axon of the squid

The mechanism of the action potential was studied intensively by Hodgkin and Huxley, using the giant axon of the squid, which is a very convenient experimental preparation on account of its large size.

1 - The amplitude of the action potential is dependent on the concentration of Na^+ in the bathing fluid

They found that the amplitude of the action potential was very dependent upon the concentration of sodium ions in the bathing fluid; following a long and very painstaking series of experiments they found that there were changes in the membrane permeabilities to several ions.

1 - When the membrane is depolarized there is a sudden increase in its permeability to Na^+

2 - This allows the Na^+ ions to flow into the cell, carrying a positive charge producing further depolarization

DEPOLARIZATION

ENTRY OF Na +

INCREASE IN PERMEABILITY

When the membrane becomes depolarized by a critical amount, there is a sudden and very large increase in the permeability to sodium ions; this allows sodium ions to flow into the cell under the influence of the large concentration gradient and electrical gradient. The entry of sodium ions carries positive charge into the cell, producing further depolarization; this depolarization causes a further increase in permeability to sodium, which causes further influx of sodium ions, further depolarization and so on. The process becomes self-reinforcing and almost explosive, and the membrane potential changes very rapidly.

The permeability to sodium varies with the membrane potential, becoming greater as the membrane is depolarized. The permeability to potassium is also potential dependent, but changes more slowly; as the membrane becomes depolarized during the action potential, the permeability to potassium gradually begins to rise, and potassium ions begin to flow out of the cell. This tends to limit and counteract the depolarization due to sodium entry, and eventually the potassium outflow exceeds the sodium inflow and the membrane potential is brought back to its resting level. Sometimes the potassium outflow is so great that the membrane is briefly hyperpolarized or made more negative than its resting potential.

Another process which limits the size and duration of the action potential is **inactivation** of the sodium permeability. This is a separate process from the activation or increase in permeability, but proceeds in parallel. It too is a potential-dependent process, and has the effect of allowing the sodium permeability to increase briefly, and then decrease.

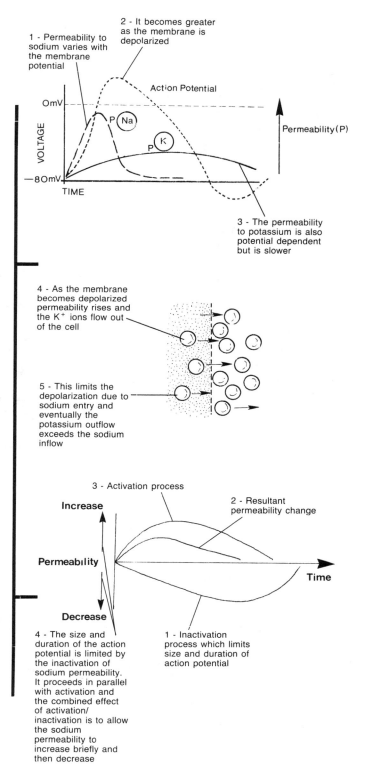

1 - Permeability to sodium varies with the membrane potential

2 - It becomes greater as the membrane is depolarized

Action Potential

OmV

VOLTAGE

P (Na)

P (K)

Permeability(P)

—8OmV

TIME

3 - The permeability to potassium is also potential dependent but is slower

4 - As the membrane becomes depolarized permeability rises and the K$^+$ ions flow out of the cell

5 - This limits the depolarization due to sodium entry and eventually the potassium outflow exceeds the sodium inflow

3 - Activation process

2 - Resultant permeability change

Increase

Permeability

Time

Decrease

4 - The size and duration of the action potential is limited by the inactivation of sodium permeability. It proceeds in parallel with activation and the combined effect of activation/inactivation is to allow the sodium permeability to increase briefly and then decrease

1 - Inactivation process which limits size and duration of action potential

The increases and decreases in permeabilities have been explained in terms of 'gates' in the membrane, which are complex molecules, probably proteins, which can undergo conformational or structural change under the influence of potential fields.

Such changes probably increase or decrease the size of a 'hole' or 'channel' in the membrane through which ions can penetrate, and it is suggested that the sodium channel has one gate which is normally closed but opens during the action potential, and another which is normally open but closes during the depolarization. No evidence has been found for inactivation of the potassium channel.

The presence of a refractory period is explained by the sodium channels being first in an open state (and thus being incapable of further opening) and then in the closed inactivated state; during the relative refractory period the sodium channels are almost back to normal, but the potassium channels are still partly open, tending to keep the membrane hyperpolarized and making it difficult to excite.

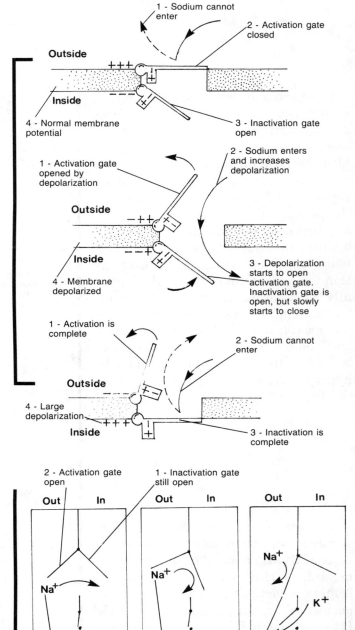

1 - Sodium cannot enter

2 - Activation gate closed

Outside

Inside

4 - Normal membrane potential

3 - Inactivation gate open

1 - Activation gate opened by depolarization

2 - Sodium enters and increases depolarization

Outside

Inside

4 - Membrane depolarized

3 - Depolarization starts to open activation gate. Inactivation gate is open, but slowly starts to close

1 - Activation is complete

2 - Sodium cannot enter

Outside

4 - Large depolarization

Inside

3 - Inactivation is complete

2 - Activation gate open

1 - Inactivation gate still open

Out   In

Out   In

Out   In

Na+

Na+

Na+

K+

3 - During the absolute refractory period the sodium channels are first fully open

4 - Then the channels are fully inactivated and cannot be opened

5 - During the relative refractory period the sodium channels are almost back to normal and available for re-opening, but the open potassium channels keep the membrane hyperpolarized

Ion pumps

During each action potential there is an inward migration of a measurable quantity of sodium ions, and an outward transfer of almost the same number of potassium ions.

It follows that if the nerve or muscle undergoes repetitive activity the ionic concentration gradients across the membrane are likely to run down, and the membrane will become permanently depolarized. This would take a long time in a large axon or muscle fibre, but could happen quickly in the finer, smaller cells.

There is a mechanism present in all cell membranes which uses energy carried by adenosine triphosphate (ATP) from the cellular metabolism to perform **active transport** of sodium ions out of the cell and potassium ions into the cell. This mechanism is known as the **sodium pump** (sometimes called the Na^+-K^+ pump) and restores the transmembrane concentration gradients, not only after action potentials in nerve but also following the passive slow leak of ions which constantly occurs in all cells because the membrane is not absolutely impermeable to ions.

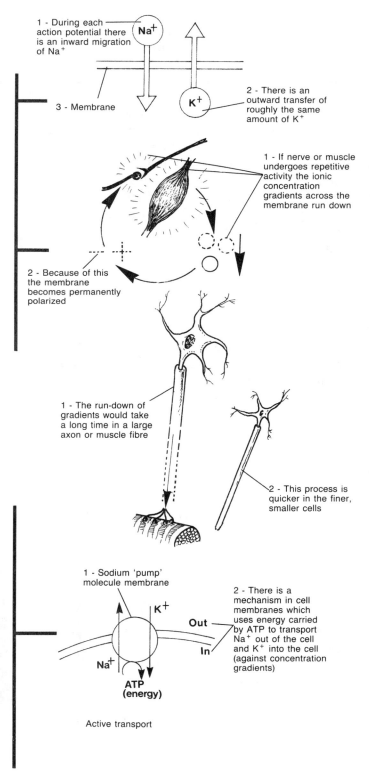

1 - During each action potential there is an inward migration of Na$^+$

2 - There is an outward transfer of roughly the same amount of K$^+$

3 - Membrane

1 - If nerve or muscle undergoes repetitive activity the ionic concentration gradients across the membrane run down

2 - Because of this the membrane becomes permanently polarized

1 - The run-down of gradients would take a long time in a large axon or muscle fibre

2 - This process is quicker in the finer, smaller cells

1 - Sodium 'pump' molecule membrane

2 - There is a mechanism in cell membranes which uses energy carried by ATP to transport Na$^+$ out of the cell and K$^+$ into the cell (against concentration gradients)

K$^+$

Out

In

Na$^+$

ATP (energy)

Active transport

In certain conditions the sodium pump transfers unequal numbers of sodium and potassium ions across the membrane, so that there is a change in the distribution of charge and therefore of membrane potential, but it must be emphasized that the Na^+-K^+ pump is **not** the primary mechanism for the generation of the resting membrane potential; it is **not** a breakdown of pump activity that accounts for the action potential, and in fact the pump has almost nothing to do with the action potential mechanism.

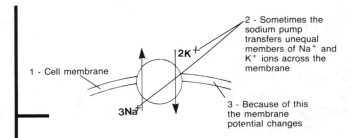

1 - Cell membrane

2 - Sometimes the sodium pump transfers unequal members of Na^+ and K^+ ions across the membrane

3 - Because of this the membrane potential changes

The chief role for the ion pump is to restore concentration gradients after membrane activity has taken place.

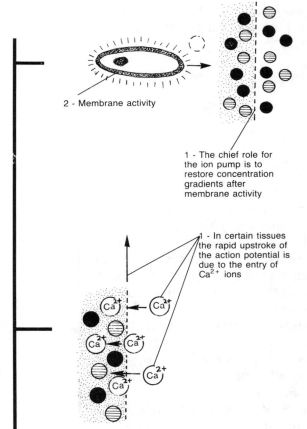

2 - Membrane activity

1 - The chief role for the ion pump is to restore concentration gradients after membrane activity

Other ions have a role in the generation and control of the action potential. In certain tissues the rapid upstroke of the action potential is due to the entry of calcium ions rather than sodium. In many tissues the concentration of calcium ions either inside or outside the membrane can influence the membrane's permeability to other ions.

1 - In certain tissues the rapid upstroke of the action potential is due to the entry of Ca^{2+} ions

A high level of extracellular calcium can lower the permeability to sodium ions, perhaps by binding to the membrane and then repelling the positive sodium ions, and a reduced level of calcium can increase sodium permeability, rendering the membrane more excitable.

An increase in **intracellular** calcium can increase potassium permeability.

Calcium ions often enter the cells through the same channels as are used by sodium ions, and in almost all tissues depolarization is accompanied by the entry of calcium ions into the cell: in certain cells this can cause contraction or the expulsion of secretory products.

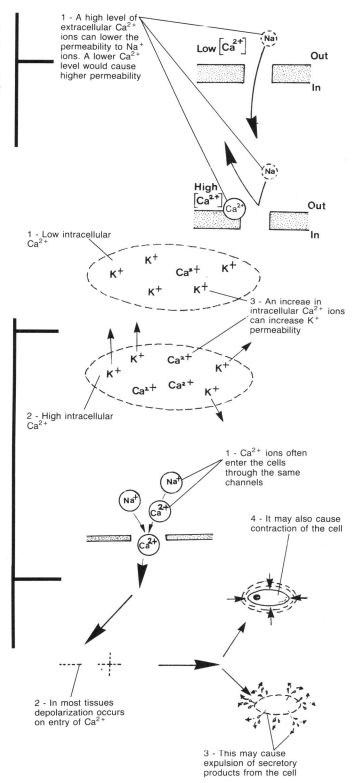

CONDUCTION OF THE IMPULSE

Once an impulse has been generated in a nerve or muscle membrane, it is necessary for that potential disturbance to be propagated or conducted along the cell surface, in order to transfer the information to another part of the body.

The process is not a simple conduction of electric current like a telephone message travelling along a wire; whilst electricity travels along wires at the speed of light (300 000 m/s), the nerve impulse travels at speeds of up to 100 m/s.

Let us imagine a nerve with a purely passive membrane, i.e. without any action potential mechanism. If we produce a potential disturbance at some point along its length, say by injecting current from some kind of stimulator, then there will be current flow between that point and neighbouring points along the membrane. Some of the current flows along the fibre through the cytoplasm, and would be detectable at a point distant from the site of current injection, but a large proportion of the current leaks out of the cell by flowing through the rather leaky membrane; this reduces the proportion of current available to be detected remotely.

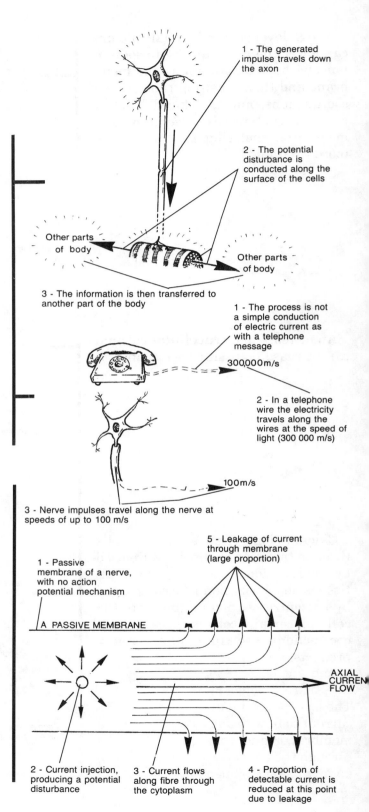

1 - The generated impulse travels down the axon

2 - The potential disturbance is conducted along the surface of the cells

Other parts of body

Other parts of body

3 - The information is then transferred to another part of the body

1 - The process is not a simple conduction of electric current as with a telephone message

300,000 m/s

2 - In a telephone wire the electricity travels along the wires at the speed of light (300 000 m/s)

100 m/s

3 - Nerve impulses travel along the nerve at speeds of up to 100 m/s

5 - Leakage of current through membrane (large proportion)

1 - Passive membrane of a nerve, with no action potential mechanism

A PASSIVE MEMBRANE

AXIAL CURRENT FLOW

2 - Current injection, producing a potential disturbance

3 - Current flows along fibre through the cytoplasm

4 - Proportion of detectable current is reduced at this point due to leakage

The flow of leakage current through the cell membrane causes a change in the voltage across the membrane; as the amount of current flowing axially along the cell declines with distance, so does the amount available to flow through the membrane.

Hence the change in voltage also declines with distance away from the site of stimulation. In a purely passive cell a potential disturbance of about the size of an action potential would decay to almost zero within a very few millimetres.

The membrane of a real nerve is not purely passive; there are spots along the membrane where action potentials can be generated. Suppose such a membrane is excited locally by current injection or some other mechanism. The local potential disturbance causes current to flow to adjacent sites on the membrane, and some current leaks through the membrane, causing a local passive change in membrane potential.

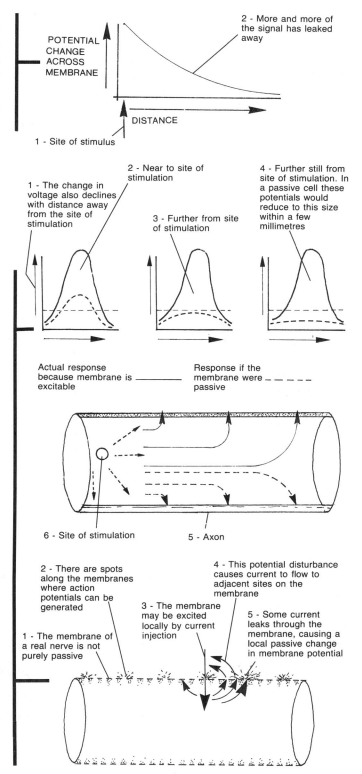

If this change is greater than the threshold then the action potential mechanism is switched on, and instead of there being a small passive voltage change there will be a large rapid change in membrane potential.

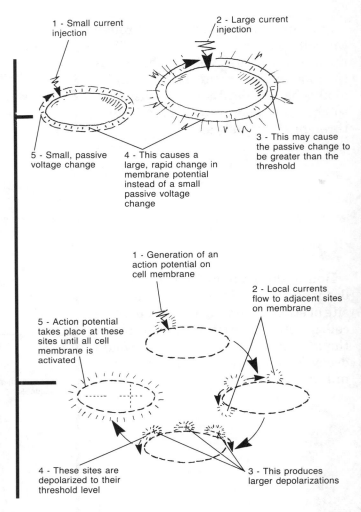

1 - Small current injection

2 - Large current injection

3 - This may cause the passive change to be greater than the threshold

4 - This causes a large, rapid change in membrane potential instead of a small passive voltage change

5 - Small, passive voltage change

The generation of an action potential at this new site causes local currents to flow to adjacent sites on the membrane, and produces larger depolarizations than would otherwise have occurred in a purely passive membrane. These new sites are then depolarized to their threshold, and generate action potentials, acting in turn as foci for further depolarization of subsequent sites on the membrane.

1 - Generation of an action potential on cell membrane

2 - Local currents flow to adjacent sites on membrane

5 - Action potential takes place at these sites until all cell membrane is activated

3 - This produces larger depolarizations

4 - These sites are depolarized to their threshold level

In this way, the potential disturbance produced by excitation at one site is propagated along the membrane without decrement. The process is rather analogous to the provision of 'repeater' stations along a submarine cable, where the signal is repeatedly amplified or 'boosted' to prevent it from decaying with distance due to leakage of current through the insulation.

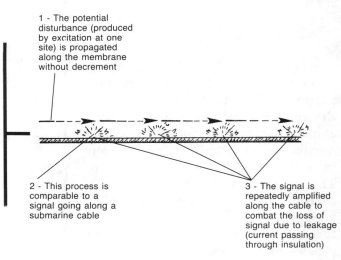

1 - The potential disturbance (produced by excitation at one site) is propagated along the membrane without decrement

2 - This process is comparable to a signal going along a submarine cable

3 - The signal is repeatedly amplified along the cable to combat the loss of signal due to leakage (current passing through insulation)

Another useful analogy is the smoking of a cigarette (a process which is thoroughly to be discouraged on health grounds!). The burning tip of a cigarette produces passive heating of the adjacent non-burning part, until the temperature is raised above the threshold level for combustion to occur. Then the passively heated part begins to burn, producing far more heat and rising to a far higher temperature than if it had not been combustible. The new area of burning material now acts as a focus for the passive heating of an adjacent area until this area, too, is heated above its threshold and begins to burn. In this way the 'wavefront' of burning is conducted along the cigarette.

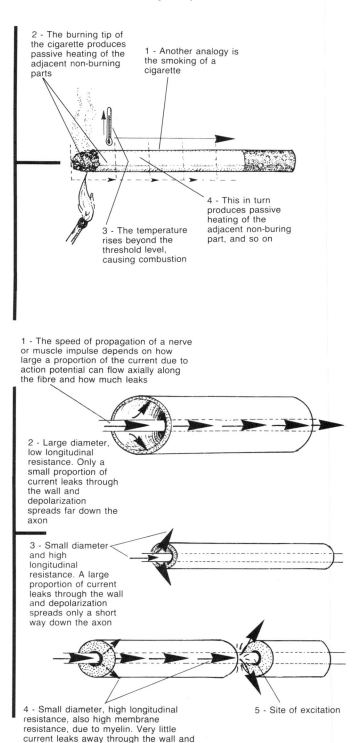

2 - The burning tip of the cigarette produces passive heating of the adjacent non-burning parts

1 - Another analogy is the smoking of a cigarette

4 - This in turn produces passive heating of the adjacent non-buring part, and so on

3 - The temperature rises beyond the threshold level, causing combustion

1 - The speed of propagation of a nerve or muscle impulse depends on how large a proportion of the current due to action potential can flow axially along the fibre and how much leaks

2 - Large diameter, low longitudinal resistance. Only a small proportion of current leaks through the wall and depolarization spreads far down the axon

3 - Small diameter and high longitudinal resistance. A large proportion of current leaks through the wall and depolarization spreads only a short way down the axon

4 - Small diameter, high longitudinal resistance, also high membrane resistance, due to myelin. Very little current leaks away through the wall and depolarization is forced to spread to the next site, where excitation is possible at the node of Ranvier

5 - Site of excitation

The speed of propagation of a nerve or muscle impulse depends upon how large a proportion of the current due to an action potential is able to flow axially along the fibre, and how much leaks across the membrane. If most of the current flows axially, then more remote parts of the cell can be passively depolarized to their thresholds, and the action potential can move rapidly along the cell. The conduction velocity depends upon the ratio of membrane resistance to axial or internal resistance, so if membrane resistance is high and axial resistance low, the conduction velocity will be high. Since axial resistance depends on the diameter of the cell, it follows that cells with large diameters will conduct rapidly.

The giant axon of the squid is about 1 mm in diameter and conducts at 50−70 m/s; many vertebrate skeletal muscles and the rapidly conducting fibres of the heart are of comparable size and conduction velocity.

The fibres of the human optic nerve conduct at about the same speed; there are about one million fibres in the optic nerve, so obviously they cannot all be 1 mm in diameter! How, then, do the very much smaller fibres of the mammalian nervous system conduct impulses?

If conduction velocity depends upon the ratio of membrane resistance to internal resistance, then instead of increasing the diameter to decrease internal resistance, we can greatly increase the membrane resistance, so that a greater proportion of the current is forced to flow along the cell.

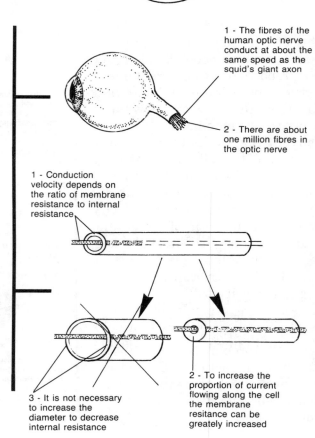

1 - The giant axon of the squid is approx 1 mm in diameter

2 - It conducts at 50−70 m/s

50−70m/s

1mm

3 - The vertebrate skeletal muscles and conducting fibres of the heart are of comparable size and conduction velocity

1 - The fibres of the human optic nerve conduct at about the same speed as the squid's giant axon

2 - There are about one million fibres in the optic nerve

1 - Conduction velocity depends on the ratio of membrane resistance to internal resistance

2 - To increase the proportion of current flowing along the cell the membrane resitance can be greatly increased

3 - It is not necessary to increase the diameter to decrease internal resistance

This has been achieved by wrapping the vertebrate nerve in a layer of insulating material, **myelin**. It is still necessary to have some areas of the membrane where action potentials can be generated, so there are periodic gaps in the myelin sheath, the **nodes of Ranvier**, where the cell membrane comes into contact with the interstitial fluid and where membrane currents can flow.

Excitation occurs at the nodes, and the resulting currents flow with very little decrement or leakage along the axis of the cell to the next node, where passive depolarization up to the threshold level initiates the generation of an action potential. The process of impulse generation 'skips' from node to node along the nerve, and has been called **saltatory** conduction.

Although the use of intracellular microelectrodes has given a great deal of information about the behaviour of excitable membranes, it is a difficult technique to apply; the function of peripheral nerves can be more easily studied by dissecting out the sciatic nerve and its associated gastrocnemius muscle from a frog's hind leg, and arranging the preparation in a muscle bath so that contraction of the muscle moves a lever which writes on a kymograph drum or activates an electronic transducer.

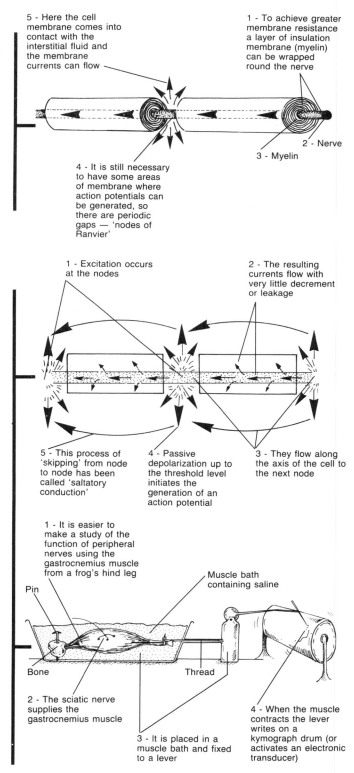

5 - Here the cell membrane comes into contact with the interstitial fluid and the membrane currents can flow

1 - To achieve greater membrane resistance a layer of insulation membrane (myelin) can be wrapped round the nerve

2 - Nerve

3 - Myelin

4 - It is still necessary to have some areas of membrane where action potentials can be generated, so there are periodic gaps — 'nodes of Ranvier'

1 - Excitation occurs at the nodes

2 - The resulting currents flow with very little decrement or leakage

5 - This process of 'skipping' from node to node has been called 'saltatory conduction'

4 - Passive depolarization up to the threshold level initiates the generation of an action potential

3 - They flow along the axis of the cell to the next node

1 - It is easier to make a study of the function of peripheral nerves using the gastrocnemius muscle from a frog's hind leg

Pin

Muscle bath containing saline

Bone

Thread

2 - The sciatic nerve supplies the gastrocnemius muscle

3 - It is placed in a muscle bath and fixed to a lever

4 - When the muscle contracts the lever writes on a kymograph drum (or activates an electronic transducer)

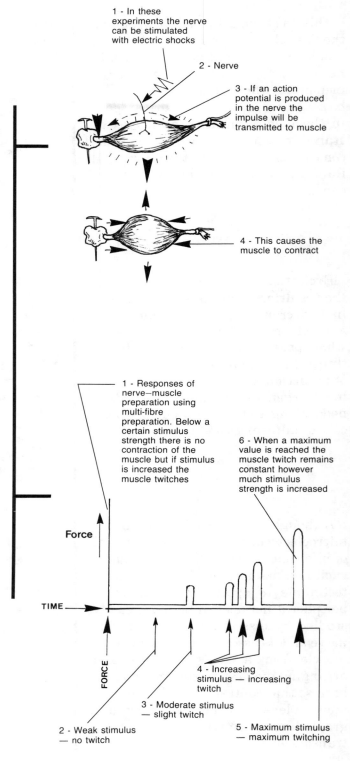

In such experiments, the nerve can be stimulated with electric shocks and if an action potential is produced in the nerve it will cause the impulse to be transmitted to the muscle with consequent contraction of the muscle.

1 - In these experiments the nerve can be stimulated with electric shocks

2 - Nerve

3 - If an action potential is produced in the nerve the impulse will be transmitted to muscle

4 - This causes the muscle to contract

Below a certain stimulus strength there is no contraction of the muscle, but if the strength is increased slightly the muscle twitches. As the stimulus strength is increased the size of the twitch increases until a maximum value is reached, above which the muscle twitch remains constant no matter how much the stimulus strength is increased.

1 - Responses of nerve—muscle preparation using multi-fibre preparation. Below a certain stimulus strength there is no contraction of the muscle but if stimulus is increased the muscle twitches

6 - When a maximum value is reached the muscle twitch remains constant however much stimulus strength is increased

Force

TIME

FORCE

2 - Weak stimulus — no twitch

3 - Moderate stimulus — slight twitch

4 - Increasing stimulus — increasing twitch

5 - Maximum stimulus — maximum twitching

If a single nerve fibre is teased out the behaviour is different; below a certain strength of stimulation (**threshold**) there is no contraction, but above the threshold level of stimulation there is a twitch which is of constant amplitude no matter how much the stimulus strength is increased.

The single fibre is said to be exhibiting **all-or-none** behaviour; either it is at rest, or it is fully activated.

A multi-fibre nerve such as the whole sciatic nerve consists of many individual nerve fibres, each one of which exhibits all-or-none behaviour, but as each fibre has a different threshold level it is possible to excite only a few fibres with a low stimulus strength, and to excite many more with a stronger stimulus. Thus it is possible to produce twitches of varying sizes from a multi-fibre nerve—muscle preparation.

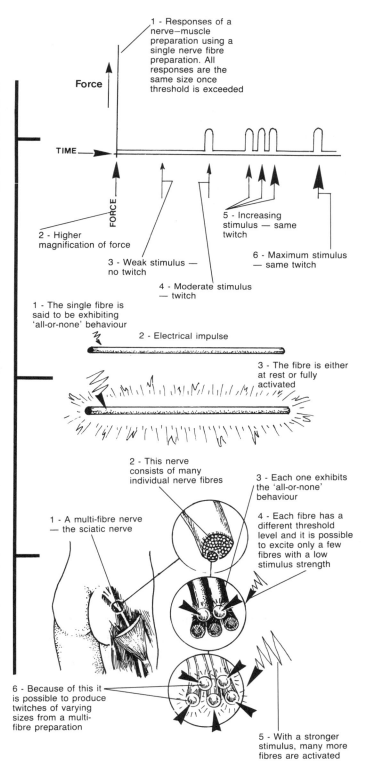

1 - Responses of a nerve—muscle preparation using a single nerve fibre preparation. All responses are the same size once threshold is exceeded

Force

TIME

FORCE

2 - Higher magnification of force

3 - Weak stimulus — no twitch

4 - Moderate stimulus — twitch

5 - Increasing stimulus — same twitch

6 - Maximum stimulus — same twitch

1 - The single fibre is said to be exhibiting 'all-or-none' behaviour

2 - Electrical impulse

3 - The fibre is either at rest or fully activated

2 - This nerve consists of many individual nerve fibres

3 - Each one exhibits the 'all-or-none' behaviour

1 - A multi-fibre nerve — the sciatic nerve

4 - Each fibre has a different threshold level and it is possible to excite only a few fibres with a low stimulus strength

6 - Because of this it is possible to produce twitches of varying sizes from a multi-fibre preparation

5 - With a stronger stimulus, many more fibres are activated

If a pair of electrodes is placed on the surface of the nerve and connected by an amplifier to an oscilloscope or other electronic recording device, it is possible to observe the passage of nerve impulses along the nerve following the application of electric shocks by a pair of stimulating electrodes.

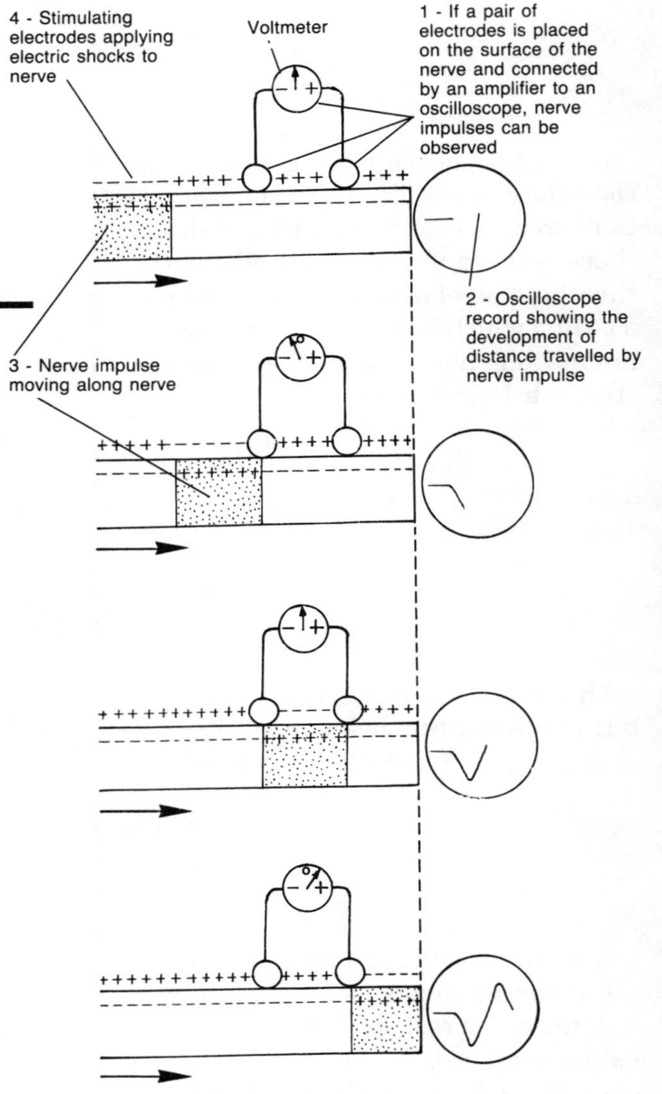

4 - Stimulating electrodes applying electric shocks to nerve

Voltmeter

1 - If a pair of electrodes is placed on the surface of the nerve and connected by an amplifier to an oscilloscope, nerve impulses can be observed

2 - Oscilloscope record showing the development of distance travelled by nerve impulse

3 - Nerve impulse moving along nerve

The **compound action potential** recorded from such a preparation has a large number of different components which represent the passage of the impulse along different types of nerve fibres.

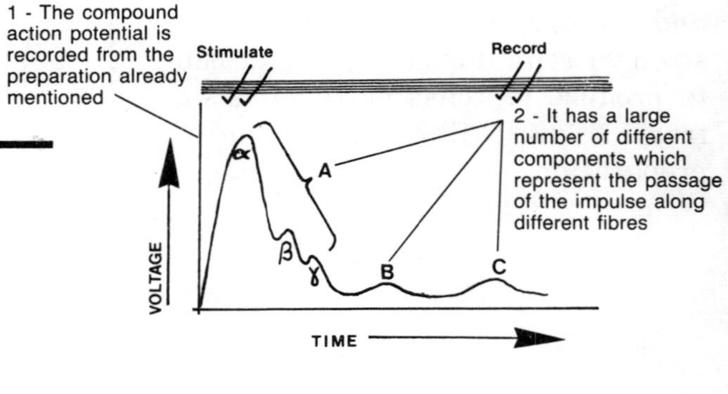

1 - The compound action potential is recorded from the preparation already mentioned

Stimulate   Record

2 - It has a large number of different components which represent the passage of the impulse along different fibres

VOLTAGE

TIME

The reason why it is possible to record electrical activity with electrodes on the surface of the nerve is that the impulse is not stationary but moves along the nerve. Thus the wavefront of activity passes under first one electrode and then the other, producing a potential difference between the electrodes first in one direction and then in the other.

The various peaks in the compound action potential have been identified as coming from different groups of sensory or motor nerves. The earliest group of peaks, corresponding to the most rapidly conducting fibres, is known as A and is subdivided into alpha, beta and gamma peaks. These fibres may be either sensory or motor in function, and either carry information about muscle position sense (proprioception) or carry the command signals making the muscles contract.

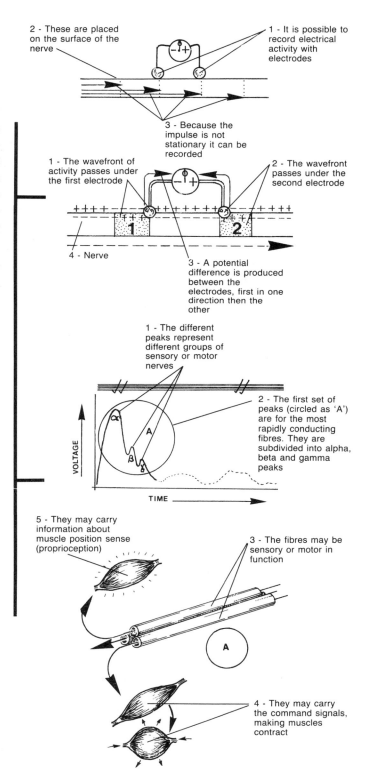

2 - These are placed on the surface of the nerve

1 - It is possible to record electrical activity with electrodes

3 - Because the impulse is not stationary it can be recorded

1 - The wavefront of activity passes under the first electrode

2 - The wavefront passes under the second electrode

4 - Nerve

3 - A potential difference is produced between the electrodes, first in one direction then the other

1 - The different peaks represent different groups of sensory or motor nerves

2 - The first set of peaks (circled as 'A') are for the most rapidly conducting fibres. They are subdivided into alpha, beta and gamma peaks

VOLTAGE

TIME

5 - They may carry information about muscle position sense (proprioception)

3 - The fibres may be sensory or motor in function

A

4 - They may carry the command signals, making muscles contract

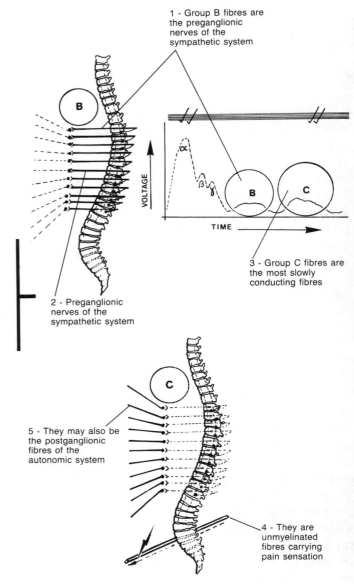

1 - Group B fibres are the preganglionic nerves of the sympathetic system

2 - Preganglionic nerves of the sympathetic system

3 - Group C fibres are the most slowly conducting fibres

5 - They may also be the postganglionic fibres of the autonomic system

4 - They are unmyelinated fibres carrying pain sensation

The B group of fibres are the preganglionic nerves of the sympathetic system, and the C group, the most slowly conducting fibres, are the unmyelinated fibres carrying pain sensation or the postganglionic fibres of the autonomic system.

Sensory nerve fibres have also been classified on the basis of their size or diameter; there is a strong correlation between fibre size and conduction velocity.

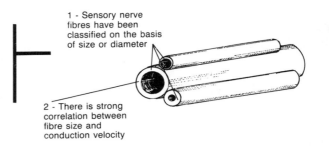

1 - Sensory nerve fibres have been classified on the basis of size or diameter

2 - There is strong correlation between fibre size and conduction velocity

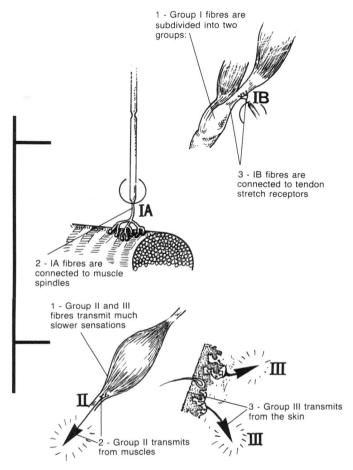

Group I fibres are subdivided into IA, connected to muscle spindles, and IB, connected to tendon stretch receptors.

1 - Group I fibres are subdivided into two groups:

3 - IB fibres are connected to tendon stretch receptors

2 - IA fibres are connected to muscle spindles

Groups II and III transmit much slower sensations from muscles and skin. The various modalities of sensation carried by the nerves are detailed in the chapter on the sensory system.

1 - Group II and III fibres transmit much slower sensations

3 - Group III transmits from the skin

2 - Group II transmits from muscles

VARIETIES OF EXCITABLE MEMBRANE

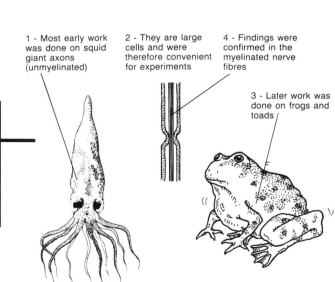

Not all excitable membranes have exactly the same action potential mechanism. Most of the early work was done on squid giant axons because they were so large and therefore convenient for experiments; many of the findings were later confirmed in the myelinated nerve fibres of frogs and toads.

1 - Most early work was done on squid giant axons (unmyelinated)

2 - They are large cells and were therefore convenient for experiments

4 - Findings were confirmed in the myelinated nerve fibres

3 - Later work was done on frogs and toads

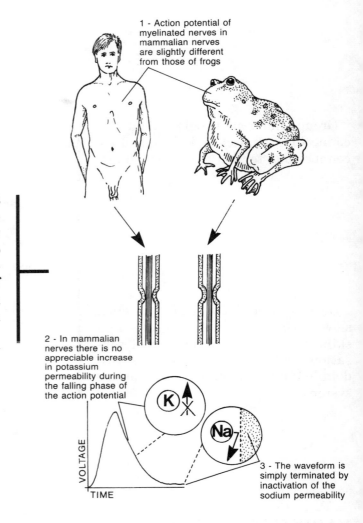

1 - Action potential of myelinated nerves in mammalian nerves are slightly different from those of frogs

Only recently has it become apparent that the action potentials of mammalian myelinated nerves are slightly different from those of frogs; there is no appreciable increase in potassium permeability during the falling phase of the action potential, and the waveform is simply termi-nated by inactivation of the sodium permeability.

2 - In mammalian nerves there is no appreciable increase in potassium permeability during the falling phase of the action potential

3 - The waveform is simply terminated by inactivation of the sodium permeability

The action potential of skeletal muscle fibres is very similar to that of the invertebrate nerve, in that sodium permeability initially increases during the upstroke, then the potassium permeability increases as sodium permeability decreases during the downstroke.

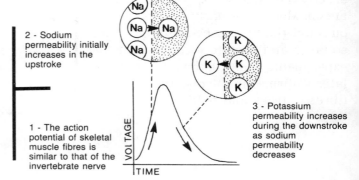

2 - Sodium permeability initially increases in the upstroke

1 - The action potential of skeletal muscle fibres is similar to that of the invertebrate nerve

3 - Potassium permeability increases during the downstroke as sodium permeability decreases

The action potential is conducted not only over the surface membrane of the muscle fibre, but also along the membranes of the transverse tubules, which penetrate deep inside the cell; this phenomenon will be discussed more fully when the contraction of muscle is described.

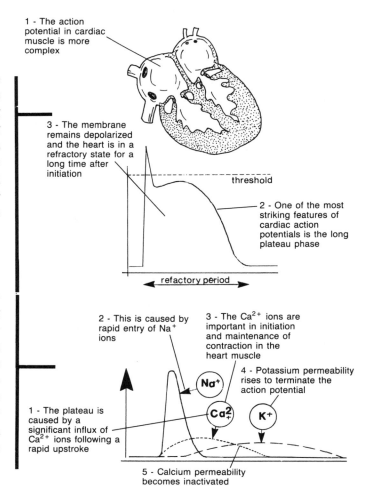

1 - The action potential is conducted over the whole surface membrane of the muscle fibre

2 - The action potential is also conducted along the membranes of the transverse tubules

5 - Action potential

4 - Cell

3 - These penetrate deep inside the cell

The action potential in cardiac muscle is much more complex, and depends upon which part of the heart is being examined. One of the most striking features of all cardiac action potentials is the long plateau phase, where the membrane remains depolarized and keeps the heart in a refractory state for a long time after the initiation of the action potential.

1 - The action potential in cardiac muscle is more complex

3 - The membrane remains depolarized and the heart is in a refractory state for a long time after initiation

threshold

2 - One of the most striking features of cardiac action potentials is the long plateau phase

refactory period

This plateau is caused by a significant influx of calcium ions following the rapid upstroke (which is caused by the very rapid entry of sodium ions); the calcium ions are important in the initiation and maintenance of contraction in the heart muscle. Following the plateau, the calcium permeability becomes inactivated and the potassium permeability rises to terminate the action potential.

2 - This is caused by rapid entry of Na^+ ions

3 - The Ca^{2+} ions are important in initiation and maintenance of contraction in the heart muscle

4 - Potassium permeability rises to terminate the action potential

1 - The plateau is caused by a significant influx of Ca^{2+} ions following a rapid upstroke

Na^+

Ca_+^{2+}

K^+

5 - Calcium permeability becomes inactivated

Heart muscle also exhibits **spontaneous activity**, especially in the pacemaker areas; instead of having a steady resting potential in the intervals between action potentials, there is a slow depolarization of the membrane, until the potential reaches threshold when another action potential is initiated.

This spontaneous diastolic depolarization occurs most rapidly at the pacemaker, so the impulse is initiated here and then conducted quickly to other parts of the heart before the cells there have an opportunity to develop spontaneous action potentials.

The so-called pacemaker potential is probably caused by a slow leakage inward of sodium ions producing depolarization, but it is a very complex phenomenon involving several other ions such as calcium, acting as controllers of this process.

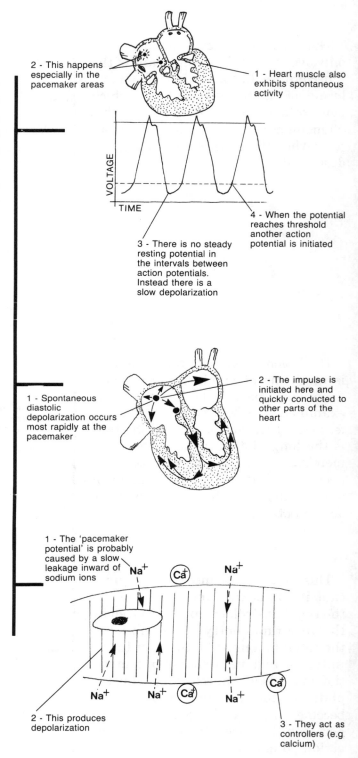

2 - This happens especially in the pacemaker areas

1 - Heart muscle also exhibits spontaneous activity

VOLTAGE

TIME

3 - There is no steady resting potential in the intervals between action potentials. Instead there is a slow depolarization

4 - When the potential reaches threshold another action potential is initiated

1 - Spontaneous diastolic depolarization occurs most rapidly at the pacemaker

2 - The impulse is initiated here and quickly conducted to other parts of the heart

1 - The 'pacemaker potential' is probably caused by a slow leakage inward of sodium ions

Na^+ Ca^+ Na^+

2 - This produces depolarization

Na^+ Na^+ Ca^+ Na^+ Ca^+

3 - They act as controllers (e.g. calcium)

Smooth muscle, which lines the internal organs and blood vessels, has action potentials with much slower upstrokes than in most nerve and muscle cells; there is strong evidence that the main ion which flows during the action potential is calcium, not sodium, and as calcium is present in much lower concentrations than sodium this explains the lower rate of depolarization.

The calcium which enters the cell helps to initiate contraction in a manner similar to the calcium flowing into heart muscle cells during the plateau, and these mechanisms will be fully described when muscle contraction is discussed.

Many types of smooth muscle exhibit spontaneous activity rather similar to that in cardiac muscle, with areas of internal organs acting as pacemaker regions.

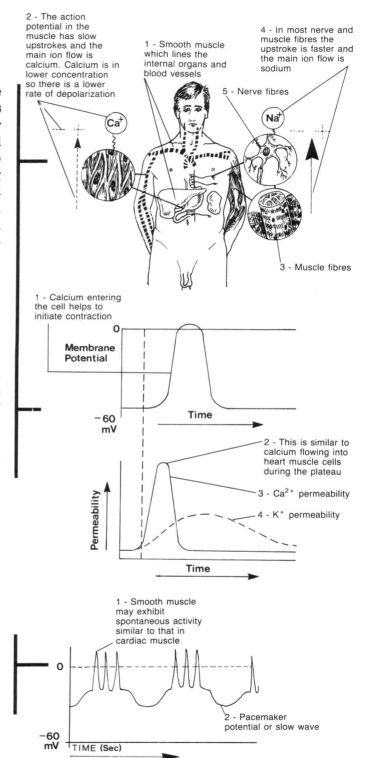

2 - The action potential in the muscle has slow upstrokes and the main ion flow is calcium. Calcium is in lower concentration so there is a lower rate of depolarization

1 - Smooth muscle which lines the internal organs and blood vessels

4 - In most nerve and muscle fibres the upstroke is faster and the main ion flow is sodium

5 - Nerve fibres

3 - Muscle fibres

1 - Calcium entering the cell helps to initiate contraction

Membrane Potential

0

−60 mV

Time

2 - This is similar to calcium flowing into heart muscle cells during the plateau

3 - Ca^{2+} permeability

4 - K^+ permeability

Permeability

Time

1 - Smooth muscle may exhibit spontaneous activity similar to that in cardiac muscle

0

2 - Pacemaker potential or slow wave

−60 mV

TIME (Sec)

The exact mechanisms involved in the spontaneous activity are still far from clear, but there may be rhythmic changes in permeability to sodium or calcium, or fluctuations in the activity of active transport mechanisms pumping ions across the cell membrane.

1 - There may be rhythmic changes in permeability to sodium or calcium

2 - There may be rhythmic changes or fluctuations in the activity of active transport

3 - Active transport mechanisms pumping ions across the cell membrane

Several others types of excitable membrane have action potentials involving calcium rather than sodium, and these include many of the cell bodies of neurones within the central nervous system and the peripheral ganglia (although the long axon processes of these cells almost always have sodium action potentials).

1 - Other excitable membranes have action potentials involving calcium. This includes the cell bodies of neurones in the CNS and peripheral ganglia

4 - Cell body

3 - Axon

2 - The axons of these cells, however, almost always have sodium action potentials

SYNAPTIC TRANSMISSION

The generation and conduction of an action potential in a cell is not a particularly useful event, unless the information can be transmitted to other cells in the body, or can produce some mechanical or chemical event in the cell such as contraction or secretion.

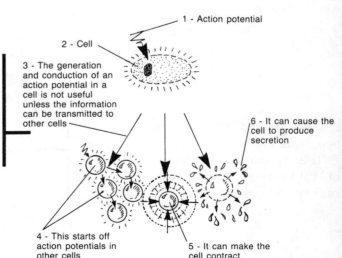

1 - Action potential

2 - Cell

3 - The generation and conduction of an action potential in a cell is not useful unless the information can be transmitted to other cells

6 - It can cause the cell to produce secretion

4 - This starts off action potentials in other cells

5 - It can make the cell contract

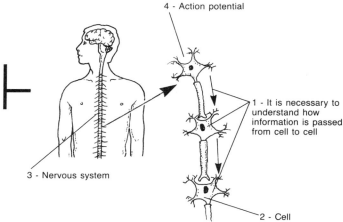

We shall now consider how information is transmitted from cell to cell within the nervous system.

4 - Action potential

1 - It is necessary to understand how information is passed from cell to cell

3 - Nervous system

2 - Cell

Convergence and divergence are two important concepts in describing neural pathways. **Convergence** is a term used to describe the input of information from many different sources on to a single neurone.

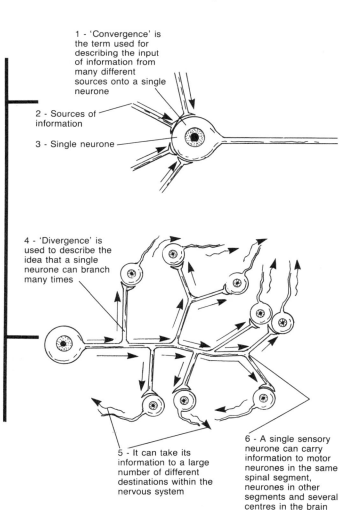

1 - 'Convergence' is the term used for describing the input of information from many different sources onto a single neurone

2 - Sources of information

3 - Single neurone

Divergence is the term used to describe the idea that a single neurone can branch many times and take its information to a large number of different destinations within the nervous system. For example, a single sensory neurone can carry information to motor neurones in the same spinal segment, to neurones in other segments, and to several centres in the brain.

4 - 'Divergence' is used to describe the idea that a single neurone can branch many times

5 - It can take its information to a large number of different destinations within the nervous system

6 - A single sensory neurone can carry information to motor neurones in the same spinal segment, neurones in other segments and several centres in the brain

The chemical nature of synapses

The terminal processes of some nerve cells come very close to the dendrites or cell bodies of other nerves; these close approaches are called **synapses**. At first it was unclear whether nerves communicated at synapses by some obscure electrical means, or whether there was some chemical agent involved.

Proof that nerves released chemicals was provided by an elegant experiment by Otto Loewi, who isolated the hearts of two frogs and arranged that the fluid perfusing the first heart flowed over the second.

Electrical stimulation of the vagus nerve to the first heart caused it to beat more slowly; the effluent fluid from this heart flowing over the second heart slowed its beat as well, showing that a chemical substance had been released during stimulation of the nerve supplying the first heart. This substance was later identified as acetylcholine.

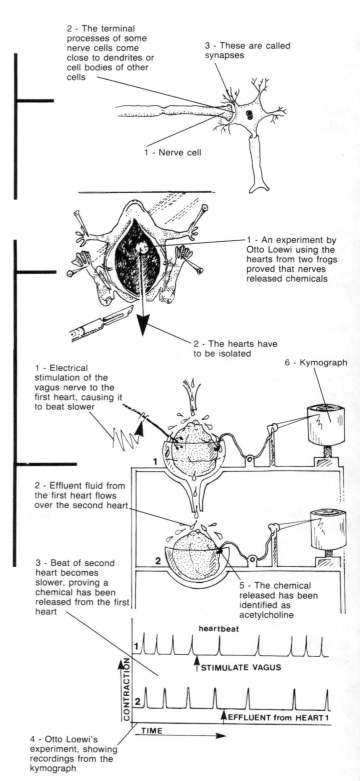

2 - The terminal processes of some nerve cells come close to dendrites or cell bodies of other cells

3 - These are called synapses

1 - Nerve cell

1 - An experiment by Otto Loewi using the hearts from two frogs proved that nerves released chemicals

2 - The hearts have to be isolated

1 - Electrical stimulation of the vagus nerve to the first heart, causing it to beat slower

6 - Kymograph

2 - Effluent fluid from the first heart flows over the second heart

3 - Beat of second heart becomes slower, proving a chemical has been released from the first heart

5 - The chemical released has been identified as acetylcholine

heartbeat

STIMULATE VAGUS

EFFLUENT from HEART 1

CONTRACTION

TIME

4 - Otto Loewi's experiment, showing recordings from the kymograph

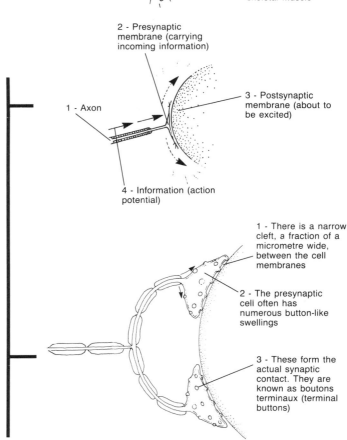

1 - A similar experiment is attempted during stimulation of the nerves supplying skeletal muscle

2 - Nerve

3 - Muscle

4 - The release of a chemical was difficult to demonstrate

5 - A drug was then added, inhibiting enzymatic breakdown of acetylcholine

6 - This showed that acetylcholine was also released during stimulation of the nerves supplying skeletal muscle

Many attempts were made to do a similar experiment during stimulation of the nerves which supply skeletal muscle, but at first it was difficult to demonstrate the release of a chemical. Later, when a drug was added which inhibits the enzymatic breakdown of acetylcholine, it was possible to show that acetylcholine was also released during stimulation of the nerves supplying skeletal muscle.

Structure of the synapse

With the electron microscope it is possible to identify the **presynaptic** membrane of the cell which is carrying the incoming information and the **postsynaptic** membrane of the cell which is about to be excited.

2 - Presynaptic membrane (carrying incoming information)

3 - Postsynaptic membrane (about to be excited)

1 - Axon

4 - Information (action potential)

There is a narrow cleft, typically a fraction of a micrometre wide, between the cell membranes. The presynaptic cell often has numerous button-like swellings which form the actual synaptic contact, and are known as **boutons terminaux** or terminal buttons.

1 - There is a narrow cleft, a fraction of a micrometre wide, between the cell membranes

2 - The presynaptic cell often has numerous button-like swellings

3 - These form the actual synaptic contact. They are known as boutons terminaux (terminal buttons)

These buttons contain many mitochondria, suggesting that intense metabolic activity occurs here; they also contain numerous vesicles close to the presynaptic membrane, which are thought to contain small 'packets' of the chemical transmitter which is to be released from the cell.

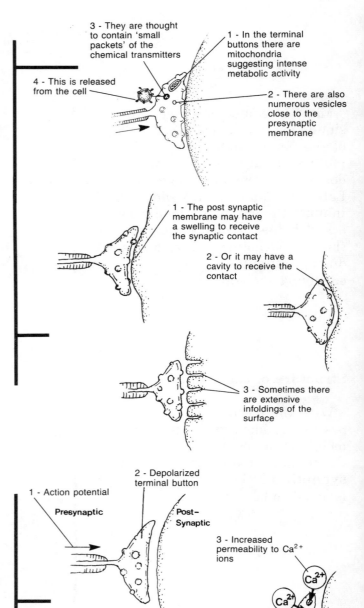

3 - They are thought to contain 'small packets' of the chemical transmitters

1 - In the terminal buttons there are mitochondria suggesting intense metabolic activity

4 - This is released from the cell

2 - There are also numerous vesicles close to the presynaptic membrane

1 - The post synaptic membrane may have a swelling to receive the synaptic contact

2 - Or it may have a cavity to receive the contact

The postsynaptic membrane may have a swelling or a cavity to receive the synaptic contact; sometimes there are extensive infoldings of the surface membrane, but often there are no specialized structures.

3 - Sometimes there are extensive infoldings of the surface

Release of neurotransmitters

When an action potential in the presynaptic nerve reaches the terminal buttons, it depolarizes the membrane, causing an increase in the permeability of the presynaptic membrane to calcium ions. These enter the cell along their electrochemical gradient (there is normally an extremely low intracellular concentration of free calcium ions) and cause the small vesicles to migrate towards the cell membrane, where the membrane of the vesicle fuses with the surface membrane of the cell, and the contents of the vesicle are liberated into the synaptic cleft.

1 - Action potential

Presynaptic

2 - Depolarized terminal button

Post-Synaptic

3 - Increased permeability to Ca^{2+} ions

4 - Ca^{2+} entry causes vesicles to migrate towards cell membrane and release their contents into the synaptic cleft

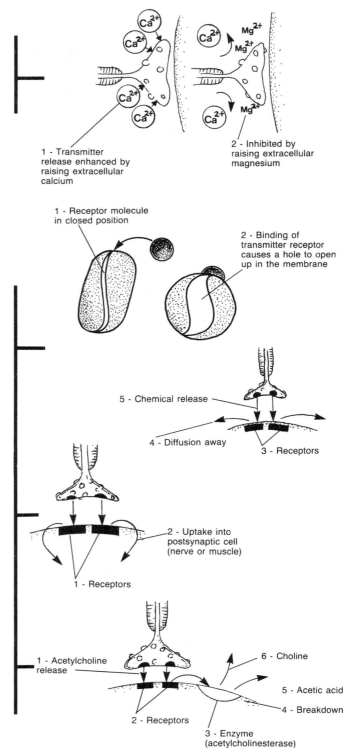

The release of transmitter is enhanced by raising the extracellular concentration of calcium ions, and inhibited by raising the concentration of magnesium.

1 - Transmitter release enhanced by raising extracellular calcium

2 - Inhibited by raising extracellular magnesium

1 - Receptor molecule in closed position

2 - Binding of transmitter receptor causes a hole to open up in the membrane

The released chemicals diffuse across the narrow cleft between cells, reaching the postsynaptic cell membrane, where they bind with specialized molecules or **receptors** and produce a change in shape in the receptor. This alters the postsynaptic membrane's permeability to certain ions.

5 - Chemical release

4 - Diffusion away

3 - Receptors

There are a number of inactivation mechanisms for rapidly terminating the action of the neurotransmitter. The simplest (and slowest) mechanism is passive diffusion of the chemical away from the receptors.

2 - Uptake into postsynaptic cell (nerve or muscle)

1 - Receptors

Many systems have a specific enzyme close to the synapse which breaks down the transmitter (the best known is acetylcholinesterase, which breaks down acetylcholine into choline and acetic acid).

1 - Acetylcholine release

2 - Receptors

3 - Enzyme (acetylcholinesterase)

4 - Breakdown

5 - Acetic acid

6 - Choline

Other systems have a specific uptake or active transport mechanism which takes the transmitter back into the nerve endings for reuse, or into a postsynaptic neurone or muscle for subsequent inactivation or degradation (this is the mechanism whereby the catecholamines such as adrenaline and noradrenaline are inactivated).

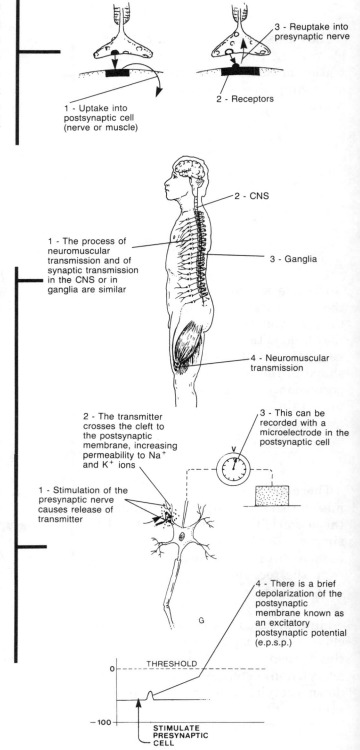

3 - Reuptake into presynaptic nerve

2 - Receptors

1 - Uptake into postsynaptic cell (nerve or muscle)

Postsynaptic actions of transmitters

The processes of neuromuscular transmission and of synaptic transmission in the central nervous system or in ganglia are rather similar.

2 - CNS

1 - The process of neuromuscular transmission and of synaptic transmission in the CNS or in ganglia are similar

3 - Ganglia

4 - Neuromuscular transmission

Stimulation of the presynaptic nerve causes release of transmitter into the synaptic cleft, with diffusion of chemical across the gap to combine with receptors on the postsynaptic membrane. This produces an increase in the membrane's permeability to sodium and potassium (and possibly chloride) ions, which results in a brief depolarization of the postsynaptic membrane, known as an **excitatory postsynaptic potential** (e.p.s.p.) which can be recorded with a microelectrode in the postsynaptic cell.

2 - The transmitter crosses the cleft to the postsynaptic membrane, increasing permeability to Na^+ and K^+ ions

3 - This can be recorded with a microelectrode in the postsynaptic cell

1 - Stimulation of the presynaptic nerve causes release of transmitter

4 - There is a brief depolarization of the postsynaptic membrane known as an excitatory postsynaptic potential (e.p.s.p.)

THRESHOLD

0

-100

STIMULATE PRESYNAPTIC CELL

The permeability change is *not* dependent upon the magnitude of the membrane potential (unlike the action potential), but only upon the concentration of transmitter molecules in contact with receptors on the membrane.

It is very unusual for a single pre-synaptic action potential at one synapse to produce an action potential in the postsynaptic cell, but if a number of impulses in the presynaptic neurone follow each other in rapid succession, then each wave of depolarization (or e.p.s.p.) can build up on top of the previous one, producing progressively increasing depolarization until the threshold of the postsynaptic membrane is reached, and an action potential is initiated.

This process of increasing depolariz-ation in response to repetitive stimu-lation is known as **temporal summation**.

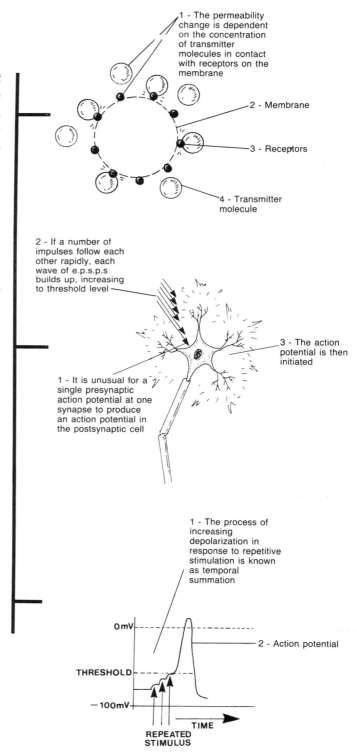

1 - The permeability change is dependent on the concentration of transmitter molecules in contact with receptors on the membrane

2 - Membrane

3 - Receptors

4 - Transmitter molecule

2 - If a number of impulses follow each other rapidly, each wave of e.p.s.p.s builds up, increasing to threshold level

3 - The action potential is then initiated

1 - It is unusual for a single presynaptic action potential at one synapse to produce an action potential in the postsynaptic cell

1 - The process of increasing depolarization in response to repetitive stimulation is known as temporal summation

2 - Action potential

0 mV

THRESHOLD

-100mV

TIME

REPEATED STIMULUS

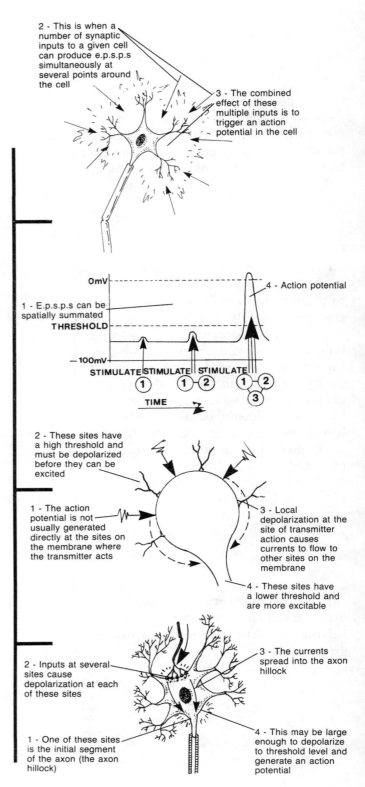

2 - This is when a number of synaptic inputs to a given cell can produce e.p.s.p.s simultaneously at several points around the cell

3 - The combined effect of these multiple inputs is to trigger an action potential in the cell

E.p.s.p.s can also be **spatially summated**, when a number of synaptic inputs to a given cell can produce e.p.s.p.s almost simultaneously at several points around the cell's circumference, and the combined effect of these multiple inputs is to trigger an action potential in the cell.

0mV

1 - E.p.s.p.s can be spatially summated

THRESHOLD

—100mV

STIMULATE STIMULATE STIMULATE

① ①② ①②③

4 - Action potential

TIME

The action potential in a postsynaptic cell is not usually generated directly at the sites on the membrane where the transmitter acts; these sites actually have quite a high threshold to which they must be depolarized before they can be excited. Instead, the local depolarization at the site of transmitter action causes currents to flow within the cell to other sites on the membrane which have a lower threshold and are more excitable; one such site is the **initial segment** of the axon, or the **axon hillock**, and if several synaptic inputs are received to different parts of the cell, causing depolarization at a number of sites, the currents spreading into the axon hillock may be large enough to depolarize it to threshold and generate an action potential.

2 - These sites have a high threshold and must be depolarized before they can be excited

1 - The action potential is not usually generated directly at the sites on the membrane where the transmitter acts

3 - Local depolarization at the site of transmitter action causes currents to flow to other sites on the membrane

4 - These sites have a lower threshold and are more excitable

2 - Inputs at several sites cause depolarization at each of these sites

3 - The currents spread into the axon hillock

1 - One of these sites is the initial segment of the axon (the axon hillock)

4 - This may be large enough to depolarize to threshold level and generate an action potential

The action potential generated at the axon hillock spreads **orthodromically** (in the normal direction) or out along the long axon process of the cell, and the excitation also spreads **antidromically** to invade the soma of the neurone, causing a soma—dendrite action potential.

The axon hillock is a site of **integration**, sensing the sum of synaptic inputs to the cell and discharging an impulse if the inputs are large enough.

For example, a neurone may require to have inputs both from segmental sensory neurones and from higher centres within the brain before it can discharge; neither input alone may be sufficient.

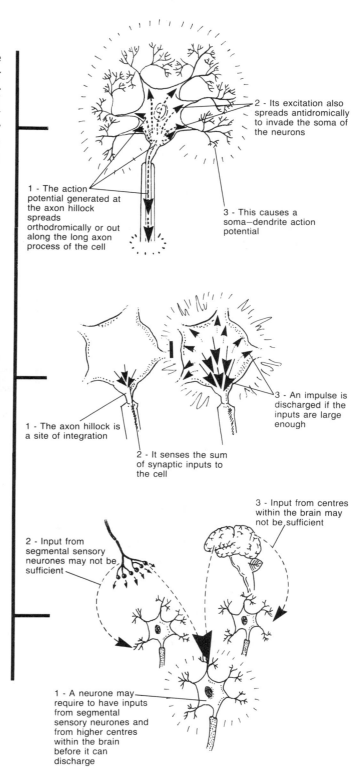

2 - Its excitation also spreads antidromically to invade the soma of the neurons

1 - The action potential generated at the axon hillock spreads orthodromically or out along the long axon process of the cell

3 - This causes a soma—dendrite action potential

1 - The axon hillock is a site of integration

2 - It senses the sum of synaptic inputs to the cell

3 - An impulse is discharged if the inputs are large enough

3 - Input from centres within the brain may not be sufficient

2 - Input from segmental sensory neurones may not be sufficient

1 - A neurone may require to have inputs from segmental sensory neurones and from higher centres within the brain before it can discharge

A typical motor neurone in the spinal cord may have many thousands of separate synaptic connections on its dendrites and soma (an example of enormous **convergence**); several of these contacts may come from the same presynaptic neurone, but there is really a very large number of inputs to the cell.

Not all of the synaptic connections are excitatory: equally important are the inhibitory inputs to the neurone, from presynaptic cells which release inhibitory transmitters. Stimulation of these presynaptic cells causes the postsynaptic membrane to be **hyperpolarized**, and a microelectrode in the postsynaptic cell would record an **inhibitory postsynaptic potential** (i.p.s.p.).

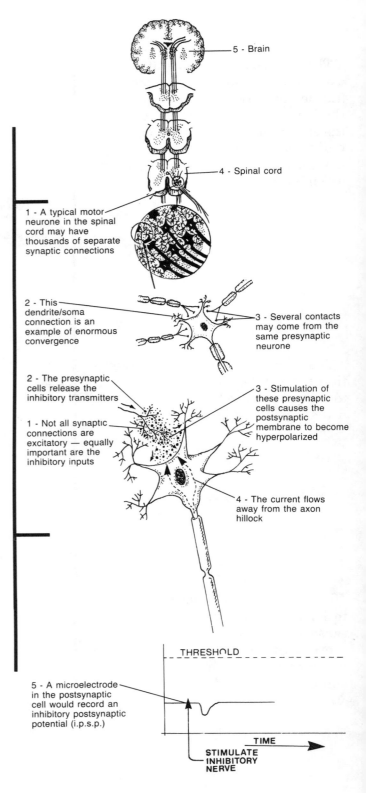

5 - Brain

4 - Spinal cord

1 - A typical motor neurone in the spinal cord may have thousands of separate synaptic connections

2 - This dendrite/soma connection is an example of enormous convergence

3 - Several contacts may come from the same presynaptic neurone

2 - The presynaptic cells release the inhibitory transmitters

1 - Not all synaptic connections are excitatory — equally important are the inhibitory inputs

3 - Stimulation of these presynaptic cells causes the postsynaptic membrane to become hyperpolarized

4 - The current flows away from the axon hillock

THRESHOLD

5 - A microelectrode in the postsynaptic cell would record an inhibitory postsynaptic potential (i.p.s.p.)

TIME

STIMULATE INHIBITORY NERVE

When an inhibitory transmitter combines with a postsynaptic receptor, it usually increases the membrane's permeability to potassium ions alone (or sometimes to potassium and chloride), and the outflow of positively charged ions along their concentration gradient causes the hyperpolarization.

If an inhibitory input coincides with an excitatory input, the hyperpolarization at one site on the membrane tends to counteract the depolarization at another site, so that the sum of the currents flowing into the axon hillock will be smaller, and the cell is less likely to discharge an action potential.

If a neurone is under heavy inhibitory bombardment, it requires a very large excitatory input indeed to excite the cell; such a large input may take the form either of large numbers of impulses along a single group of pathways (temporal summation) or a large number of simultaneous inputs along parallel pathways (spatial summation).

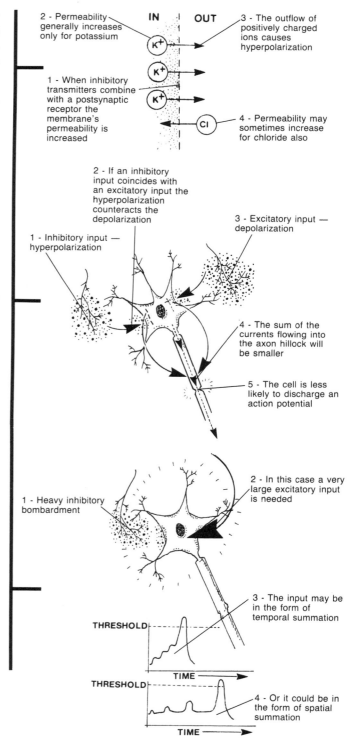

2 - Permeability generally increases only for potassium

IN   OUT

3 - The outflow of positively charged ions causes hyperpolarization

1 - When inhibitory transmitters combine with a postsynaptic receptor the membrane's permeability is increased

4 - Permeability may sometimes increase for chloride also

2 - If an inhibitory input coincides with an excitatory input the hyperpolarization counteracts the depolarization

3 - Excitatory input — depolarization

1 - Inhibitory input — hyperpolarization

4 - The sum of the currents flowing into the axon hillock will be smaller

5 - The cell is less likely to discharge an action potential

2 - In this case a very large excitatory input is needed

1 - Heavy inhibitory bombardment

3 - The input may be in the form of temporal summation

THRESHOLD

TIME

THRESHOLD

4 - Or it could be in the form of spatial summation

TIME

The neuromuscular junction

One of the most convenient preparations for studying the effects of neurotransmitters is the neuromuscular junction of skeletal muscle.

A microelectrode inserted into the muscle cell close to the site where the nerve terminal makes contact (**motor endplate**) can be used to follow the voltage changes in the postsynaptic membrane in response to stimulation of the presynaptic nerve.

When the presynaptic nerve is stimulated, acetylcholine is released and diffuses across the neuromuscular cleft to reach the postsynaptic membrane.

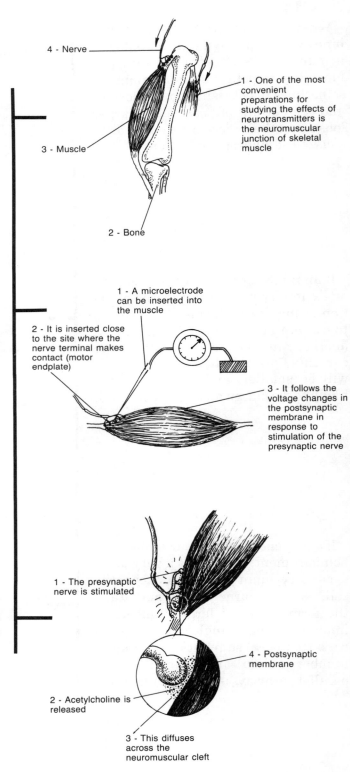

4 - Nerve

1 - One of the most convenient preparations for studying the effects of neurotransmitters is the neuromuscular junction of skeletal muscle

3 - Muscle

2 - Bone

1 - A microelectrode can be inserted into the muscle

2 - It is inserted close to the site where the nerve terminal makes contact (motor endplate)

3 - It follows the voltage changes in the postsynaptic membrane in response to stimulation of the presynaptic nerve

1 - The presynaptic nerve is stimulated

4 - Postsynaptic membrane

2 - Acetylcholine is released

3 - This diffuses across the neuromuscular cleft

2 - This produces an increase in the membrane's permeability to sodium and potassium

There it combines with receptors to produce an increase in the membrane's permeability to sodium and potassium ions, which results in a brief depolarization of the postsynaptic membrane, known as an **endplate potential** (e.p.p.), which is similar to the e.p.s.p.

1 - There the acetylcholine combines with receptors

3 - This results in a brief depolarization of the postsynaptic membrane

0mV

Threshold

−100mV

4 - This is known as an endplate potential (e.p.p.)

STIMULATE NERVE   STIMULATE NERVE   REPETITIVE STIMULATION

Normally the endplate potential in response to a single presynaptic impulse is large enough to depolarize the postsynaptic membrane to threshold and initiate an action potential in the muscle; this is then conducted along the whole surface of the muscle cell and causes contraction.

1 - The e.p.p. in response to a single presynaptic impulse

2 - It is normally large enough to depolarize the postsynaptic membrane to threshold

3 - This initiates an action potential along the muscle cell

4 - This causes contraction

This makes the details of the endplate potential difficult to study, as it becomes obscured by the much larger action potential, and the contraction may dislodge the microelectrode from the cell.

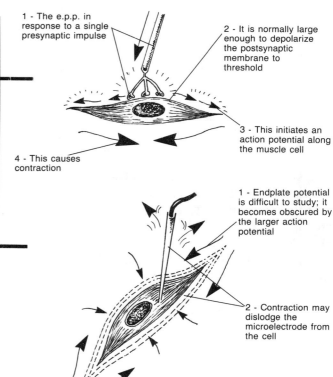

1 - Endplate potential is difficult to study; it becomes obscured by the larger action potential

2 - Contraction may dislodge the microelectrode from the cell

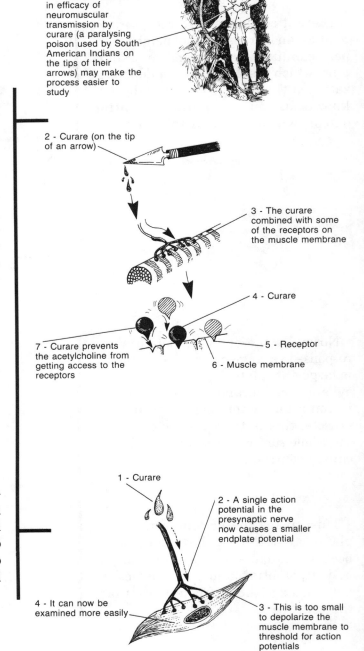

1 - Artificial reduction in efficacy of neuromuscular transmission by curare (a paralysing poison used by South American Indians on the tips of their arrows) may make the process easier to study

Researchers have often taken steps to reduce artificially the efficacy of neuromuscular transmission, so that the individual events may be studied more easily. It is usual to apply some *curare* (a paralysing poison originally used by South American Indians on the tips of their blow-pipe darts or arrows), which combines with some of the receptors on the muscle membrane, preventing acetylcholine from getting access to some of the receptors and hence reducing its efficacy.

2 - Curare (on the tip of an arrow)

3 - The curare combined with some of the receptors on the muscle membrane

4 - Curare

5 - Receptor

6 - Muscle membrane

7 - Curare prevents the acetylcholine from getting access to the receptors

A single action potential in the presynaptic nerve now causes a much smaller endplate potential — too small to depolarize the muscle membrane to threshold. It now becomes possible to examine the properties of individual (attenuated) e.p.p.s in more detail.

1 - Curare

2 - A single action potential in the presynaptic nerve now causes a smaller endplate potential

3 - This is too small to depolarize the muscle membrane to threshold for action potentials

4 - It can now be examined more easily

The membrane of skeletal muscle cells is not uniformly sensitive to acetylcholine. It is possible to use an extremely fine micropipette filled with the transmitter to eject minute quantities of the drug in the vicinity of the cell membrane; it is found that drug ejected at points away from the motor endplate is ineffective at depolarising the membrane, but small amounts of the drug ejected near the endplate are extremely effective at producing depolarization. This suggests that the receptors for acetylcholine are concentrated at the endplate region, with very few receptors on other parts of the cell membrane.

If a microelectrode is inserted into a muscle cell near the endplate and the membrane potential recorded at high amplifier gain, it is possible to observe rapid, tiny fluctuations in potential; these are probably due to the random spontaneous release of individual vesicles of acetylcholine from the presynaptic nerve ending, and are known as **miniature endplate potentials** (m.e.p.p.s).

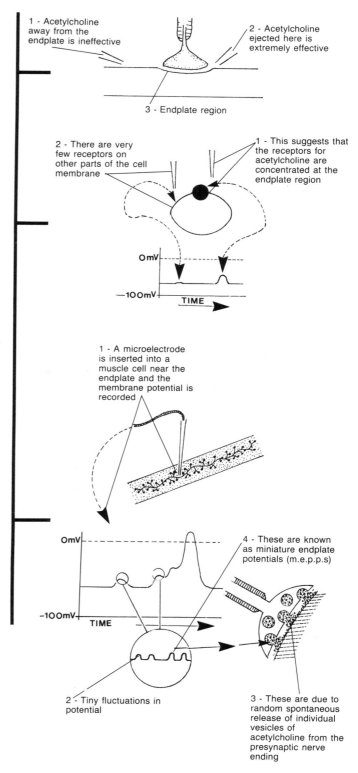

1 - Acetylcholine away from the endplate is ineffective

2 - Acetylcholine ejected here is extremely effective

3 - Endplate region

2 - There are very few receptors on other parts of the cell membrane

1 - This suggests that the receptors for acetylcholine are concentrated at the endplate region

0 mV

−100 mV TIME

1 - A microelectrode is inserted into a muscle cell near the endplate and the membrane potential is recorded

0 mV

−100 mV TIME

4 - These are known as miniature endplate potentials (m.e.p.p.s)

2 - Tiny fluctuations in potential

3 - These are due to random spontaneous release of individual vesicles of acetylcholine from the presynaptic nerve ending

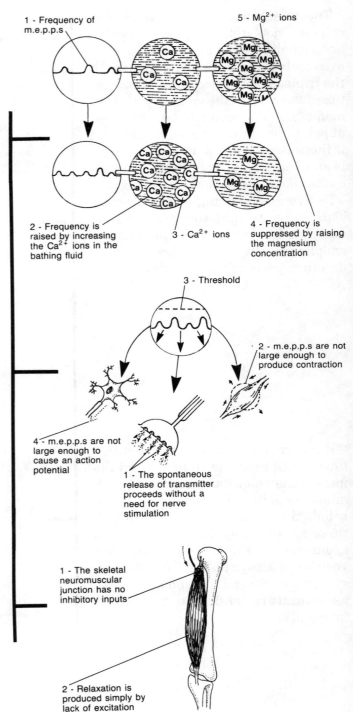

The frequency of m.e.p.p.s is increased by raising the concentration of calcium ions in the bathing fluid, and suppressed by raising the magnesium concentration.

The spontaneous release of transmitter proceeds without any need for nerve stimulation, but the m.e.p.p.s are not large enough to produce action potentials or cause contraction of the muscle.

The skeletal neuromuscular junction has no inhibitory inputs, and relaxation is provided simply by lack of excitation.

1 - Frequency of m.e.p.p.s

5 - Mg^{2+} ions

2 - Frequency is raised by increasing the Ca^{2+} ions in the bathing fluid

3 - Ca^{2+} ions

4 - Frequency is suppressed by raising the magnesium concentration

3 - Threshold

2 - m.e.p.p.s are not large enough to produce contraction

4 - m.e.p.p.s are not large enough to cause an action potential

1 - The spontaneous release of transmitter proceeds without a need for nerve stimulation

1 - The skeletal neuromuscular junction has no inhibitory inputs

2 - Relaxation is produced simply by lack of excitation

The identity of neurotransmitters

A number of criteria must be satisfied before a particular chemical can be identified as the neurotransmitter at a particular synapse or junction:

1. It must be released from the presynaptic nerve during stimulation.

2. The artificially applied chemical must produce the same effect on the postsynaptic membrane as does the transmitter naturally released during nerve stimulation.

3. There must be metabolic pathways in the presynaptic cell for manufacture of the transmitter.

4. There must be a mechanism demonstrated for inactivation or removal of the transmitter.

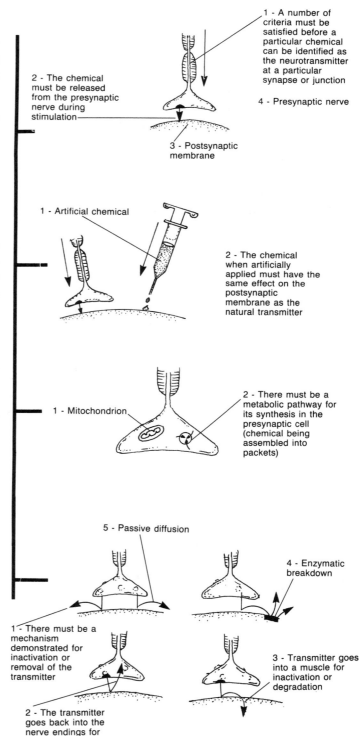

1 - A number of criteria must be satisfied before a particular chemical can be identified as the neurotransmitter at a particular synapse or junction

2 - The chemical must be released from the presynaptic nerve during stimulation

4 - Presynaptic nerve

3 - Postsynaptic membrane

1 - Artificial chemical

2 - The chemical when artificially applied must have the same effect on the postsynaptic membrane as the natural transmitter

1 - Mitochondrion

2 - There must be a metabolic pathway for its synthesis in the presynaptic cell (chemical being assembled into packets)

5 - Passive diffusion

4 - Enzymatic breakdown

1 - There must be a mechanism demonstrated for inactivation or removal of the transmitter

2 - The transmitter goes back into the nerve endings for reuse

3 - Transmitter goes into a muscle for inactivation or degradation

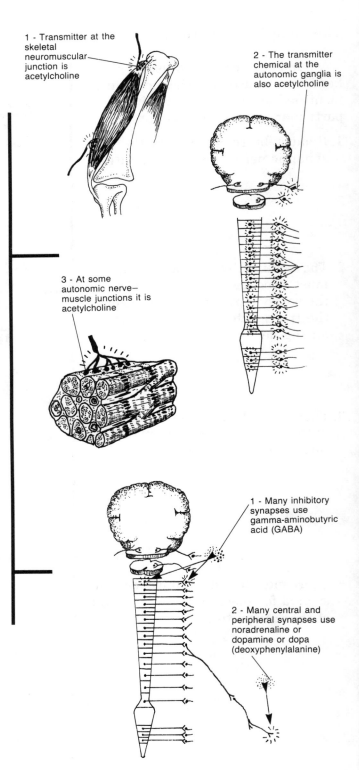

1 - Transmitter at the skeletal neuromuscular junction is acetylcholine

2 - The transmitter chemical at the autonomic ganglia is also acetylcholine

3 - At some autonomic nerve—muscle junctions it is acetylcholine

1 - Many inhibitory synapses use gamma-aminobutyric acid (GABA)

2 - Many central and peripheral synapses use noradrenaline or dopamine or dopa (deoxyphenylalanine)

If these criteria are applied, there are very few synaptic junctions at which the chemical identity of the transmitter is fully known. The evidence is complete for the skeletal neuromuscular junction, where the transmitter is known to be acetylcholine; at many autonomic ganglia the excitatory transmitter is also acetylcholine; at some autonomic nerve—muscle junctions the transmitter is acetylcholine, and at others it is noradrenaline. The inhibitory transmitters have been harder to identify, and there is still considerable doubt about the precise identity of the transmitters at many central synapses. However, many central synapses almost certainly use acetylcholine.

Many inhibitory synapses use gamma-aminobutyric acid (GABA), and many central synapses use noradrenaline or its close relations dopamine or dopa (deoxyphenylalanine).

Some central and peripheral synapses use a variety of polypeptide transmitters, such as vasoactive intestinal peptide (VIP), bombesin and the enkephalins, some of which are excitatory and some inhibitory.

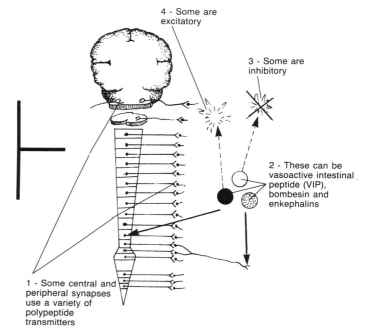

4 - Some are excitatory

3 - Some are inhibitory

2 - These can be vasoactive intestinal peptide (VIP), bombesin and enkephalins

1 - Some central and peripheral synapses use a variety of polypeptide transmitters

Motor Functions and Pathways

All activity in the brain is eventually translated into some form of motor activity, whether it be muscular movement (locomotion), linguistic communication (such as speech or writing, expressing simple or complex ideas) or autonomic activity (secretion from glands, or contraction or relaxation of smooth muscle in blood vessels or viscera). This chapter is concerned with the control of movement, and a later chapter will consider the control of visceral function.

THE MAIN MOTOR PATHWAY

Voluntary movement is initiated in large cells found in the pre-central gyrus of the cerebral cortex, the motor area. The various parts of the body are controlled by specific parts of the motor cortex, and the size of the area of cortex responsible for each organ is often out of proportion to the size of the organ controlled. For example, the hand and face areas in the motor cortex are very large, while a much smaller area is devoted to the foot.

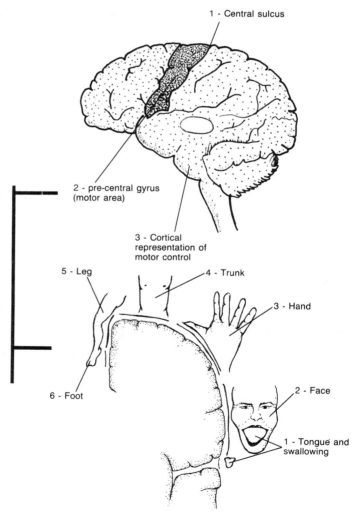

1 - Central sulcus

2 - pre-central gyrus (motor area)

3 - Cortical representation of motor control

5 - Leg

4 - Trunk

3 - Hand

6 - Foot

2 - Face

1 - Tongue and swallowing

The giant cells in the motor cortex, the pyramidal cells of Betz, have large axons which pass through the white matter of the cerebral hemisphere (the **internal capsule**), down through the brain stem in a clearly identifiable band, and cross the midline in the medulla oblongata as the dramatic **decussation of the pyramids**. Thus most pyramidal neurones control muscles on the opposite (**contralateral**) side of the body: a small proportion of axons do not cross, but control muscles on the same (**ipsilateral**) side.

Below the decussation, the axons of the **pyramidal tract** (or corticospinal tract) continue down the anterior part of the spinal cord in the white matter until they reach the level in the spinal cord which they are destined to control. At the appropriate level the axons enter the anterior horn of the spinal grey matter, and synapse with large cells known as anterior horn cells or alpha motor neurones (motorneurones).

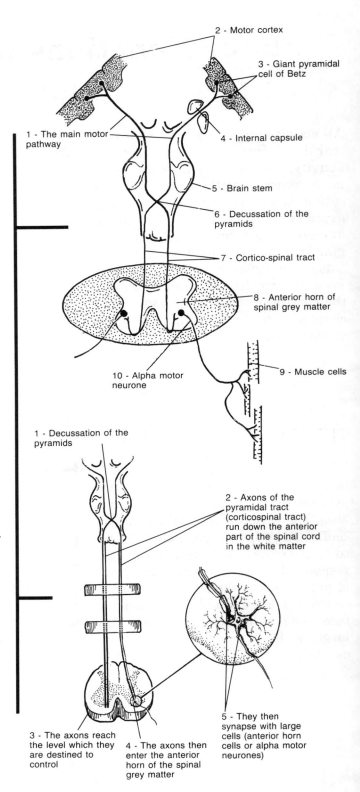

2 - Motor cortex

3 - Giant pyramidal cell of Betz

1 - The main motor pathway

4 - Internal capsule

5 - Brain stem

6 - Decussation of the pyramids

7 - Cortico-spinal tract

8 - Anterior horn of spinal grey matter

9 - Muscle cells

10 - Alpha motor neurone

1 - Decussation of the pyramids

2 - Axons of the pyramidal tract (corticospinal tract) run down the anterior part of the spinal cord in the white matter

5 - They then synapse with large cells (anterior horn cells or alpha motor neurones)

3 - The axons reach the level which they are destined to control

4 - The axons then enter the anterior horn of the spinal grey matter

The axons from the anterior horn cells leave the spinal cord in the anterior or ventral roots, enter the mixed spinal nerve and radiate out to the muscles.

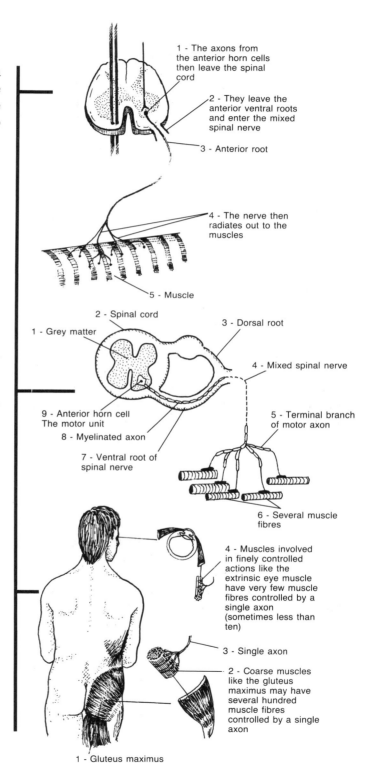

1 - The axons from the anterior horn cells then leave the spinal cord

2 - They leave the anterior ventral roots and enter the mixed spinal nerve

3 - Anterior root

4 - The nerve then radiates out to the muscles

5 - Muscle

2 - Spinal cord

1 - Grey matter

3 - Dorsal root

4 - Mixed spinal nerve

9 - Anterior horn cell The motor unit

8 - Myelinated axon

7 - Ventral root of spinal nerve

5 - Terminal branch of motor axon

6 - Several muscle fibres

Within the muscle each axon splits up into a number of terminal branches, controlling a number of individual muscle fibres. A single axon together with the group of muscle fibres which it controls is known as a **motor unit**.

The number of muscle fibres in a motor unit varies greatly from muscle to muscle: coarse muscles like the gluteus maximus, with a simple, rather stereotyped anti-gravity function, may have several hundred muscle fibres controlled by a single axon, while muscles involved in finely controlled actions, like the small muscles in the hand or the extrinsic eye muscles, have a very few (sometimes less than ten) muscle cells activated by each axon.

4 - Muscles involved in finely controlled actions like the extrinsic eye muscle have very few muscle fibres controlled by a single axon (sometimes less than ten)

3 - Single axon

2 - Coarse muscles like the gluteus maximus may have several hundred muscle fibres controlled by a single axon

1 - Gluteus maximus

Just after the axon leaves the cell body of the alpha motor neurone, it has a short collateral branch which synapses with an interneurone known as the **Renshaw cell**.

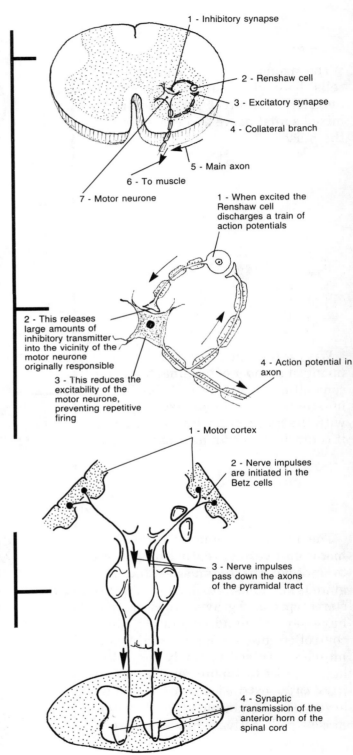

1 - Inhibitory synapse

2 - Renshaw cell

3 - Excitatory synapse

4 - Collateral branch

5 - Main axon

6 - To muscle

7 - Motor neurone

When excited by an action potential occurring in the main motor axon the Renshaw cell discharges a train of action potentials, releasing large amounts of inhibitory transmitter into the vicinity of the motor neurone responsible for the original impulse. This has the effect of reducing motor neurone excitability immediately after the successful initiation of an action potential, and prevents prolonged or repetitive firing of the neurone.

1 - When excited the Renshaw cell discharges a train of action potentials

2 - This releases large amounts of inhibitory transmitter into the vicinity of the motor neurone originally responsible

3 - This reduces the excitability of the motor neurone, preventing repetitive firing

4 - Action potential in axon

Nerve impulses initiated in the Betz cells of the motor cortex (the **upper motor neurone**) travel down the axons of the pyramidal tract and cause synaptic transmission to occur in the anterior horn of the spinal cord.

1 - Motor cortex

2 - Nerve impulses are initiated in the Betz cells

3 - Nerve impulses pass down the axons of the pyramidal tract

4 - Synaptic transmission of the anterior horn of the spinal cord

Impulses excited in the anterior horn cells (the **lower motor neurones**) pass along the motor axons and cause the release of acetylcholine at the neuro-muscular junctions with striated muscle fibres; this depolarizes the membrane of the muscle cells at the motor end-plate, and an action potential is pro-duced in the muscle fibre membrane.

1 - Impulses excited in anterior horn cells

2 - They pass along the motor axons and cause release of acetylcholine at the neuromuscular junctions

3 - Striated muscle fibres

4 - An action potential is produced and the cells are depolarized

EXCITATION–CONTRACTION COUPLING

The surface membrane of the muscle cell is connected to an extensive series of tubules, the **transverse tubule system**, and an action potential passing along the surface membrane is con-ducted down the tubules, so that excita-tion is carried deep into the substance of the muscle fibre.

1 - Action potential

2 - Release of acetylcholine

4 - Action potential along surface membrane

3 - Action potential along transverse tubule carrying excitation deep into the muscle

There is a second series of tubules, close to the transverse tubules but not making any direct contact with them, and completely isolated from the sur-face of the muscle cell. They are called the **sarcoplasmic reticulum** (which is simply the name for endoplasmic reti-culum, as applied to muscle cells) and its vesicles or **cisternae** are capable of being influenced by electric currents flowing in the transverse tubular system.

1 - The sarcoplasmic reticulum is a second series of tubules

2 - They are close to the transverse tubules with no direct contact and isolated from the cell surface

3 - Its vesicles (or cisternae) are capable of being influenced by electric currents flowing in the transverse tubular system

4 - Transverse tubules

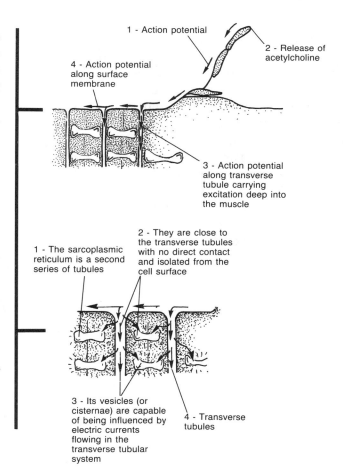

The sarcoplasmic reticulum contains large quantities of calcium, while the cytoplasm (or sarcoplasm) of the muscle fibre normally has a very low concentration of free calcium ions — typically less than 10^{-9} mol/l. There are enzyme systems in the walls of the sarcoplasmic reticulum which actively transport calcium ions out of the cytoplasm and into the sarcoplasmic reticulum, which acts as a calcium store.

Excitation of the transverse tubule system causes the sarcoplasmic reticulum to release stored calcium ions into the sarcoplasm, and there they interact with specialized proteins, the **contractile proteins**, to cause the muscle cell to shorten or to develop contractile force or tension. As soon as the excitation is removed from the muscle cell the calcium ions are actively transported from the sarcoplasm back into the sarcoplasmic reticulum and the muscle relaxes.

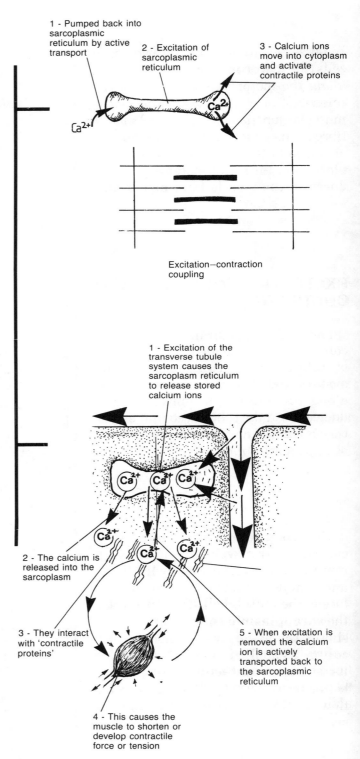

1 - Pumped back into sarcoplasmic reticulum by active transport

2 - Excitation of sarcoplasmic reticulum

3 - Calcium ions move into cytoplasm and activate contractile proteins

Ca^{2+}

Ca^{2+}

Excitation—contraction coupling

1 - Excitation of the transverse tubule system causes the sarcoplasm reticulum to release stored calcium ions

2 - The calcium is released into the sarcoplasm

3 - They interact with 'contractile proteins'

4 - This causes the muscle to shorten or develop contractile force or tension

5 - When excitation is removed the calcium ion is actively transported back to the sarcoplasmic reticulum

MUSCLE CONTRACTION

The proteins of striated muscle are highly specialized for contraction. The main contractile proteins are **actin** and **myosin**, which are long molecules arranged in a highly organized and registered way which gives the cells their striped appearance when they are viewed under polarized light or after the use of certain histological stains.

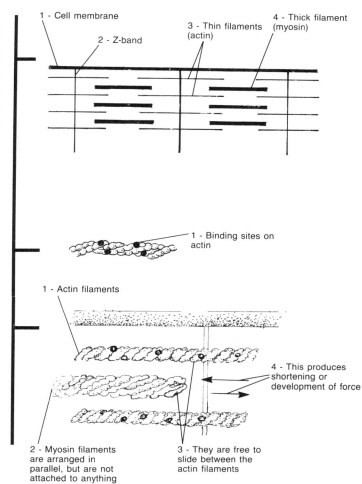

1 - Cell membrane

2 - Z-band

3 - Thin filaments (actin)

4 - Thick filament (myosin)

1 - Binding sites on actin

1 - Actin filaments

2 - Myosin filaments are arranged in parallel, but are not attached to anything

3 - They are free to slide between the actin filaments

4 - This produces shortening or development of force

The molecules of myosin form thick filaments (when viewed with the electron microscope), and actin forms thin filaments. Actin filaments are arranged in parallel and attached to fine proteins connected to the surface membrane at the Z-bands. Myosin filaments are also arranged in parallel, but are not attached to anything; they are free to slide between the actin filaments, producing shortening or the development of force.

The myosin filaments are made up of bundles of individual molecules which have a long shaft and a club-like head. There are two points where the molecule can bend or pivot, and the head has an active site which can bind to a corresponding active site on the actin molecule.

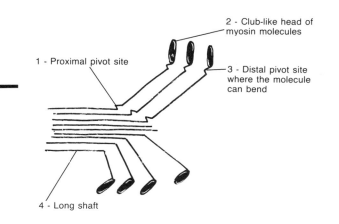

1 - Proximal pivot site

2 - Club-like head of myosin molecules

3 - Distal pivot site where the molecule can bend

4 - Long shaft

The active site in the actin filament is usually covered by an inhibitory molecule, tropomyosin, which prevents the myosin molecule from binding to actin. Tropomyosin is connected to another molecule, troponin, which has a high affinity for free calcium ions, and when these ions enter the cytoplasm from the sarcoplasmic reticulum they become bound to troponin. This inactivates the inhibitory action of tropomyosin; in other words, calcium ions inhibit the inhibition!

Once tropomyosin is inactivated, the heads of the myosin molecules are enabled to bind to the active sites of actin, forming cross-bridges between actin and myosin. The chemical action of binding produces stresses in the myosin molecule, making the head pivot about its nearest 'hinge', with the release of stored energy. This rotation moves the point of attachment, producing relative sliding of the filaments.

The rotation of the head weakens the link between actin and myosin, so that eventually the head disengages from the binding site; in its rotated state the head has very strong ATPase activity, enzymatically cleaving adenosine triphosphate (ATP) to the diphosphate (ADP) and releasing a large amount of energy. This energy is used to reset the myosin head back into its original 'cocked' state, ready to bind to another active site on the actin molecule and produce further movement. Thus the cellular energy released from breaking down ATP is stored in the reset myosin head and is available to produce the 'power stroke' of the cross-bridge cycle.

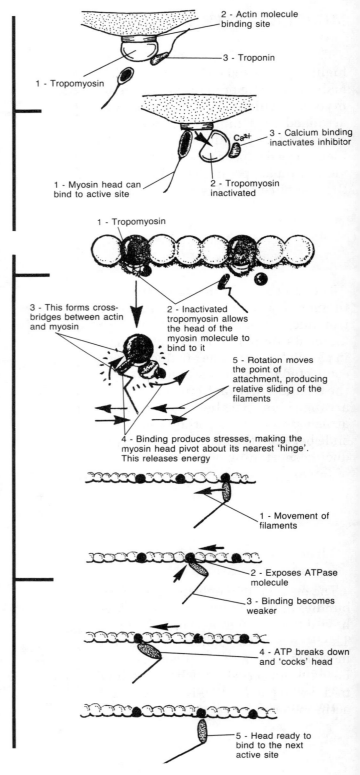

2 - Actin molecule binding site
3 - Troponin
1 - Tropomyosin

3 - Calcium binding inactivates inhibitor
1 - Myosin head can bind to active site
2 - Tropomyosin inactivated

1 - Tropomyosin

3 - This forms cross-bridges between actin and myosin
2 - Inactivated tropomyosin allows the head of the myosin molecule to bind to it
5 - Rotation moves the point of attachment, producing relative sliding of the filaments
4 - Binding produces stresses, making the myosin head pivot about its nearest 'hinge'. This releases energy

1 - Movement of filaments

2 - Exposes ATPase molecule
3 - Binding becomes weaker

4 - ATP breaks down and 'cocks' head

5 - Head ready to bind to the next active site

So long as calcium ions are present in the cytoplasm, the process of binding, bending and unbinding of myosin and actin (cross-bridge cycling) takes place repeatedly, producing movement of the muscle or the generation of force.

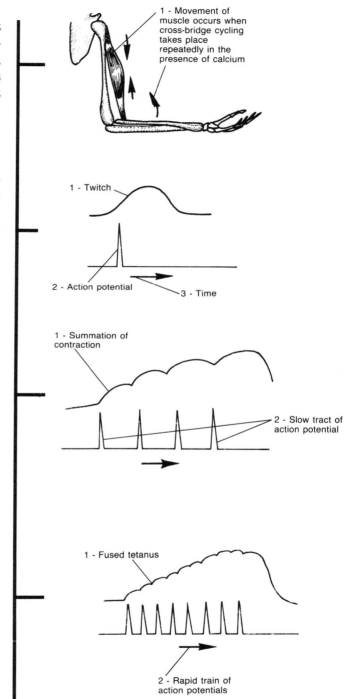

1 - Movement of muscle occurs when cross-bridge cycling takes place repeatedly in the presence of calcium

The action potential which initiates contraction in muscle lasts for only a few milliseconds, and then the muscle cell membrane is ready to be excited again. The release and subsequent re-uptake of calcium is a rather slower process, so that the contraction in response to a single action potential ('twitch') is a more prolonged event.

1 - Twitch

2 - Action potential

3 - Time

If a subsequent action potential occurs before the muscle has had a chance to relax from the previous twitch, the second twitch can summate with the previous one.

1 - Summation of contraction

2 - Slow tract of action potential

If action potentials follow one another in rapid succession, the individual twitches become fused to form a smooth 'tetanus'. The amplitude of the tetanic contraction can be several times larger than the individual twitch, and is determined by the frequency of action potentials, which is usually the same as the rate of firing in the motor neurone.

1 - Fused tetanus

2 - Rapid train of action potentials

There are two kinds of result from activation of the contractile machinery: the muscle may shorten or it may develop force (or of course it may do both). If it shortens without developing tension the contraction is known as **isotonic**, and if it develops force (or tension) without shortening it is known as an **isometric** contraction.

The magnitude of an isometric contraction (in response to a maximal tetanic stimulation of the nerve) depends upon the length of the muscle fibre; more particularly it depends upon the **sarcomere length** or the distance between one Z-band and the next.

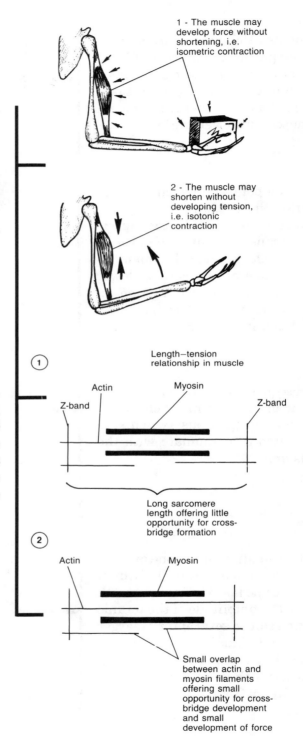

1 - The muscle may develop force without shortening, i.e. isometric contraction

2 - The muscle may shorten without developing tension, i.e. isotonic contraction

① Length–tension relationship in muscle

Actin Myosin

Z-band Z-band

Long sarcomere length offering little opportunity for cross-bridge formation

② Actin Myosin

Small overlap between actin and myosin filaments offering small opportunity for cross-bridge development and small development of force

At long sarcomere lengths, the actin and myosin filaments are pulled far apart so that there is very little overlap between filaments and therefore very little opportunity for cross-bridge formation and cycling; the maximum force which can be developed is rather small.

If the sarcomere length is a little less there is a greater degree of overlap between the filament types, with more opportunity for cross-bridge interaction.

There is an optimal length at which the greatest opportunity for cross-bridge formation occurs.

If the muscle is shortened beyond this length then the ends of the actin filaments overlap one another, preventing myosin from forming cross-bridges with actin at these sites. With still further shortening the ends of the myosin molecules come up against the Z-bands and start to become distorted and crinkled. At these lengths the muscle's ability to form cross-bridges and develop force is greatly impaired.

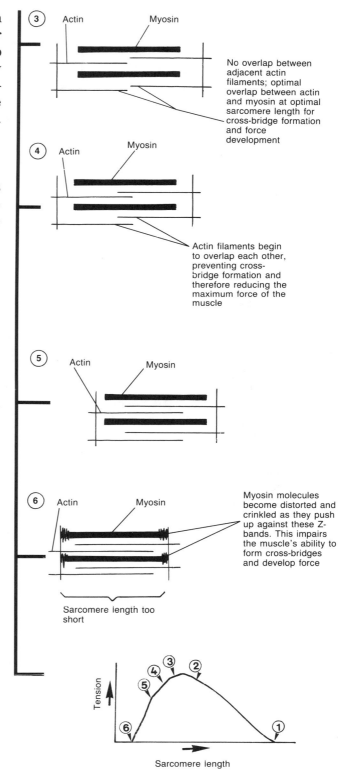

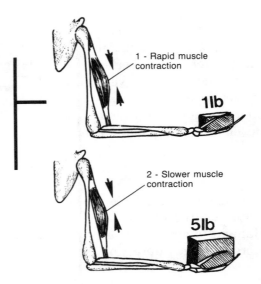

1 - Rapid muscle contraction

1lb

2 - Slower muscle contraction

5lb

If a contracting muscle is allowed to shorten, the velocity of shortening depends upon the initial load which was placed on the muscle. If the load is small the muscle can contract rapidly; at higher loads the velocity of contraction is much lower.

CARDIAC MUSCLE

The mechanism of contraction in cardiac muscle is very similar to that in skeletal muscle, as cardiac muscle is also striated. The tissues differ in their electrophysiology, with cardiac muscle relying not on nerves but on its spontaneous rhythmicity for its excitation. Impulses initiated in pacemaker regions and propagated from cell to cell through the intercalated discs cause depolarization of the surface membrane and the spread of excitation down the transverse tubules.

The cardiac cell has a prolonged action potential, which lasts almost as long as the twitch-like contraction. The refractory period of heart muscle is thus very long, and it is not normally possible to initiate a second action potential or contraction until the heart has recovered and relaxed from the first.

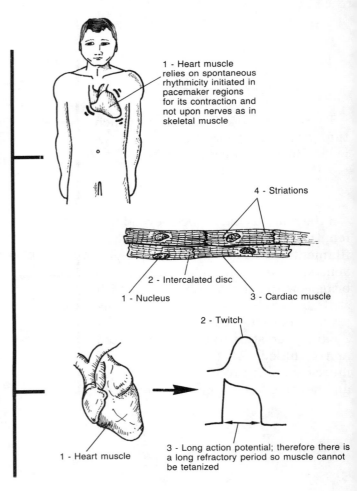

1 - Heart muscle relies on spontaneous rhythmicity initiated in pacemaker regions for its contraction and not upon nerves as in skeletal muscle

4 - Striations

2 - Intercalated disc

1 - Nucleus

3 - Cardiac muscle

2 - Twitch

1 - Heart muscle

3 - Long action potential; therefore there is a long refractory period so muscle cannot be tetanized

It is not possible to tetanize normal cardiac muscle; this is an advantage, as the function of the heart as a pump requires the rhythmic contraction and relaxation of its muscle.

1 - It is not possible to tetanize normal cardiac muscle

4 - Relaxation

2 - The function of the heart as a pump requires the rhythmic contraction and relaxation of its muscle

3 - Contraction

There is a significant inward current of calcium during the plateau phase of the prolonged cardiac action potential, and this calcium acts as the trigger for the release of further calcium from the sarcoplasmic reticulum.

1 Second

0

Voltage

-90mV

INa

ICa

IK

Current

1 - Calcium during plateau acts as a trigger for calcium release from sarcoplasmic reticulum

1 - The mechanism whereby calcium activates the myofilaments is identical to that in skeletal muscle

The mechanism whereby calcium activates the myofilaments is identical to that in skeletal muscle. The length–tension relationship for cardiac muscle is very similar to that for skeletal muscle, because cardiac muscle is striated and its filaments are arranged in a very similar way.

2 - Cardiac muscle

4 - Skeletal muscle

3 - Cardiac and skeletal muscle are both striated and their filaments are arranged in a similar way

SMOOTH MUSCLE

Visceral and vascular smooth muscle are organized very differently from skeletal muscle. Like cardiac muscle, the cells have low-resistance contacts which allow excitation to spread from cell to cell.

Some smooth muscle tissues are densely innervated by autonomic nerves and behave rather like skeletal muscles, being normally relaxed and only contracting when neuromuscular transmission takes place; other tissues may be sparsely innervated but have pacemaker areas, spontaneously discharging rhythmic action potentials which spread through the tissue and cause contraction.

The action potentials in smooth muscle are carried by calcium ions rather than sodium; sometimes enough calcium enters the cell during an action potential to cause contraction, but more often a small amount of calcium crossing the membrane acts as a trigger for the release of much more calcium from the sarcoplasmic reticulum (which is not nearly as extensive or as organized as in striated muscles but is nevertheless an important calcium store).

Smooth muscle has no structure analogous to the transverse tubule system, but the cells are so narrow that most points are relatively close to the surface membrane and can be influenced by substances diffusing in from outside.

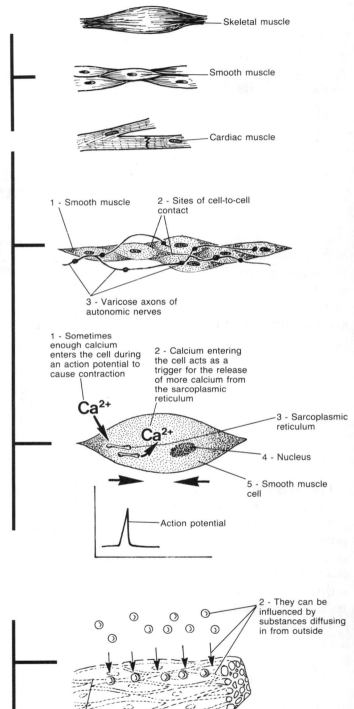

Skeletal muscle

Smooth muscle

Cardiac muscle

1 - Smooth muscle

2 - Sites of cell-to-cell contact

3 - Varicose axons of autonomic nerves

1 - Sometimes enough calcium enters the cell during an action potential to cause contraction

2 - Calcium entering the cell acts as a trigger for the release of more calcium from the sarcoplasmic reticulum

Ca^{2+}

Ca^{2+}

3 - Sarcoplasmic reticulum

4 - Nucleus

5 - Smooth muscle cell

Action potential

2 - They can be influenced by substances diffusing in from outside

1 - Cells are so narrow that most points are close to the surface membrane

The contractile proteins in smooth muscle are not as regularly arranged as in striated muscle (that is why it is 'smooth' or 'unstriated' muscle) but actin and myosin filaments are present nonetheless. There are no Z-bands, but some of the actin filaments are attached to the surface membrane, which provides a point of tethering for the filament system when sliding takes place; the filaments are arranged somewhat obliquely.

The mechanism whereby calcium triggers contraction in smooth muscle is different from that described in for striated muscles. There is no inhibitory protein which has to be inhibited; instead calcium ions **activate** a special protein, **myosin light-chain kinase**, and this enzyme in turn triggers the binding of myosin to actin. The cyclic binding and unbinding of cross-bridges then proceeds just as in striated muscle.

Smooth muscle has superficially similar length–tension properties to striated muscle, but as there are no Z-bands there is no structure which limits the sliding of the filaments; thus the smooth muscle cells are capable of shortening to a very much smaller fraction of their resting length (**supercontraction**), though at very short muscle lengths the opportunities for cross-bridge formation are reduced by the overlapping of adjacent actin filaments.

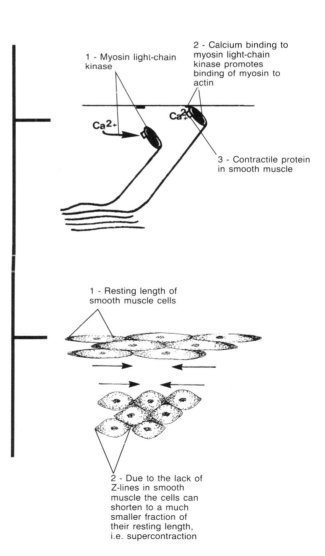

2 - Thin filaments (actin) attached to surface membrane

1 - Smooth muscle cell

3 - Nucleus

4 - Thick filaments (myosin)

1 - Myosin light-chain kinase

2 - Calcium binding to myosin light-chain kinase promotes binding of myosin to actin

Ca2+

Ca2+

3 - Contractile protein in smooth muscle

1 - Resting length of smooth muscle cells

2 - Due to the lack of Z-lines in smooth muscle the cells can shorten to a much smaller fraction of their resting length, i.e. supercontraction

MUSCLE RECEPTORS

Skeletal muscles contain a series of sensory receptors which inform the central nervous system about their state of contraction or relaxation; this enables the motor system to execute very finely controlled movements. Some receptors, the **muscle spindles**, are present in the fleshy part of the muscle; others, the **Golgi tendon organs**, are located in the tendons.

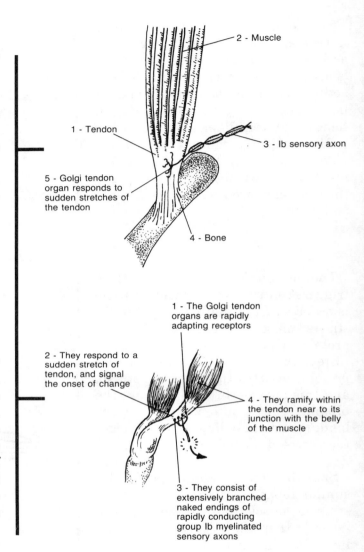

2 - Muscle

1 - Tendon

3 - Ib sensory axon

5 - Golgi tendon organ responds to sudden stretches of the tendon

4 - Bone

The Golgi tendon organs are rapidly adapting receptors which respond to a sudden stretch of the tendon; they are dynamic or acceleration receptors, signalling the onset of change. The sensory receptors consist simply of the extensively branched naked endings of rapidly conducting group Ib myelinated sensory axons, ramifying within the tendon near to its junction with the belly of the muscle.

1 - The Golgi tendon organs are rapidly adapting receptors

2 - They respond to a sudden stretch of tendon, and signal the onset of change

4 - They ramify within the tendon near to its junction with the belly of the muscle

3 - They consist of extensively branched naked endings of rapidly conducting group Ib myelinated sensory axons

If a muscle starts to contract, or a tendon is passively stretched by an external force, the Golgi tendon organ fires, but otherwise it remains silent.

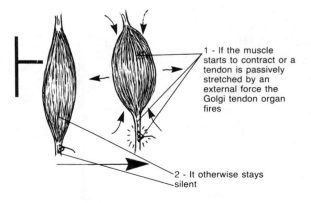

1 - If the muscle starts to contract or a tendon is passively stretched by an external force the Golgi tendon organ fires

2 - It otherwise stays silent

The muscle spindles are found **in parallel** with the ordinary muscle fibres, unlike the tendon organs, which are **in series**.

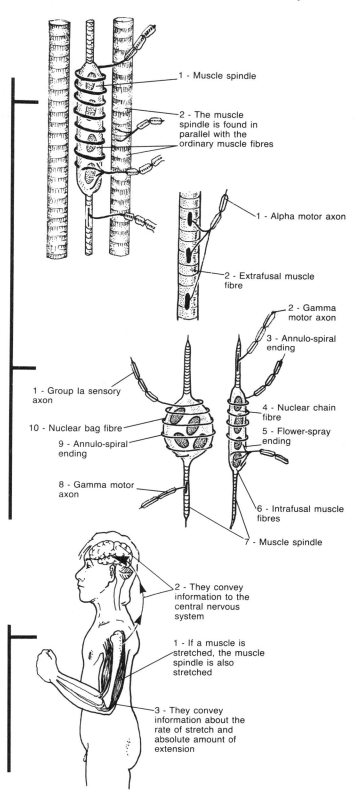

1 - Muscle spindle

2 - The muscle spindle is found in parallel with the ordinary muscle fibres

1 - Alpha motor axon

2 - Extrafusal muscle fibre

Each spindle is a bundle of fine modified muscle cells, some of which are called **nuclear bag** fibres and some **nuclear chain** fibres. The nuclear bag fibres have a sensory nerve ending wound around their middle region, the **annulo-spiral** ending of a group Ia axon; the nuclear chain fibres are innervated by **'flower-spray'** endings of group II sensory axons, as well as annulo-spiral endings of group Ia axons. The flower-spray endings are relatively rapidly adapting stretch receptors; the annulo-spiral endings adapt to stretch much more slowly.

2 - Gamma motor axon

3 - Annulo-spiral ending

1 - Group Ia sensory axon

4 - Nuclear chain fibre

5 - Flower-spray ending

10 - Nuclear bag fibre

9 - Annulo-spiral ending

8 - Gamma motor axon

6 - Intrafusal muscle fibres

7 - Muscle spindle

2 - They convey information to the central nervous system

1 - If a muscle is stretched, the muscle spindle is also stretched

If a muscle is stretched, the muscle spindles also become stretched and the sensory nerves become excited. They convey information to the central nervous system both about the rate of stretch (dynamic response of rapidly adapting receptors) and about the absolute amount of extension (static response of slowly adapting receptors).

3 - They convey information about the rate of stretch and absolute amount of extension

On the other hand, if a muscle is excited to contract by stimulation of its alpha motor neurones, the tension on the muscle spindles is removed and their sensory nerves become silent.

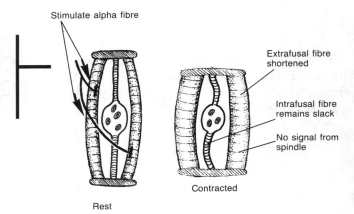

As well as having a sensory innervation, the muscle spindles have a motor nerve supply. The end portions of each cell, on either side of the nuclear region, are contractile and are supplied with synaptic input from gamma motor neurones (which lie, like the alpha motor neurone, in the anterior horn of the spinal cord).

If the **extrafusal** muscle fibres (those in the bulk of the muscle, not in the spindle) are relaxed but the **intrafusal** fibres (those within the spindle) are made to contract by excitation of the gamma motor neurones, then the central areas of the spindle become stretched and excite the annulo-spiral and flower-spray endings exactly as if the whole muscle had been passively stretched.

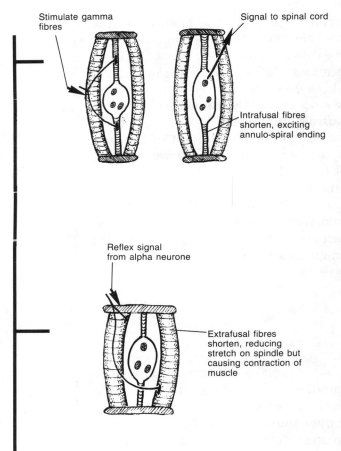

THE STRETCH REFLEX

Stretching a muscle excites the spindle sensors, and the proprioceptive fibres making synapse with the alpha motor neurones cause the muscle to contract. This is the basis of the stretch reflex, which is a major postural mechanism. If a person is standing upright in a given posture, and tends to fall forward, then the muscles along the back of his legs and spine become stretched and reflexly shorten, restoring him to the upright posture.

There are two pathways by which a higher centre can make a skeletal muscle contract. The first is by directly activating its alpha motor neurones, in which case there is a brisk contraction and the spindles become unstretched so that the central nervous system receives no feedback information from the muscle (except for a little from the Golgi tendon organs). The second is by activating the gamma motor neurones supplying the intrafusal muscle fibres of the spindles; these contract and stretch their receptor endings, initiating a discharge in the sensory nerve fibre and producing reflex contraction by synaptic activation of the alpha motor neurones.

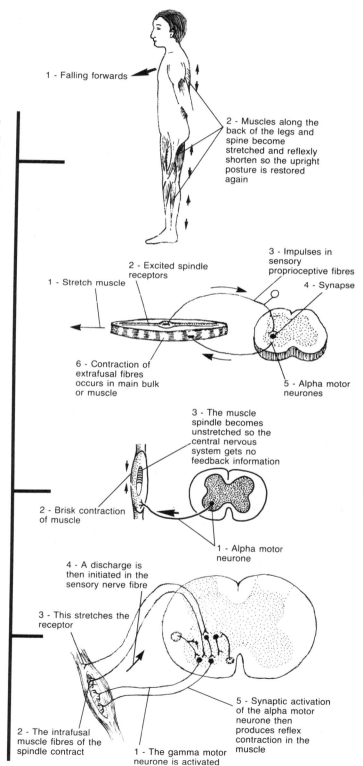

1 - Falling forwards

2 - Muscles along the back of the legs and spine become stretched and reflexly shorten so the upright posture is restored again

1 - Stretch muscle

2 - Excited spindle receptors

3 - Impulses in sensory proprioceptive fibres

4 - Synapse

5 - Alpha motor neurones

6 - Contraction of extrafusal fibres occurs in main bulk or muscle

3 - The muscle spindle becomes unstretched so the central nervous system gets no feedback information

2 - Brisk contraction of muscle

1 - Alpha motor neurone

4 - A discharge is then initiated in the sensory nerve fibre

3 - This stretches the receptor

2 - The intrafusal muscle fibres of the spindle contract

1 - The gamma motor neurone is activated

5 - Synaptic activation of the alpha motor neurone then produces reflex contraction in the muscle

Although this second pathway is more complicated and takes longer, it can produce a smoother and more controlled movement since the central nervous system is receiving information all the time from the spindles about the state of contraction.

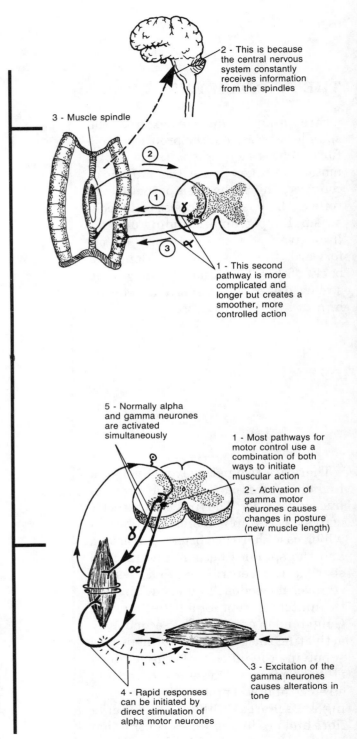

2 - This is because the central nervous system constantly receives information from the spindles

3 - Muscle spindle

1 - This second pathway is more complicated and longer but creates a smoother, more controlled action

5 - Normally alpha and gamma neurones are activated simultaneously

1 - Most pathways for motor control use a combination of both ways to initiate muscular action

2 - Activation of gamma motor neurones causes changes in posture (new muscle length)

3 - Excitation of the gamma neurones causes alterations in tone

4 - Rapid responses can be initiated by direct stimulation of alpha motor neurones

Most of the pathways and mechanisms for motor control use a combination of these two ways of initiating muscular action. Changes in posture can be caused by activating gamma motor neurones in order to set a new muscle length at which the stretch reflex is to operate; alterations in tone can be brought about by changing the degree of excitation of the gamma neurones; rapid responses can be initiated by direct stimulation of alpha motor neurones.

During a normal voluntary movement initiated by the pyramidal system the alpha and gamma motor neurones supplying a muscle are activated simultaneously.

The alpha axon conducts faster, so the direct activation of extrafusal fibres occurs first, but very shortly afterwards the slack is taken up by the intrafusal fibres and thereafter the action is continuously monitored by feedback information from the spindles. The rate and force of contraction can be constantly adjusted through the mechanism of the stretch reflex to suit the load applied and the task being performed.

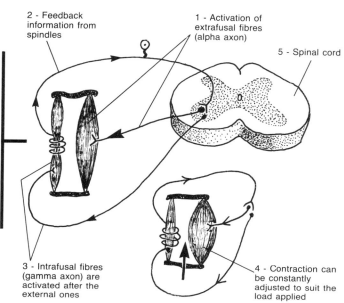

2 - Feedback information from spindles

1 - Activation of extrafusal fibres (alpha axon)

5 - Spinal cord

3 - Intrafusal fibres (gamma axon) are activated after the external ones

4 - Contraction can be constantly adjusted to suit the load applied

OTHER SIMPLE SPINAL REFLEXES

The stretch reflex is an example of a simple spinal reflex; it can take place even if the spinal cord has been transected above the level at which the muscles are innervated, so that there is no connection with the brain. It is a particularly simple reflex in that the input and output occur in the same segment, on the same side of the body, and involve only one central synapse.

A more complex response is the **flexor** or **withdrawal** reflex. If an area of skin on a limb is subjected to a noxious stimulus such as a pin-prick or contact with a hot object, the limb is rapidly withdrawn from the stimulus by flexion at one or more of the joints of that limb. The more intense or painful the stimulus, the more vigorous is the response; a very painful stimulus causes flexion at several joints as well as extension of joints of the contralateral limb or limbs to maintain rigidity and support in the rest of the body.

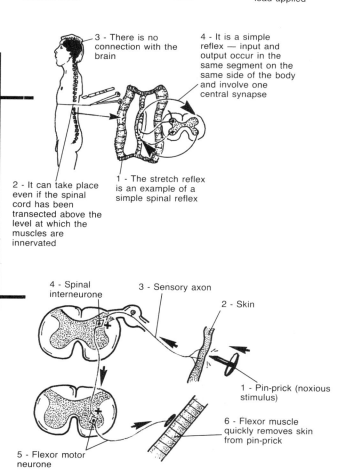

3 - There is no connection with the brain

4 - It is a simple reflex — input and output occur in the same segment on the same side of the body and involve one central synapse

2 - It can take place even if the spinal cord has been transected above the level at which the muscles are innervated

1 - The stretch reflex is an example of a simple spinal reflex

4 - Spinal interneurone

3 - Sensory axon

2 - Skin

1 - Pin-prick (noxious stimulus)

6 - Flexor muscle quickly removes skin from pin-prick

5 - Flexor motor neurone

1 - The painful stimulus excites pain receptors

4 - Skin

2 - This produces a train of impulses along the nociceptive nerve fibres (mostly 'C' fibres)

3 - Nociceptive 'C' nerve fibre

The painful stimulus excites pain receptors in the skin and produces a train of impulses along the nociceptive nerve fibres (mostly 'C' fibres) which enter the spinal cord in the dorsal or posterior root.

5 - Nerve pathway

4 - Grey matter

3 - White matter

1 - The 'C' fibres enter the spinal cord in the dorsal or posterior root

2 - Segment of spinal cord

These fibres synapse with a number of **interneurones** which run up or down within the spinal cord carrying information to different levels in the cord. This is necessary because the muscles which produce flexion of the limb are often innervated at a different spinal level from the area of skin which detected the noxious stimulus.

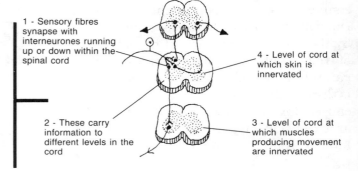

1 - Sensory fibres synapse with interneurones running up or down within the spinal cord

4 - Level of cord at which skin is innervated

2 - These carry information to different levels in cord

3 - Level of cord at which muscles producing movement are innervated

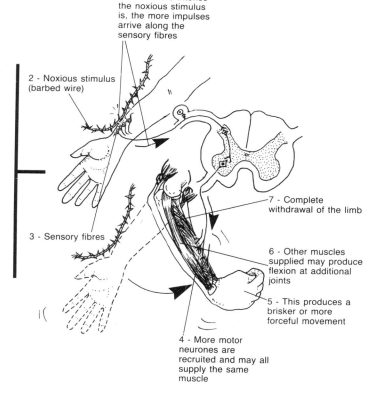

1 - The interneurones may synapse with a series of other interneurones

2 - This produces extremely complex possible pathways for information processing

3 - Eventually synaptic contact is made with alpha motor neurones, responsible for activating the appropriate flexor muscles

The interneurones may synapse with a series of other interneurones, to produce extremely complex possible pathways for information processing, but eventually synaptic contact is made with alpha motor neurones which are responsible for activating the appropriate flexor muscles.

1 - The more intense the noxious stimulus is, the more impulses arrive along the sensory fibres

2 - Noxious stimulus (barbed wire)

3 - Sensory fibres

4 - More motor neurones are recruited and may all supply the same muscle

5 - This produces a brisker or more forceful movement

6 - Other muscles supplied may produce flexion at additional joints

7 - Complete withdrawal of the limb

If the noxious stimulus is more intense then more impulses arrive along the sensory fibres, or more sensory fibres are activated, and more of the motor neurones are eventually **recruited** to take part in the movement. The additional neurones may supply the same muscle, producing a brisker or more forceful movement, or they may supply other muscles producing flexion at additional joints and causing a more complete withdrawal of the limb.

While the flexor muscles are contracting to cause withdrawal of the limb, the **antagonistic** extensor muscles must relax, otherwise the movement would be impeded.

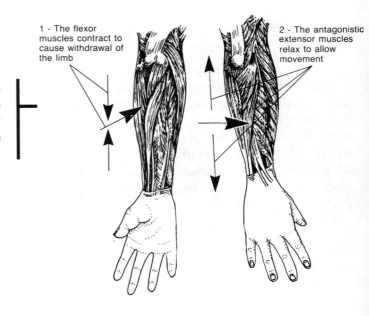

1 - The flexor muscles contract to cause withdrawal of the limb

2 - The antagonistic extensor muscles relax to allow movement

As additional flexor motor neurones become recruited, interneurones also cause inhibition at synapses with the motor neurones of antagonistic muscles; this phenomenon is an example of **reciprocal innervation** in which excitation of one group of neurones is accompanied by simultaneous inhibition of another.

As the stimulus is increased and recruitment proceeds further, the muscles of the opposite side become involved as well. While the ipsilateral flexors are excited and the extensors are inhibited, on the contralateral side it is the extensors which become excited by reciprocal innervation and the flexors which become inhibited. This is known as the **crossed extensor response**, and ensures that the body is firmly supported during the vigorous withdrawal of a limb.

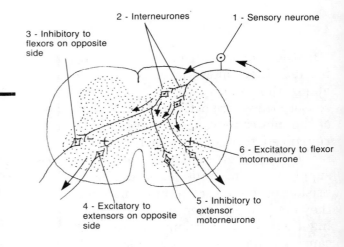

2 - Interneurones

1 - Sensory neurone

3 - Inhibitory to flexors on opposite side

6 - Excitatory to flexor motorneurone

4 - Excitatory to extensors on opposite side

5 - Inhibitory to extensor motorneurone

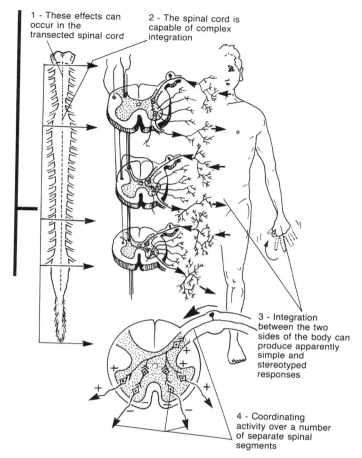

1 - These effects can occur in the transected spinal cord

2 - The spinal cord is capable of complex integration

3 - Integration between the two sides of the body can produce apparently simple and stereotyped responses

4 - Coordinating activity over a number of separate spinal segments

All of these effects can occur in the transected spinal cord; it is obvious that the spinal cord is capable of very complex integration, coordinating activity over a number of separate spinal segments and between the two sides of the body, to produce such apparently simple and stereotyped responses.

HIGHER CONTROL OF MOTOR FUNCTION

We have already described the initiation of voluntary movements by the motor cortex along the pyramidal pathway. This is the most direct pathway for activating the motor neurones of the spinal cord, but there are many other influences which are brought to bear upon these motor neurones and several pathways for conveying information to them.

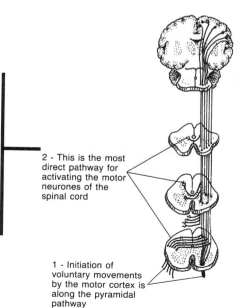

2 - This is the most direct pathway for activating the motor neurones of the spinal cord

1 - Initiation of voluntary movements by the motor cortex is along the pyramidal pathway

LESIONS IN THE SPINAL CORD OR BRAIN STEM

If the spinal cord is removed from the influence of higher centres, the stretch reflexes become highly exaggerated and very brisk.

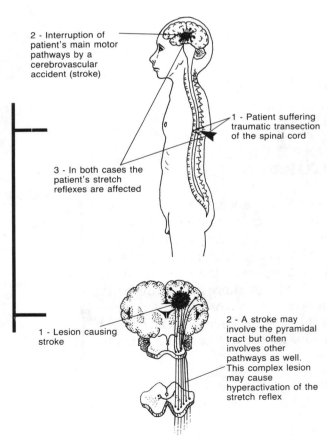

1 - The spinal cord is removed from the influences of higher centres

2 - Stretch reflexes become highly exaggerated and very brisk

2 - Interruption of patient's main motor pathways by a cerebrovascular accident (stroke)

1 - Patient suffering traumatic transection of the spinal cord

3 - In both cases the patient's stretch reflexes are affected

1 - Lesion causing stroke

2 - A stroke may involve the pyramidal tract but often involves other pathways as well. This complex lesion may cause hyperactivation of the stretch reflex

This is seen in patients suffering traumatic transection of the spinal cord or interruption of their main motor pathways by a cerebrovascular accident ('stroke'); in experimental lesions involving only the pyramidal tract this does not happen, but few strokes involve only one pathway, and this hyperactivity of the stretch reflex is very often associated with loss of function in the pyramidal tract. It illustrates the fact that simple spinal reflexes are capable of modification by influences, often inhibitory, from higher centres.

If the brain stem is transected at a high level, the resultant patient or animal is often capable of considerable motor activity and postural control. The amount of control available to the lower body depends upon the site of the lesion, but provided the brain stem centres for respiratory and cardiovascular control are still attached to the spinal cord the individual can survive for quite some time.

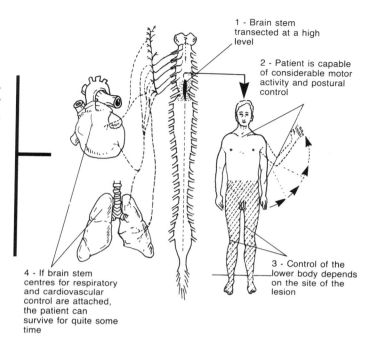

1 - Brain stem transected at a high level

2 - Patient is capable of considerable motor activity and postural control

3 - Control of the lower body depends on the site of the lesion

4 - If brain stem centres for respiratory and cardiovascular control are attached, the patient can survive for quite some time

If the lesion is high in the midbrain, so that the red nucleus is still attached to the brain stem and spine, but the thalamus and cortex are disconnected, a state of **decerebrate rigidity** is observed. The limbs become stiff and extended, so that the animal or person can stand firmly upright, and has certain primitive righting reflexes.

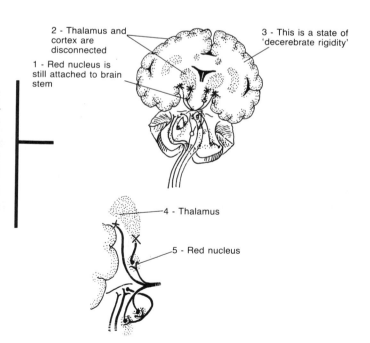

2 - Thalamus and cortex are disconnected

1 - Red nucleus is still attached to brain stem

3 - This is a state of 'decerebrate rigidity'

4 - Thalamus

5 - Red nucleus

1 - If the head is moved relative the body, input from neck proprioceptors produces tonic neck reflexes

If the head is moved relative to the body, the input from neck proprioceptors produces **tonic neck reflexes**; for instance, if the head of a decerebrate cat is tilted upwards and backwards the hind limbs become flexed and the animal sits down; if the head is tilted down the forelegs bend and the animal adopts a posture reminiscent of feeding; if the head is rotated upon the neck the ipsilateral forelimb flexes and the contralateral forelimb extends.

2 - If the head is tilted upwards and backwards the hind limbs become flexed

3 - The animal sits down

4 - If head is tilted forwards, forelegs bend

5 - The animal adopts a posture reminiscent of feeding

6 - If the head is rotated upon the neck, the ipsilateral forelimb flexes

7 - Contralateral forelimb extends

1 - Decerebrate animal is placed on its back or side or (as shown) allowed to drop from a moderate height

If the decerebrate animal is placed on its back or side, or is allowed to drop from a moderate height, its vestibular apparatus initiates turning movements of the head. These stretch the neck muscles, initiating tonic neck reflexes and producing movements of the limb which cause the body to turn and roll the animal into the correct posture.

2 - Vestibular apparatus initiates turning movements of the head

3 - Neck muscles are stretched, initiating tonic neck reflexes

4 - Movements of the limbs are produced, causing body to turn and roll animal to correct posture

The decerebrate patient or animal is capable of certain primitive locomotor actions, and can even walk in a crude manner.

This type of locomotion and the righting reflexes are composed of several simple building blocks which are controlled by the brain stem and contribute to the rather stereotyped reaction. It is possible that the complex motor activity in the intact nervous system is built up from a number of such simple components.

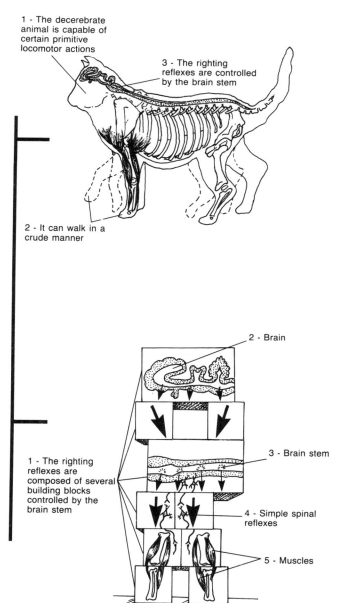

1 - The decerebrate animal is capable of certain primitive locomotor actions

3 - The righting reflexes are controlled by the brain stem

2 - It can walk in a crude manner

2 - Brain

3 - Brain stem

1 - The righting reflexes are composed of several building blocks controlled by the brain stem

4 - Simple spinal reflexes

5 - Muscles

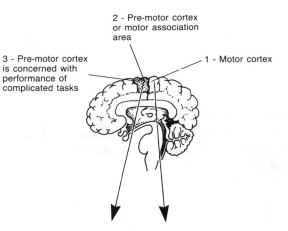

2 - Pre-motor cortex or motor association area

3 - Pre-motor cortex is concerned with performance of complicated tasks

1 - Motor cortex

OTHER HIGHER MOTOR CENTRES

Just in front of the pre-central gyrus (the motor cortex) is an area known as the **pre-motor** cortex or the motor association area. While the neurones of the main motor cortex are concerned with activating individual muscles or groups of muscles, with an accurate mapping of cortical area to spinal motor neurone, the pre-motor cortex is more concerned with the performance of complex tasks.

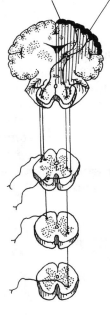

4 - Neurones of main motor cortex are concerned with activating individual muscles or groups of muscles

5 - It has an accurate mapping of cortical area to spinal motor neurone

The actions of waving the arm or walking or screwing up a nut and bolt are all manoeuvres which require several muscle groups to move accurately in sequence, and the pre-motor cortex contains coded instructions for such actions. At the appropriate time the right set of instructions in the sequence is passed to the correct part of the motor cortex to make the proper muscle move, in order to execute the complex task required.

The motor and pre-motor areas of the cortex are connected to a number of nuclei of grey matter deep within the cerebral hemisphere (the **basal ganglia**) as well as a number of centres high in the midbrain. These include part of the thalamus, the caudate and lentiform nuclei, the red nucleus and the substantia nigra.

These basal ganglia receive inputs from the motor cortex, are highly interconnected and send outputs back to the cortex. They also send descending fibres to the spinal motor neurones and to the reticular formation.

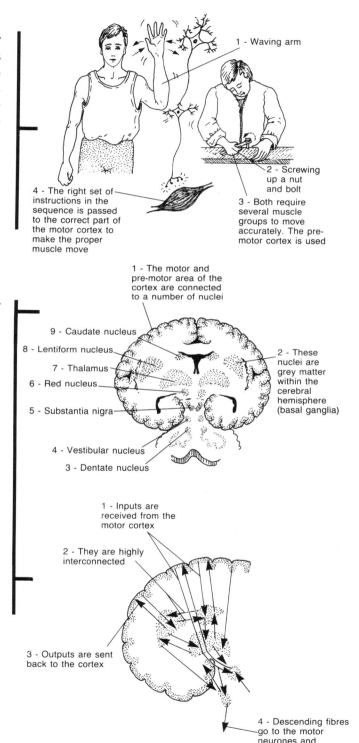

1 - Waving arm

2 - Screwing up a nut and bolt

3 - Both require several muscle groups to move accurately. The pre-motor cortex is used

4 - The right set of instructions in the sequence is passed to the correct part of the motor cortex to make the proper muscle move

1 - The motor and pre-motor area of the cortex are connected to a number of nuclei

9 - Caudate nucleus
8 - Lentiform nucleus
7 - Thalamus
6 - Red nucleus
5 - Substantia nigra

2 - These nuclei are grey matter within the cerebral hemisphere (basal ganglia)

4 - Vestibular nucleus

3 - Dentate nucleus

1 - Inputs are received from the motor cortex

2 - They are highly interconnected

3 - Outputs are sent back to the cortex

4 - Descending fibres go to the motor neurones and reticular formation

The function of these extensively interlinked centres (the **extrapyramidal system**) is to regulate the level of activity in muscle groups throughout the body, producing a suitable posture and a baseline level of muscle tone against which voluntary movements can take place.

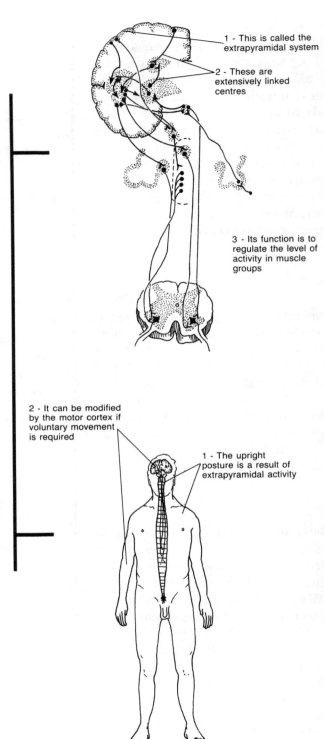

1 - This is called the extrapyramidal system

2 - These are extensively linked centres

3 - Its function is to regulate the level of activity in muscle groups

2 - It can be modified by the motor cortex if voluntary movement is required

1 - The upright posture is a result of extrapyramidal activity

Thus the upright posture is produced as a result of extrapyramidal activity, and then this posture can be modified by the motor cortex to produce purposeful voluntary movement.

Patients with damage to the basal ganglia have marked abnormalities of posture and muscle tone; they tend to be rather crouched over with many of their limb joints flexed, and their muscle tone is slightly increased, with a rigidity which has been likened to a lead pipe. They also have a characteristic tremor, particularly in the hands.

They tend to have much less spontaneous movement than most people, they have difficulty in starting voluntary movements and difficulty in stopping movements once they are started. It is hard to explain all of these changes in terms of the known functions of the extrapyramidal system, but it is not an easy part of the brain to study, and much of our knowledge is based upon the study of patients with damage to these nuclei.

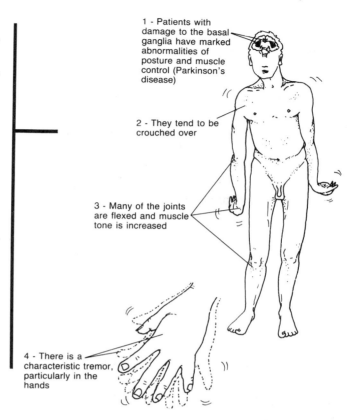

1 - Patients with damage to the basal ganglia have marked abnormalities of posture and muscle control (Parkinson's disease)

2 - They tend to be crouched over

3 - Many of the joints are flexed and muscle tone is increased

4 - There is a characteristic tremor, particularly in the hands

THE CEREBELLUM

Behind the brain stem, forming the roof of the fourth ventricle, is the cerebellum, which is the largest part of the brain after the cerebral hemispheres. Indeed in primitive vertebrates like fish it is far bigger than the cerebrum.

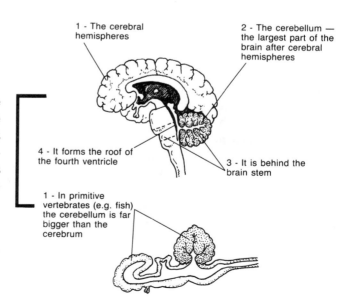

1 - The cerebral hemispheres

2 - The cerebellum — the largest part of the brain after cerebral hemispheres

4 - It forms the roof of the fourth ventricle

3 - It is behind the brain stem

1 - In primitive vertebrates (e.g. fish) the cerebellum is far bigger than the cerebrum

Like the cerebrum, the cerebellum has a cortex of grey matter surrounding a large amount of white matter with a number of nuclei of grey matter embedded within. The structure of the cerebellar cortex, which is thrown into large numbers of parallel folds or folia (analogous to the gyri in the cerebral cortex), is very uniform, with three clearly recognizable layers.

1 - The cerebellum has a cortex of grey matter

2 - This surrounds a large amount of white matter

3 - In the white matter is a large number of nuclei of grey matter embedded within

4 - The cortex is thrown into large numbers of parallel folds or folia

5 - The cortex is very uniform, with three clearly recognizable layers

The outer layer, the **molecular layer**, contains few cell bodies but houses the extensive dendritic trees of the cells of the next layer, the **Purkinje cell layer**. Internal to this is the **granular cell layer**.

1 - The outer layer: the molecular layer

2 - It contains very few cell bodies but many dendritic trees

3 - The dendrites are from the cells of the next layer — the Purkinje cell layer

4 - Internal to this is the granular cell layer

The axons from the granular cells ascend into the molecular layer, where they split into two branches which run in both directions parallel to the long axis of the folia, and cross the dendritic trees (which lie at right angles to the axis of the folia) of the Purkinje cells. The parallel fibres of the granular cells synapse extensively with the Purkinje dendrites as they go past.

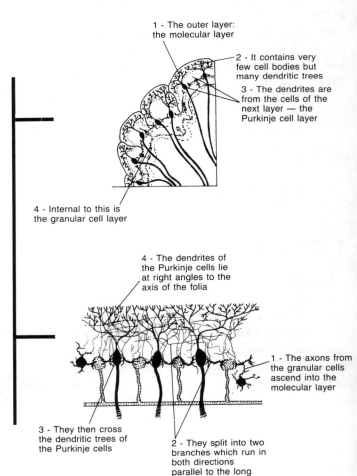

4 - The dendrites of the Purkinje cells lie at right angles to the axis of the folia

1 - The axons from the granular cells ascend into the molecular layer

3 - They then cross the dendritic trees of the Purkinje cells

2 - They split into two branches which run in both directions parallel to the long axis of the folia

The cerebellum receives inputs from the motor and pre-motor cortex via collaterals of axons of the major motor pathways, relaying in the **pontine nuclei**.

The neurones originating in these nuclei give rise to **mossy fibres** which synapse with the granular cells as well as going to some of the cerebellar nuclei such as the **dentate nucleus**. The excited granular cells cause synaptic activation of a number of Purkinje cells, causing quite a widespread area of cerebellar cortex to become activated.

The Purkinje cell axons also make synaptic connection with neurones in the deep cerebellar nuclei, but they have a strong inhibitory effect. A given motor input to the cerebellum causes both a direct excitatory and an indirect inhibitory input to the nuclear cells, which act as **integrators**.

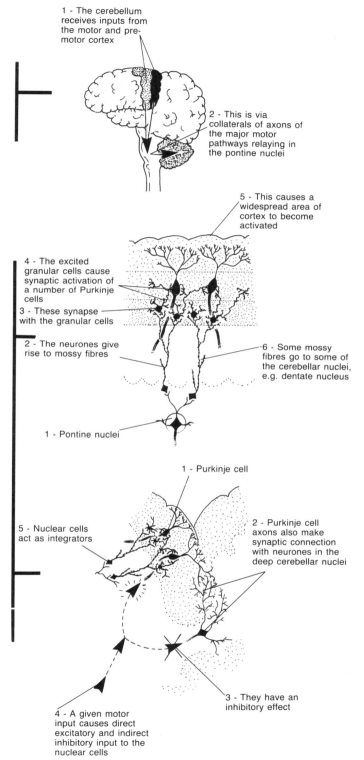

1 - The cerebellum receives inputs from the motor and pre-motor cortex

2 - This is via collaterals of axons of the major motor pathways relaying in the pontine nuclei

5 - This causes a widespread area of cortex to become activated

4 - The excited granular cells cause synaptic activation of a number of Purkinje cells

3 - These synapse with the granular cells

2 - The neurones give rise to mossy fibres

6 - Some mossy fibres go to some of the cerebellar nuclei, e.g. dentate nucleus

1 - Pontine nuclei

1 - Purkinje cell

5 - Nuclear cells act as integrators

2 - Purkinje cell axons also make synaptic connection with neurones in the deep cerebellar nuclei

3 - They have an inhibitory effect

4 - A given motor input causes direct excitatory and indirect inhibitory input to the nuclear cells

The cerebellum also receives inputs from the proprioceptive sensory pathways and the vestibular nuclei, informing it about the actual performance of muscles and about the body's orientation and movement. This information enters via the **olivary nuclei** in the brain stem, and the neurones originating here give rise to **climbing fibres** which enter the cerebellar cortex and synapse with the Purkinje cell dendrites as well as exciting the neurones of the deep cerebellar nuclei. Thus there is a second source of excitation for the Purkinje cells, and a further source of both excitatory and inhibitory influence on the deep nuclear neurones.

The cerebellar nuclear cells receive a copy of the motor instructions issued by the cerebral cortex; they also receive information about the actual performance of the muscles, and they receive inhibitory integrative information from the Purkinje cells.

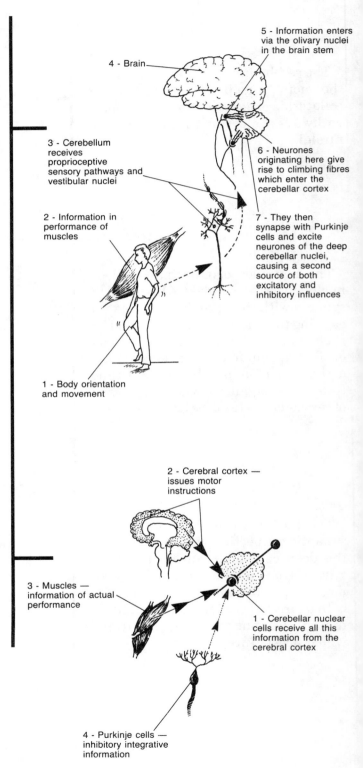

5 - Information enters via the olivary nuclei in the brain stem

4 - Brain

3 - Cerebellum receives proprioceptive sensory pathways and vestibular nuclei

6 - Neurones originating here give rise to climbing fibres which enter the cerebellar cortex

2 - Information in performance of muscles

7 - They then synapse with Purkinje cells and excite neurones of the deep cerebellar nuclei, causing a second source of both excitatory and inhibitory influences

1 - Body orientation and movement

2 - Cerebral cortex — issues motor instructions

3 - Muscles — information of actual performance

1 - Cerebellar nuclear cells receive all this information from the cerebral cortex

4 - Purkinje cells — inhibitory integrative information

They are thus able to compare the intention with the performance, and detect any error. If corrective action is necessary a signal is fed back to the motor cortex via the output pathway through the red nucleus and the thalamus; if too large a movement has been produced, the cerebellum reduces the amount of drive by the motor cortex, and if too little movement has occurred then the cerebellum instructs the motor cortex to increase its drive.

It is important to appreciate that the output of the cerebellum goes back to the motor centres of the brain, and not to the spinal cord. It is the commands which are monitored and modified, not the executive apparatus.

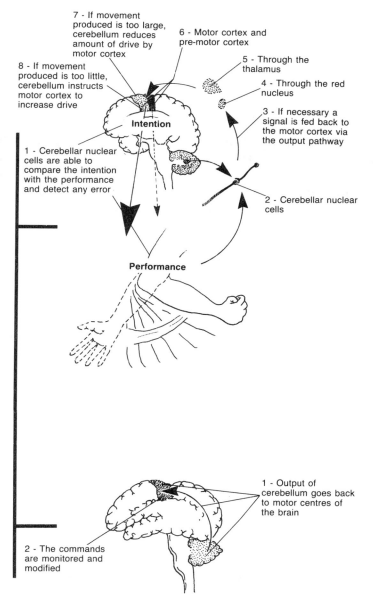

7 - If movement produced is too large, cerebellum reduces amount of drive by motor cortex

6 - Motor cortex and pre-motor cortex

5 - Through the thalamus

4 - Through the red nucleus

8 - If movement produced is too little, cerebellum instructs motor cortex to increase drive

3 - If necessary a signal is fed back to the motor cortex via the output pathway

Intention

1 - Cerebellar nuclear cells are able to compare the intention with the performance and detect any error

2 - Cerebellar nuclear cells

Performance

1 - Output of cerebellum goes back to motor centres of the brain

2 - The commands are monitored and modified

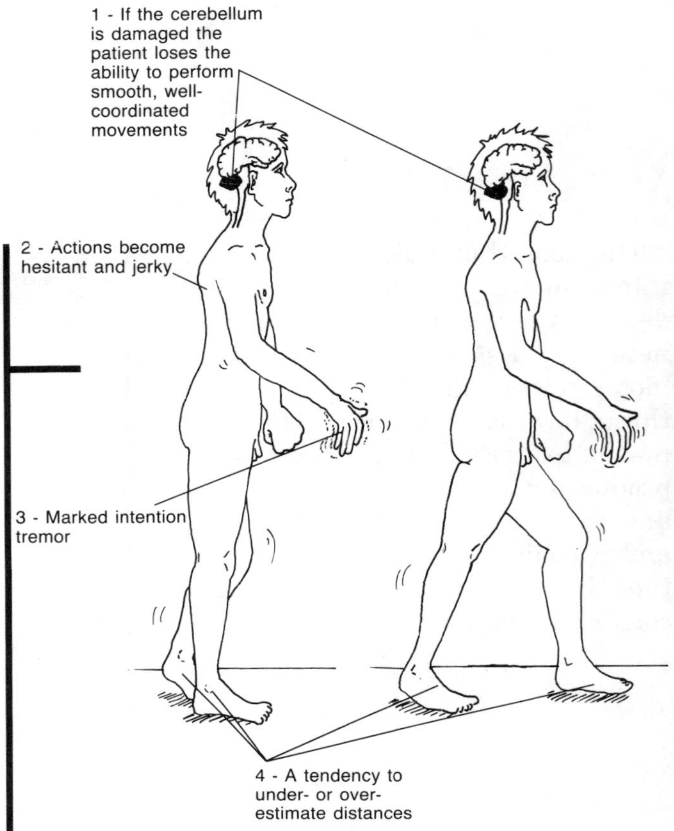

If the cerebellum is damaged, the patient loses the ability to perform smooth, well-coordinated movements; his actions become hesitant and jerky, with a marked intention tremor and a tendency to over- or under-estimate distances or the amount of force necessary to execute motor actions.

1 - If the cerebellum is damaged the patient loses the ability to perform smooth, well-coordinated movements

2 - Actions become hesitant and jerky

3 - Marked intention tremor

4 - A tendency to under- or over-estimate distances

Other parts of the cerebellum, particularly the **floccular-nodular node**, are concerned with maintaining the body's upright balance, and lesions in this part cause unsteadiness.

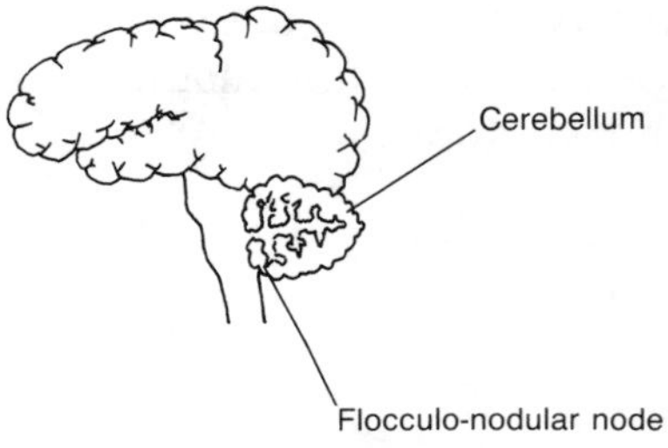

Cerebellum

Flocculo-nodular node

THE RETICULAR FORMATION

There is a series of diffuse clumps of grey matter interlaced with tracts of white matter, distributed throughout the central part of the brain stem, which forms a poorly defined network known as the reticular formation. The clumps of grey matter are extensively interconnected in such a way that excitation of one part of the network is capable of spreading widely through the system to cause excitation of most of the other parts; eventually the excitation may spread back to the part of the system whence it started, producing recurrent and self-reinforcing activation. A single input into the system can produce very long-lasting and widespread effects throughout the network.

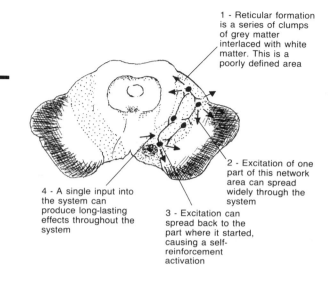

1 - Reticular formation is a series of clumps of grey matter interlaced with white matter. This is a poorly defined area

2 - Excitation of one part of this network area can spread widely through the system

3 - Excitation can spread back to the part where it started, causing a self-reinforcement activation

4 - A single input into the system can produce long-lasting effects throughout the system

This system receives a very large number of inputs at all levels. Almost all sensory tracts send collaterals to the reticular system as they ascend towards the thalamus, and almost all motor tracts send branches to the system as they descend through the brain stem. Thus any activity in the nervous system, whether motor or sensory, can cause input to the reticular formation; once such excitation enters the system at any level, it can produce an increase in the total amount of neural activity within the reticular formation, causing a greater probability of any given neurone firing.

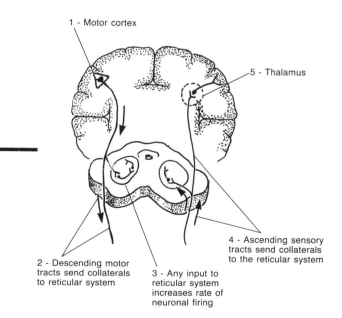

1 - Motor cortex

5 - Thalamus

2 - Descending motor tracts send collaterals to reticular system

3 - Any input to reticular system increases rate of neuronal firing

4 - Ascending sensory tracts send collaterals to the reticular system

Section of central part of brain stem

The activity of the reticular system is not directed towards any particular purpose; rather it represents a pool of neurones which are maintained in a greater or lesser state of excitability depending on activity elsewhere in the brain, and can influence the excitability of other neurones throughout the nervous system. For instance, some of the outputs from the reticular formation descend in the spinal cord to make synaptic contact with the motor neurones.

If the reticular system as a whole is in a state of high activity, caused perhaps by some intense sensory bombardment, then the output to the spinal motor neurones will be correspondingly high, and the neurones will be partially depolarized and therefore more easily excited by some more specific synaptic input. The **arousal** state of the spinal cord has been non-specifically increased.

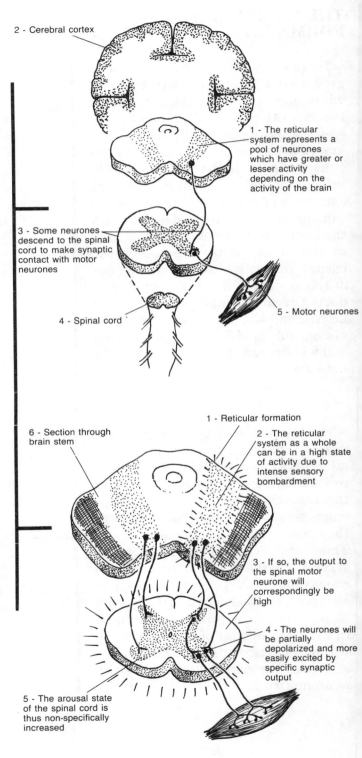

2 - Cerebral cortex

1 - The reticular system represents a pool of neurones which have greater or lesser activity depending on the activity of the brain

3 - Some neurones descend to the spinal cord to make synaptic contact with motor neurones

4 - Spinal cord

5 - Motor neurones

6 - Section through brain stem

1 - Reticular formation

2 - The reticular system as a whole can be in a high state of activity due to intense sensory bombardment

3 - If so, the output to the spinal motor neurone will correspondingly be high

4 - The neurones will be partially depolarized and more easily excited by specific synaptic output

5 - The arousal state of the spinal cord is thus non-specifically increased

Another important output from the reticular system goes to the thalamus. We have already seen how the thalamus acts as a major relay station for the main sensory pathways on their way to the sensory cortex. There is also a non-specific **diffuse thalamocortical** pathway in which the thalamus sends signals to all parts of the cortex in order to increase or decrease the average level of activity throughout the brain. The reticular formation is the main source of input to the diffuse thalamocortical pathway, and activity in this pathway accurately reflects the activity of the reticular system. Thus the reticular formation can influence the general level of excitability or arousal of neurones throughout the cerebral cortex.

If there is a large amount of activity in the reticular formation, then all parts of the brain will be placed in a state of high arousal, with the neurones partially depolarized and ready to receive synaptic inputs. If there is not much activity in the reticular formation, then the other parts of the brain will be in a state of low arousal, and the neurones will be partly hyperpolarized and harder to excite.

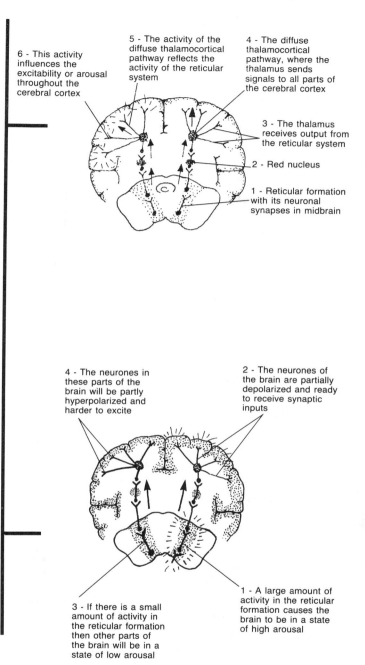

6 - This activity influences the excitability or arousal throughout the cerebral cortex

5 - The activity of the diffuse thalamocortical pathway reflects the activity of the reticular system

4 - The diffuse thalamocortical pathway, where the thalamus sends signals to all parts of the cerebral cortex

3 - The thalamus receives output from the reticular system

2 - Red nucleus

1 - Reticular formation with its neuronal synapses in midbrain

4 - The neurones in these parts of the brain will be partly hyperpolarized and harder to excite

2 - The neurones of the brain are partially depolarized and ready to receive synaptic inputs

3 - If there is a small amount of activity in the reticular formation then other parts of the brain will be in a state of low arousal

1 - A large amount of activity in the reticular formation causes the brain to be in a state of high arousal

When a person sleeps, the activity in his reticular formation reaches a low ebb, but if any major sensory input occurs such as a loud noise or vigorous shaking or a painful stimulus, then there is input to the reticular system, its activity increases and causes arousal and the brain wakes up. On the other hand, if an individual feels sleepy he can often prevent himself from falling asleep by walking around; the motor activity produces extra input to the reticular formation and increases the general level of arousal.

THE ELECTROENCEPHALOGRAPH

The electrical activity of the brain can be examined in man by placing surface electrodes on the scalp, amplifying the tiny signals and displaying or writing them on the **electroencephalograph** (**EEG**).

The signals which are the easiest to pick up are those arising from the most superficial layers of the cerebral cortex near to the electrodes; this is where the dendrites of the cortical neurones lie, receiving synaptic input from the diffuse thalamocortical system. Thus the electrical activity of the most superficial layers reflects the activity of this system and indirectly of the reticular system. In other words, the EEG is really a device for monitoring the activity of the reticular formation.

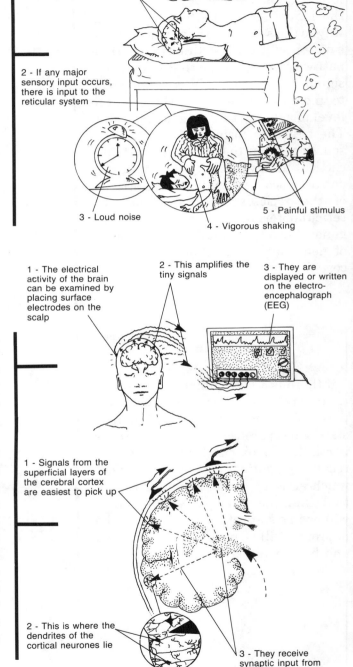

1 - When a person sleeps, activity in reticular formation reaches a low ebb

2 - If any major sensory input occurs, there is input to the reticular system

3 - Loud noise

4 - Vigorous shaking

5 - Painful stimulus

1 - The electrical activity of the brain can be examined by placing surface electrodes on the scalp

2 - This amplifies the tiny signals

3 - They are displayed or written on the electroencephalograph (EEG)

1 - Signals from the superficial layers of the cerebral cortex are easiest to pick up

2 - This is where the dendrites of the cortical neurones lie

3 - They receive synaptic input from the diffuse thalamocortical system

When the EEG is recorded from an awake individual whose eyes are open, the signal is very irregular and it is difficult to discern much from the waveform. This is because a large amount of activity is going on in the brain, with bombardment of the senses from all directions.

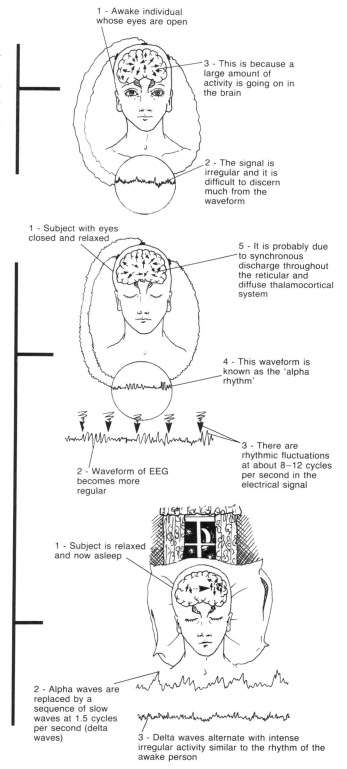

When the eyes are closed and the subject relaxes, the waveform of the EEG becomes much more regular, and we observe rhythmic fluctuations at about 8–12 cycles per second in the electrical signal from all parts of the brain. This regular waveform is known as the **alpha rhythm** and is probably due to synchronous discharge throughout the reticular and diffuse thalamocortical system.

If the relaxed subject now goes to sleep, the regular alpha waves of the awake person become replaced by a number of different waveforms, notably a sequence of **slow waves** at 1.5 cycles per second (delta waves) which occur in bouts during the night, alternating with periods of intense irregular activity which are very similar to the waveform of the awake person, except that the subject is deeply asleep (paradoxical sleep).

During these periods there are rapid eye movements and this type of sleep is known as REM sleep; there may also be tachycardia, increased movement of the body and even erection of the penis. If the person is awakened at this stage he recalls vivid dreams.

In a typical night there may be three or four periods of REM sleep alternating with periods of slow wave sleep. We do not yet know the neurophysiological basis of these types of sleep, but it appears that both kinds of sleep are necessary to give a satisfying night's rest.

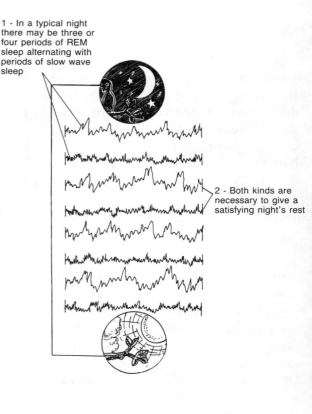

1 - In a typical night there may be three or four periods of REM sleep alternating with periods of slow wave sleep

2 - Both kinds are necessary to give a satisfying night's rest

If a person who is asleep becomes disturbed by a noise or other stimulus, or even awakes spontaneously, then the EEG waveform is seen to become very irregular, with an increase in the amount of activity indicating **arousal**. The EEG is truly reflecting the influence of the reticular system on the cerebral cortex.

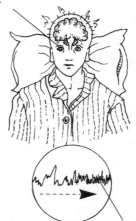

1 - If the person who is asleep becomes disturbed or is awakened, the EEG waveform becomes very irregular

2 - There is an increase in the amount of activity

The EEG is also used to detect abnormal discharges in the brain, such as **epilepsy**. This is manifest as localized or generalized bizarre electrical activity in the brain which is accompanied by abnormal jerking movements of the body, peculiar sensations, or less frequently unusual psychic experiences or disturbed behaviour.

We are still a long way from a full understanding of the complexity of motor activity; we have analysed a few simple reflexes and a small number of more complex movements. We have obtained some clues about the brain's electrical activity, but at present can only easily observe the impulses in the outermost layers, in the most distal dendrites of the cortical neurones.

There are still large tracts of the cerebral cortex about whose function we can only guess. As techniques for investigation become more refined, we shall undoubtedly learn more about this important aspect of physiology.

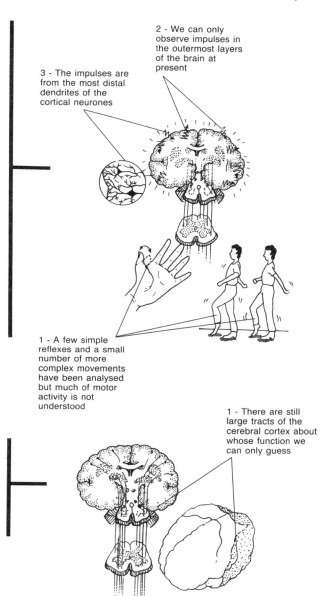

2 - We can only observe impulses in the outermost layers of the brain at present

3 - The impulses are from the most distal dendrites of the cortical neurones

1 - A few simple reflexes and a small number of more complex movements have been analysed but much of motor activity is not understood

1 - There are still large tracts of the cerebral cortex about whose function we can only guess

Sensory Mechanisms and Pathways

RECEPTORS

In this chapter we shall consider the properties of **receptors**, specialized neural elements or organs which sense events outside or inside the body, and start the process of transferring the information to the central nervous system.

We shall also deal with the nervous pathways connecting receptors with higher centres in the central nervous system, where the information is processed and causes reflex activity or produces conscious awareness of the sensation.

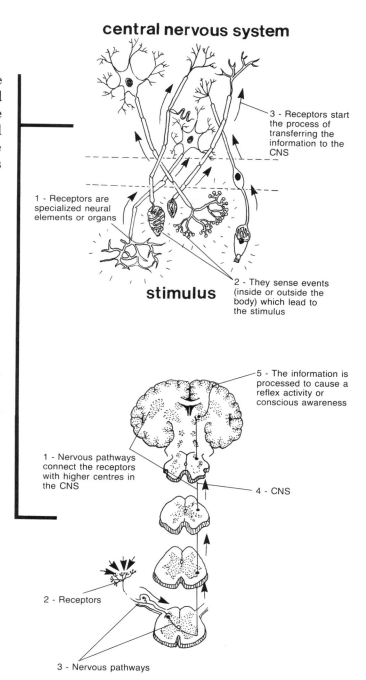

central nervous system

3 - Receptors start the process of transferring the information to the CNS

1 - Receptors are specialized neural elements or organs

2 - They sense events (inside or outside the body) which lead to the stimulus

stimulus

5 - The information is processed to cause a reflex activity or conscious awareness

1 - Nervous pathways connect the receptors with higher centres in the CNS

4 - CNS

2 - Receptors

3 - Nervous pathways

Receptors may be classified according to the type of sensation which they subserve: they are either **exteroceptors** responding to events in the external environment, or **interoceptors** responding to internal events or signals within the body. Touch or pressure receptors in the skin are typical simple exteroceptors; the eyes and ears are rather more complex receptors responding to the outside environment. The muscle spindles which sense the tension in contracted or relaxed muscles, or the carotid sinus which senses the arterial blood pressure, are examples of interoceptors.

The function of a receptor is to act as a **transducer**: a device which converts one type of energy to another. Two everyday examples of transducers are the microphone which converts sound (mechanical) energy into electrical signals which can be transmitted along wires, and the loudspeaker which converts electrical signals back into sound waves.

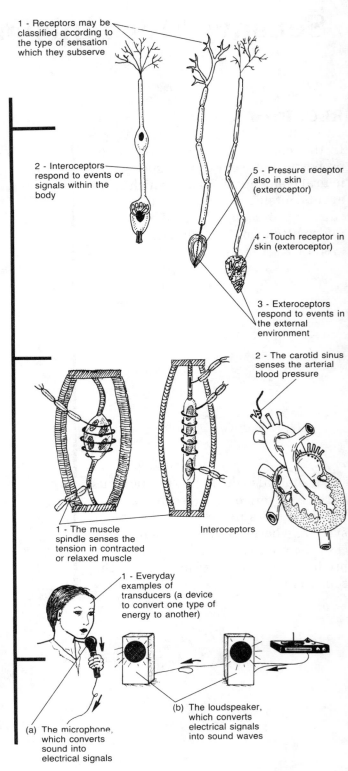

1 - Receptors may be classified according to the type of sensation which they subserve

2 - Interoceptors respond to events or signals within the body

5 - Pressure receptor also in skin (exteroceptor)

4 - Touch receptor in skin (exteroceptor)

3 - Exteroceptors respond to events in the external environment

2 - The carotid sinus senses the arterial blood pressure

1 - The muscle spindle senses the tension in contracted or relaxed muscle

Interoceptors

1 - Everyday examples of transducers (a device to convert one type of energy to another)

(a) The microphone, which converts sound into electrical signals

(b) The loudspeaker, which converts electrical signals into sound waves

In the body there are transducers which convert many types of signal into nerve impulses: there are **mechano-receptors** like pressure, touch and stretch receptors and the organs of hearing and balance in the internal ear; **chemoreceptors** like the cells responsible for taste and smell, or the carotid body which senses the amount of oxygen in the blood, or the osmo-receptors in the hypothalamus which sense the salinity of the plasma; **photo-receptors** like the rods and cones in the retina of the eye.

Receptors show **specificity** towards one particular type of stimulus, i.e. they are most easily excited by one form of energy. This does not mean that they cannot be excited by other sorts of stimulus; while the cells of the retina are most easily excited by light, they can also be stimulated by pressure. If a finger is poked in one corner of a closed eye, a sensation of light is perceived, illustrating the fact that the brain interprets information reaching it along a particular pathway as being caused by one specific form of energy, no matter what is the actual mechanism of initiation.

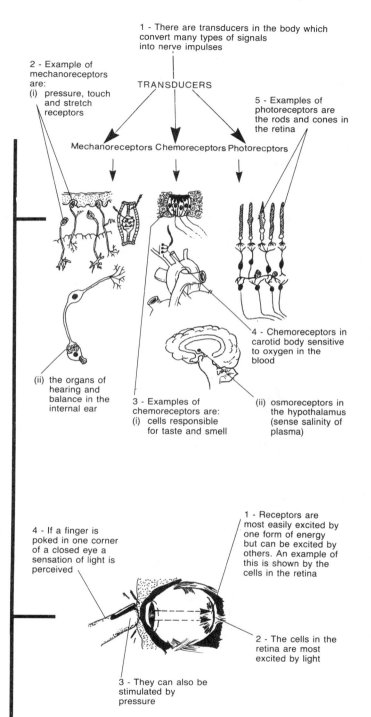

1 - There are transducers in the body which convert many types of signals into nerve impulses

TRANSDUCERS

2 - Example of mechanoreceptors are:
(i) pressure, touch and stretch receptors

5 - Examples of photoreceptors are the rods and cones in the retina

Mechanoreceptors Chemoreceptors Photoreceptors

4 - Chemoreceptors in carotid body sensitive to oxygen in the blood

(ii) the organs of hearing and balance in the internal ear

3 - Examples of chemoreceptors are:
(i) cells responsible for taste and smell

(ii) osmoreceptors in the hypothalamus (sense salinity of plasma)

1 - Receptors are most easily excited by one form of energy but can be excited by others. An example of this is shown by the cells in the retina

4 - If a finger is poked in one corner of a closed eye a sensation of light is perceived

2 - The cells in the retina are most excited by light

3 - They can also be stimulated by pressure

Similarly, the application of pressure or a sharp tap to sensory nerve trunks such as the ulnar nerve behind the elbow (the 'funny bone') causes the perception of a variety of sensations appropriate to the type of receptor found at the end of the nerve. Electric shocks applied to nerves (for instance in the clinical measurement of conduction velocity) produce a variety of sensations which are interpreted as coming from the extremities, not the site of stimulus.

The specificity of receptors means that their **threshold** is lowest for the type of energy which they are designed to transduce; they can be excited by other stimuli, but the threshold is much higher. For instance, it takes quite firm pressure on the eyeball to produce a sensation of light, whereas the photoreceptors of the retina are capable of responding to a single quantum of incident light.

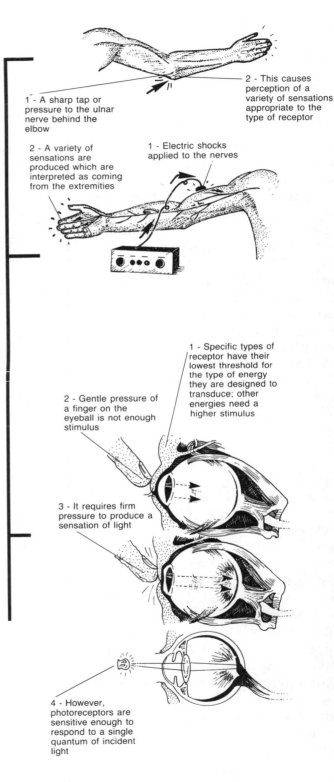

1 - A sharp tap or pressure to the ulnar nerve behind the elbow

2 - This causes perception of a variety of sensations appropriate to the type of receptor

1 - Electric shocks applied to the nerves

2 - A variety of sensations are produced which are interpreted as coming from the extremities

1 - Specific types of receptor have their lowest threshold for the type of energy they are designed to transduce; other energies need a higher stimulus

2 - Gentle pressure of a finger on the eyeball is not enough stimulus

3 - It requires firm pressure to produce a sensation of light

4 - However, photoreceptors are sensitive enough to respond to a single quantum of incident light

Organization of receptors

Many receptors or sense organs have one or more **accessory structures** which can modify the incident energy in some way before it reaches the transducing element. In some cases the accessory structures are very simple, consisting of only a covering capsule; in other cases like the eye and ear the accessory structures are very complex indeed.

All types of receptor systems consist of a **sensitive** part, responding to the specific incident energy, and a **conducting** part which takes the information to the central nervous system.

There is wide variation in the organization of the connections between these two parts. In the simplest type of organization, the sensitive part is no more than the modified end portion of the primary sensory neurone; for instance, many pain receptors are simply the naked ends of sensory nerves embedded within the tissues.

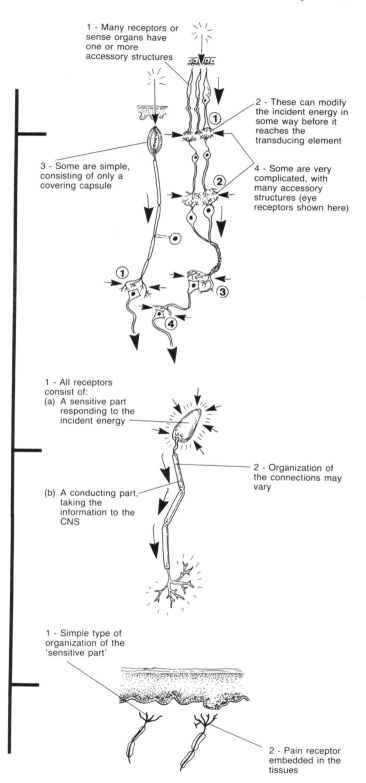

1 - Many receptors or sense organs have one or more accessory structures

2 - These can modify the incident energy in some way before it reaches the transducing element

3 - Some are simple, consisting of only a covering capsule

4 - Some are very complicated, with many accessory structures (eye receptors shown here)

1 - All receptors consist of:
(a) A sensitive part responding to the incident energy

2 - Organization of the connections may vary

(b) A conducting part, taking the information to the CNS

1 - Simple type of organization of the 'sensitive part'

2 - Pain receptor embedded in the tissues

In more elaborate types of organization, the sensitive part may be a separate receptor cell, in which incident energy produces electrical changes which must then be transmitted across a synapse to the sensory neurone, and in still more complex systems there may be one or more interneurones in the pathway, allowing a certain amount of **integration** to take place before the information is conducted to the central nervous system.

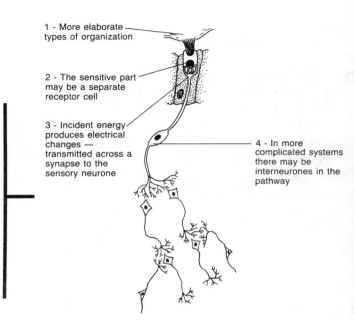

1 - More elaborate types of organization

2 - The sensitive part may be a separate receptor cell

3 - Incident energy produces electrical changes — transmitted across a synapse to the sensory neurone

4 - In more complicated systems there may be interneurones in the pathway

Electrophysiology of receptors

The application of specific incident energy to a receptor causes an area of the cell membrane to undergo a permeability change which usually results in a change in membrane potential, known as the **generator potential**, or sometimes the **receptor potential**.

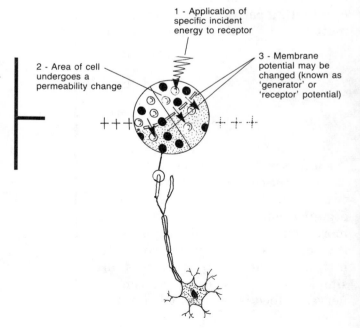

1 - Application of specific incident energy to receptor

2 - Area of cell undergoes a permeability change

3 - Membrane potential may be changed (known as 'generator' or 'receptor' potential)

This potential is rather similar to a synaptic potential; the permeability change in the cell membrane is determined by the intensity of the incident energy rather than the level of the membrane potential, and it is a graded response rather than an all-or-none phenomenon.

If the generator potential is large enough, the nerve is depolarized to threshold and action potentials are initiated and conducted, or synaptic transmission occurs with excitation of the postsynaptic cell.

If the generator potential is larger or more prolonged, it produces a train of action potentials rather than a single spike, and the frequency of spikes is determined by the amplitude of the generator potential. Thus the intensity of a stimulus is converted into a **number** of impulses rather than a **size** of signal.

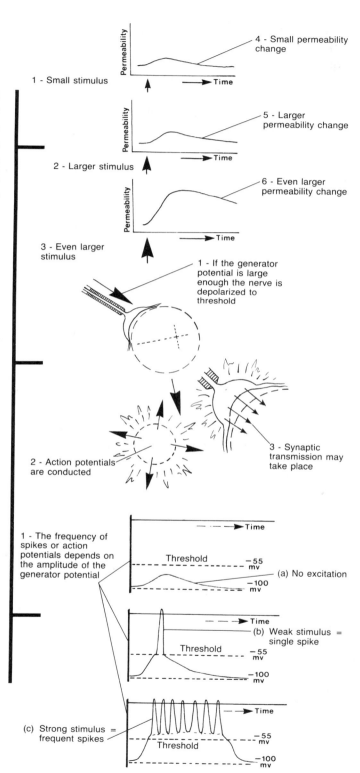

Many sensory systems have a **logarithmic** relationship between the incident stimulus and the signal reaching the nervous system; in other words, the amplitude of the generator potential is proportional to the logarithm of the stimulus intensity, and the frequency of action potentials (which depends upon the size of the generator potential) is also proportional to the logarithm of the stimulus size.

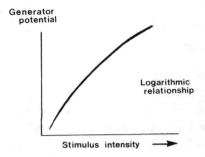

This means that if we can just perceive the difference between one stimulus and one twice as large, then in order to be able to perceive a further increase the stimulus intensity would have to be doubled again.

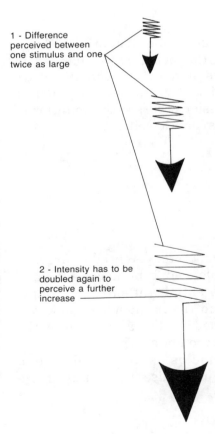

1 - Difference perceived between one stimulus and one twice as large

2 - Intensity has to be doubled again to perceive a further increase

Adaptation of receptors

Once a sensation has been registered, its perception is often diminished although the intensity of the actual stimulus remains constant. This phenomenon is called **adaptation**.

For instance, people who live near to a glue factory, rubbish dump or similar source of offensive odours soon stop noticing the smell, though anyone coming to visit them immediately remarks upon it; when we first put our clothes on in the morning we are aware of the contact between clothes and skin, but we soon cease to notice this contact — in fact life would become intolerable if all of our senses continuously bombarded the cen-tral nervous system with an unmodified barrage of sensory information.

Some of the adaptation occurs at the receptor itself: either in the accessory structures or in the neural elements. Some of the adaptation is in sensory pathways, where interneurones on the way to the higher centres act as selective filters or integrators of the incoming sensory activity. Some of the adaptation is a function of the highest brain centres, which may choose to ignore a certain train of incoming sensory information while the main attention of the conscious brain is being directed elsewhere.

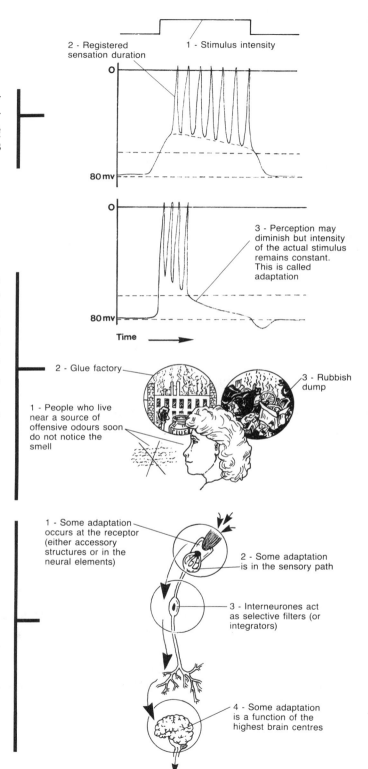

2 - Registered sensation duration

1 - Stimulus intensity

3 - Perception may diminish but intensity of the actual stimulus remains constant. This is called adaptation

Time

2 - Glue factory

3 - Rubbish dump

1 - People who live near a source of offensive odours soon do not notice the smell

1 - Some adaptation occurs at the receptor (either accessory structures or in the neural elements)

2 - Some adaptation is in the sensory path

3 - Interneurones act as selective filters (or integrators)

4 - Some adaptation is a function of the highest brain centres

1 - Competitors in sports (or military personnel in combat) can ignore extreme degrees of pain or discomfort

2 - The person is capable of doing this whilst trying to achieve an important goal or objective

For instance, competitors in sports or military personnel in combat can ignore extreme degrees of discomfort or pain while trying to achieve an important goal or objective.

Adaptation at the receptor level is well demonstrated in the Pacinian corpuscle, a pressure sensor widely distributed through the tissues and found in particularly large numbers in the mesentery. The sensitive nerve ending is embedded in a series of concentric layers of gelatinous material, arranged rather like the layers of an onion.

5 - Sensitive nerve ending

1 - Adaptation at the receptor level is well demonstrated in the Pacinian corpuscle

2 - It is widely distributed through the tissues

4 - Series of concentric layers of gelatinous material

3 - It is found in large numbers in the mesentery

Deformation of the ending produces a rapid discharge of action potentials in the nerve, but the discharge soon gets slower and stops despite the continued application of pressure. Release of the pressure, allowing the corpuscle to resume its former position, results in another burst of action potentials which once again slows down and stops.

2 - Original position (no action potential)

3 - Deformation of the ending (action potential)

1 - Deformation of the ending produces a rapid discharge of action potentials in the nerve, which slow and stop despite continued pressure

4 - Corpuscle resumes former position (release of pressure)

5 - Release of the pressure results in another burst of action potentials

6 - The discharge gets slower and stops

If the concentric layers of the capsule are removed and pressure is applied directly to the naked nerve ending, then the discharge of action potentials remains constant so long as the pressure is applied, and ceases as soon as the pressure is removed.

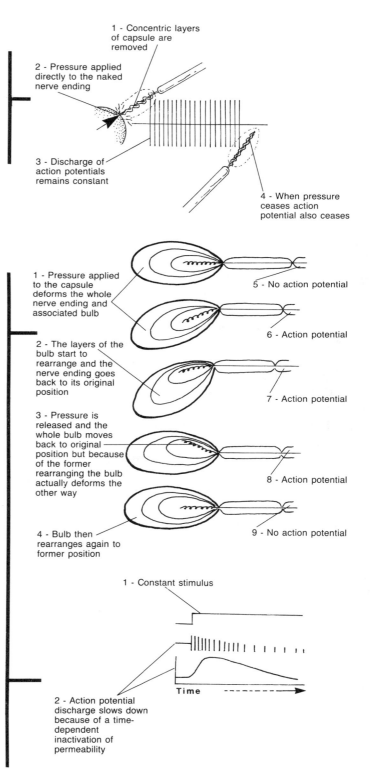

1 - Concentric layers of capsule are removed

2 - Pressure applied directly to the naked nerve ending

3 - Discharge of action potentials remains constant

4 - When pressure ceases action potential also ceases

The explanation for this behaviour is that pressure applied to the capsule deforms the whole nerve ending and associated bulb, but gradually the layers of the bulb rearrange themselves and allow the nerve ending to 'creep' back to its original straight, undeformed position. When the pressure is released the whole bulb moves back to its original position, but as the internal layers had been rearranged the nerve ending actually becomes deformed again in the opposite direction, causing another discharge of action potentials until the internal layers of the bulb rearrange themselves to the original position.

1 - Pressure applied to the capsule deforms the whole nerve ending and associated bulb

5 - No action potential

6 - Action potential

2 - The layers of the bulb start to rearrange and the nerve ending goes back to its original position

7 - Action potential

3 - Pressure is released and the whole bulb moves back to original position but because of the former rearranging the bulb actually deforms the other way

8 - Action potential

4 - Bulb then rearranges again to former position

9 - No action potential

In some cases it is the actual sensory nerve ending or receptor cell which manifests the adaptation, and in these cases we have to suppose that the ionic permeabilities which contribute to the generator potential are subject to time-dependent inactivation; thus the generator potential declines with time, and so does the rate of action potential discharge.

1 - Constant stimulus

Time

2 - Action potential discharge slows down because of a time-dependent inactivation of permeability

Receptors which adapt rapidly are sensitive to **changes** in the intensity of stimulus; the **absolute magnitude** of the stimulus is sensed by receptors which adapt slowly or not at all. Both types of sensor are necessary in the body to allow accurate control of movement and homeostatic mechanisms; almost all receptors show some adaptation, but can be broadly separated into rapidly adapting and slowly adapting receptors.

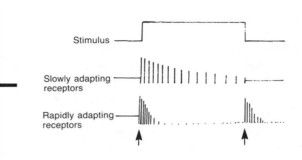

Some simple peripheral receptors

The Pacinian corpuscle, a pressure receptor, has already been discussed. Other mechanoreceptors include the free nerve endings which are found in all parts of the body and are mainly pain receptors; the hair end-organs which are wound around the base of hair follicles and sense movement of the hairs; Ruffini's endings and Merkel's discs which are expanded tip nerve endings; and Meissner's and Krause's corpuscles which have capsules around the sensitive nerve endings. Many of these are found in both the skin and deeper tissues, and detect pressure, stretch, vibration or light touch.

Some receptors in the capsules of joints detect the position of the limbs in space.

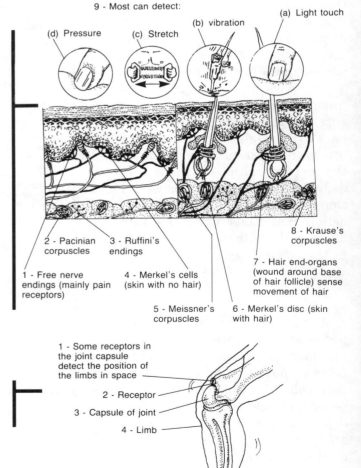

9 - Most can detect:
(a) Light touch
(b) vibration
(c) Stretch
(d) Pressure

1 - Free nerve endings (mainly pain receptors)
2 - Pacinian corpuscles
3 - Ruffini's endings
4 - Merkel's cells (skin with no hair)
5 - Meissner's corpuscles
6 - Merkel's disc (skin with hair)
7 - Hair end-organs (wound around base of hair follicle) sense movement of hair
8 - Krause's corpuscles

1 - Some receptors in the joint capsule detect the position of the limbs in space
2 - Receptor
3 - Capsule of joint
4 - Limb

The muscle spindle and the Golgi tendon organ are more complex mechanoreceptors which detect the level of contraction of muscles; these are so complicated and so intimately bound up with movement that they are described in the chapter dealing with the motor system.

1 - Mechanoreceptors

(a) Golgi tendon organ

(b) Muscle spindle

2 - These detect the level of contraction of muscles

Temperature receptors respond either to warmth or to cold; some pain receptors also respond to changes in temperature. Most thermoreceptors in the skin are free nerve endings, and produce their maximal rate of discharge at a characteristic temperature.

1 - Temperature receptors respond to either:

(a) Warmth, or   (b) Cold

HOT   COLD

2 - Temperature receptors

3 - Some receptors can also respond to changes in temperature

Each type of receptor is capable of response over a wide range of temperature, and the ranges of the various types overlap, but the brain determines the actual temperature by analysing the pattern of response of the different receptors.

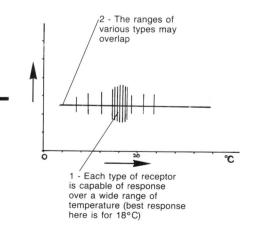

2 - The ranges of various types may overlap

°C

1 - Each type of receptor is capable of response over a wide range of temperature (best response here is for 18°C)

Each type of receptor is very sensitive to small temperature changes but adapts very quickly; if there is a sudden change in temperature the discharge rate is greatly altered but settles to a new steady level very rapidly.

This behaviour gives the brain rapid early warning of important changes in the temperature of the skin and of the environment.

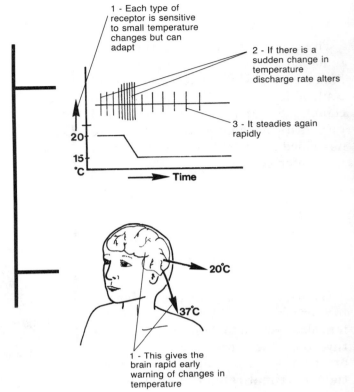

1 - Each type of receptor is sensitive to small temperature changes but can adapt

2 - If there is a sudden change in temperature discharge rate alters

3 - It steadies again rapidly

1 - This gives the brain rapid early warning of changes in temperature

THE SENSORY PATHWAYS

Peripheral sensory neurones carry signals back to the spinal cord, and the cell bodies of the primary sensory neurones are in the dorsal root ganglia. Axons entering each spinal segment send branches to the same and other segments in the spine, to synapse with local interneurones and motor neurones, causing local or segmental reflexes. There are also branches which ascend along specific sensory pathways to reach higher centres in the brain.

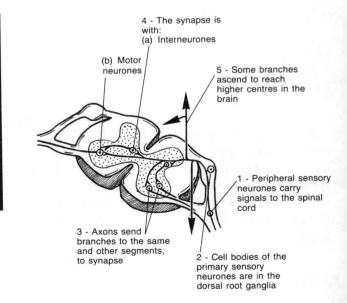

4 - The synapse is with:
(a) Interneurones

(b) Motor neurones

5 - Some branches ascend to reach higher centres in the brain

1 - Peripheral sensory neurones carry signals to the spinal cord

3 - Axons send branches to the same and other segments, to synapse

2 - Cell bodies of the primary sensory neurones are in the dorsal root ganglia

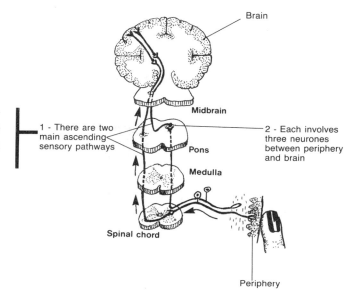

There are two main ascending sensory pathways, and each involves three neurones in the pathway between periphery and brain.

The first pathway carries information mainly from proprioceptors, i.e. muscle spindles, Golgi tendon organs and joint position receptors, together with pressure, vibration and some light touch sensation. The axons of the **primary** or first sensory neurones enter the cord, and pass straight up in the dorsal columns of the white matter to the medulla oblongata, the lowest part of the brain stem.

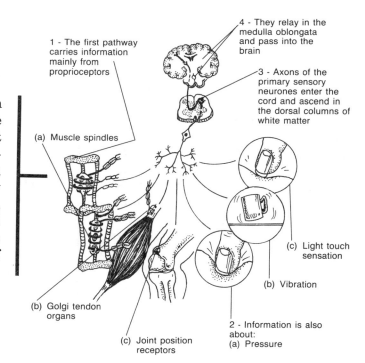

In the medulla are two major relay stations, the **nucleus cuneatus** and the **nucleus gracilis**, where the primary neurones form synapses with the **secondary** sensory neurones. The axons from these neurones ascend through the brain stem, crossing the midline to reach the other side and passing to the **thalamus**, a large aggregation of grey matter at the centre of each cerebral hemisphere. The thalamus is a major relay station, where secondary sensory neurones synapse with the **tertiary** or third neurones whose axons radiate to the cerebral cortex, where the sensory information impinges upon conscious awareness.

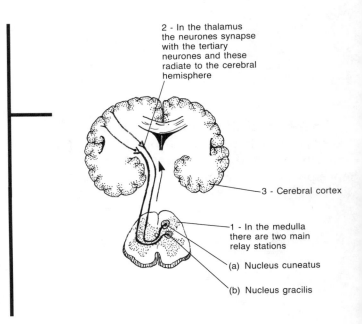

2 - In the thalamus the neurones synapse with the tertiary neurones and these radiate to the cerebral hemisphere

3 - Cerebral cortex

1 - In the medulla there are two main relay stations

(a) Nucleus cuneatus

(b) Nucleus gracilis

The second pathway carries most of the unpleasant sensations such as pain and temperature as well as some light touch. The **primary** sensory neurones enter the cord and pass directly to the dorsal grey matter, where they form synapses with the **secondary** neurones. The axons of the secondary sensory neurones cross the midline immediately, i.e. in the spinal cord itself, and then ascend in the **lateral spinothalamic tract** to relay in the thalamus. The **tertiary** sensory neurone again originates in the thalamus and projects to the cerebral cortex.

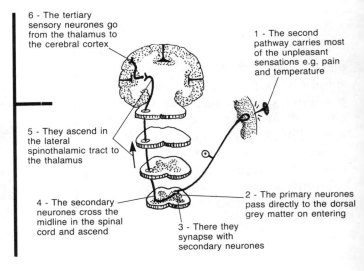

6 - The tertiary sensory neurones go from the thalamus to the cerebral cortex

1 - The second pathway carries most of the unpleasant sensations e.g. pain and temperature

5 - They ascend in the lateral spinothalamic tract to the thalamus

4 - The secondary neurones cross the midline in the spinal cord and ascend

3 - There they synapse with secondary neurones

2 - The primary neurones pass directly to the dorsal grey matter on entering

Note that both pathways cross the midline so that sensory information from one side of the body is processed in the opposite side of the brain. In both cases it is the secondary neurone that crosses the midline, either in the medulla or in the spinal cord itself. In the mechanosensitive pathway the secondary neurone originates in the medulla, but in the **nociceptive** (or unpleasant sensation) pathway the secondary neurone originates in the cord and does not relay in the brain stem. In both pathways the final neurone originates in the thalamus.

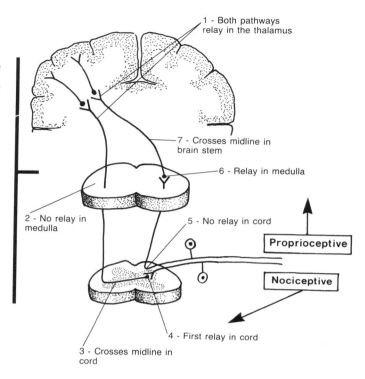

Sensations from the viscera follow essentially similar pathways to sensations from the more superficial organs and tissues. However, some sensory nerve fibres travel along the same nerve trunks as the sympathetic motor fibres, joining the mixed spinal nerves where the autonomic fibres leave them; some visceral sensory fibres run with parasympathetic nerves like the vagus, entering the brain stem in the same place. Some of the visceral sensory fibres are from specific organs like the carotid sinus baroreceptors or the carotid and aortic body chemoreceptors, or from stretch receptors in the lung. Others are from rather non-specific irritant receptors (found, for instance, in the pulmonary airways) or pressure receptors such as the Pacinian corpuscles in the mesentery. Yet others are from pain receptors.

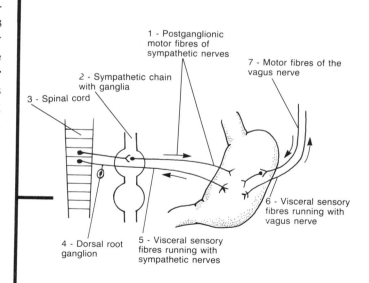

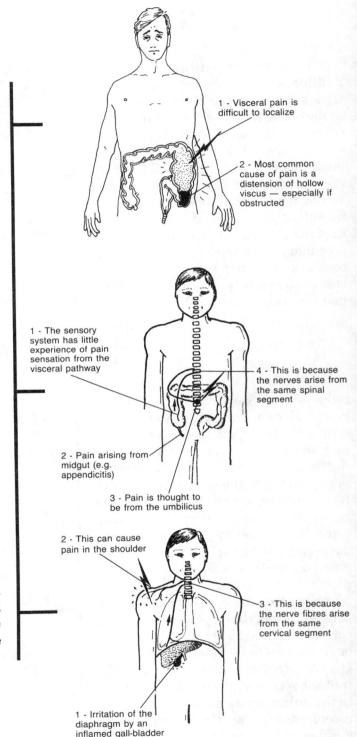

Visceral sensation, and especially visceral pain, is rather difficult to localize. The most common cause of visceral pain is distension of a hollow viscus, especially if it is obstructed.

1 - Visceral pain is difficult to localize

2 - Most common cause of pain is a distension of hollow viscus — especially if obstructed

Since the sensory system has little experience of pain sensation arriving along the visceral pathway, the brain often misinterprets the pain as arising from skin, muscle or joints which are innervated by the same spinal segment as the viscus which is being irritated. Thus pain arising from the mid-gut, such as in appendicitis, is often 'referred' to the umbilicus.

1 - The sensory system has little experience of pain sensation from the visceral pathway

4 - This is because the nerves arise from the same spinal segment

2 - Pain arising from midgut (e.g. appendicitis)

3 - Pain is thought to be from the umbilicus

Irritation of the diaphragm by an inflamed gall-bladder can cause pain in the shoulder, whose nerve fibres arise from the same cervical segments as the phrenic nerve.

2 - This can cause pain in the shoulder

3 - This is because the nerve fibres arise from the same cervical segment

1 - Irritation of the diaphragm by an inflamed gall-bladder

The pathway for pain sensation is interesting because the perception of pain can be modified by stimulating nerve fibres which do not carry pain impulses. The pain of an insect sting or a violent blow can be reduced by rubbing the part; the pain of arthritic joints or strained muscles can be eased by massage or local heat, and many types of pain can be relieved by vibrating very fine needles inserted into the skin in various parts of the body (acupuncture).

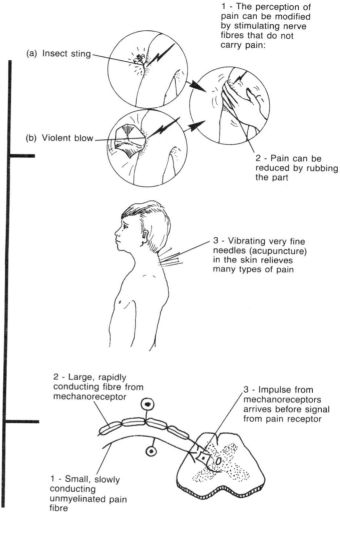

1 - The perception of pain can be modified by stimulating nerve fibres that do not carry pain:

(a) Insect sting

(b) Violent blow

2 - Pain can be reduced by rubbing the part

3 - Vibrating very fine needles (acupuncture) in the skin relieves many types of pain

The major site of relay for pain fibres is the **substantia gelatinosa** in the grey matter of the spinal cord, and it is postulated that simultaneous excitation of large-diameter fast-conducting nerve fibres (from mechanoreceptors) can cause presynaptic inhibition of the slowly conducting fine 'C' fibres from pain receptors as they relay in the cord. It is also possible that large fast fibres can inhibit other parts of the pain pathway.

2 - Large, rapidly conducting fibre from mechanoreceptor

3 - Impulse from mechanoreceptors arrives before signal from pain receptor

1 - Small, slowly conducting unmyelinated pain fibre

The part of the cerebral cortex which receives the tertiary sensory neurones is known as the **sensory cortex**, and is situated in the parietal lobe just posterior to the central sulcus, in the post-central gyrus.

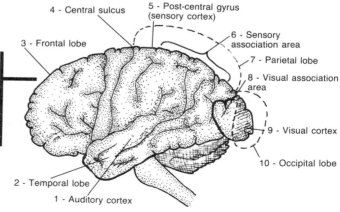

4 - Central sulcus
5 - Post-central gyrus (sensory cortex)
3 - Frontal lobe
6 - Sensory association area
7 - Parietal lobe
8 - Visual association area
9 - Visual cortex
10 - Occipital lobe
2 - Temporal lobe
1 - Auditory cortex

Each part of the body can be mapped on to a specific area of the sensory cortex, but the pattern of cortical representation is often grossly disproportionate to the size of the actual part. For instance, the face (particularly the tongue) and hands have a very large area devoted to them, as have the genitalia, whereas the legs and trunk have only a small cortical representation.

The neurones of this part of the cortex are interconnected with neurones of the opposite side through the corpus callosum, and are also connected with neurones on the same side in the motor cortex as well as with the **sensory association area** in the parietal lobe (just posterior to the main sensory cortex).

The function of the sensory association area is to process the sensory information in order to assist in its interpretation; incoming sensory information is compared with previously experienced patterns of information, to allow, for example, the shape and texture of an object to be recognized from its tactile qualities.

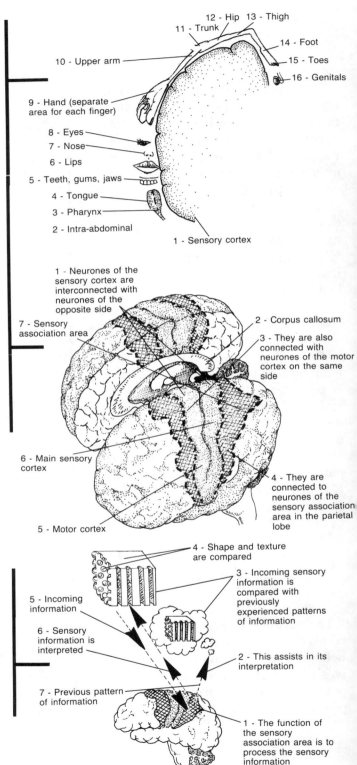

12 - Hip   13 - Thigh
11 - Trunk
14 - Foot
10 - Upper arm
15 - Toes
16 - Genitals
9 - Hand (separate area for each finger)
8 - Eyes
7 - Nose
6 - Lips
5 - Teeth, gums, jaws
4 - Tongue
3 - Pharynx
2 - Intra-abdominal
1 - Sensory cortex

1 - Neurones of the sensory cortex are interconnected with neurones of the opposite side
7 - Sensory association area
2 - Corpus callosum
3 - They are also connected with neurones of the motor cortex on the same side
6 - Main sensory cortex
4 - They are connected to neurones of the sensory association area in the parietal lobe
5 - Motor cortex

4 - Shape and texture are compared
3 - Incoming sensory information is compared with previously experienced patterns of information
5 - Incoming information
6 - Sensory information is interpreted
2 - This assists in its interpretation
7 - Previous pattern of information
1 - The function of the sensory association area is to process the sensory information

SPECIAL SENSES: TASTE AND SMELL

The receptors for smell (**olfaction**) are located in the nose; those for the sense of taste (**gustation**) are on the tongue, the palate and in the pharynx.

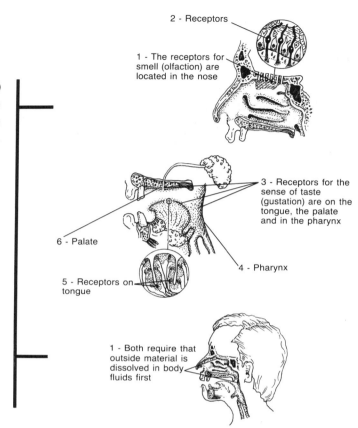

2 - Receptors

1 - The receptors for smell (olfaction) are located in the nose

3 - Receptors for the sense of taste (gustation) are on the tongue, the palate and in the pharynx

6 - Palate

4 - Pharynx

5 - Receptors on tongue

Both of these chemical special senses require that material from the outside environment is dissolved in body fluids before coming into contact with a sensitive epithelium and exciting the receptor cells.

1 - Both require that outside material is dissolved in body fluids first

The sensory receptors in the nose are **hair cells** embedded in the nasal epithelium, supported by **sustentacular cells**. Contact of specific chemicals with the hairs causes excitation of the receptor, which is part of the primary sensory neurone whose axons form the first cranial nerve and terminate in the olfactory bulb. The secondary neurones start in the olfactory bulb and run in the olfactory tract to the olfactory cortex at the base of the brain.

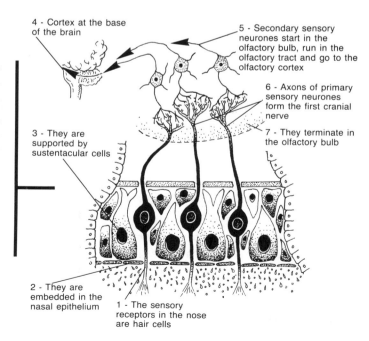

4 - Cortex at the base of the brain

5 - Secondary sensory neurones start in the olfactory bulb, run in the olfactory tract and go to the olfactory cortex

6 - Axons of primary sensory neurones form the first cranial nerve

3 - They are supported by sustentacular cells

7 - They terminate in the olfactory bulb

2 - They are embedded in the nasal epithelium

1 - The sensory receptors in the nose are hair cells

About fifty different types of olfactory sensation have been described, and there may actually be this many separate types of smell receptor. Some smelly substances may irritate other nasal receptors in addition to the olfactory hair cells; for instance, strong ammonia almost certainly irritates pain fibres as well as the receptors specific to its pungent smell. The sensation of smell is difficult to study experimentally and to test clinically, and so we are still largely ignorant about its mechanisms.

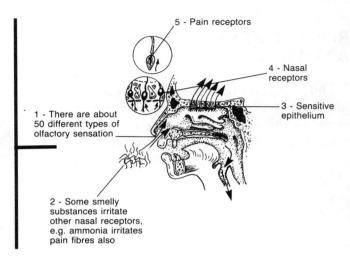

5 - Pain receptors

4 - Nasal receptors

3 - Sensitive epithelium

1 - There are about 50 different types of olfactory sensation

2 - Some smelly substances irritate other nasal receptors, e.g. ammonia irritates pain fibres also

The sense of taste is transduced by the **taste buds** found in papillae over the surface of the tongue, mouth and pharynx.

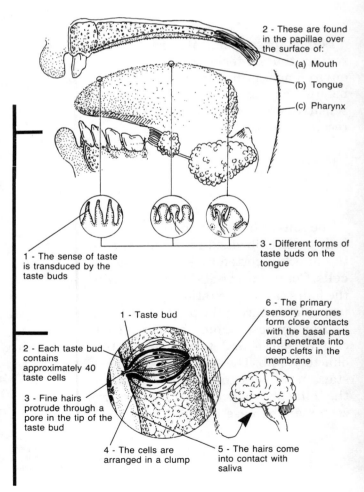

2 - These are found in the papillae over the surface of:

(a) Mouth

(b) Tongue

(c) Pharynx

1 - The sense of taste is transduced by the taste buds

3 - Different forms of taste buds on the tongue

Each taste bud consists of about forty taste cells arranged in a clump, with the primary sensory neurones forming very close contacts with their basal parts and penetrating into deep clefts in their membranes. The sensory cells have fine hairs which protrude through a pore in the tip of the taste bud and come into contact with the fine layer of fluid (saliva) covering the inner surface of the mouth.

6 - The primary sensory neurones form close contacts with the basal parts and penetrate into deep clefts in the membrane

1 - Taste bud

2 - Each taste bud contains approximately 40 taste cells

3 - Fine hairs protrude through a pore in the tip of the taste bud

4 - The cells are arranged in a clump

5 - The hairs come into contact with saliva

There are only four types of taste sensation: salt, sweet, bitter and sour. All of the complex flavours of food are made up from these basic tastes, although the odour of the food also contributes greatly to its total sensory impact.

In addition, some substances such as **capsaicin**, found in peppers and chillies, cause stimulation of irritant receptors in the mucosa and the mild pain sensation can actually enhance the pleasure of spicy meals.

The taste buds for sweetness are located on the front and tip of the tongue, those for salty and sour sensations along the sides of the tongue, and those for bitterness at the back of the tongue.

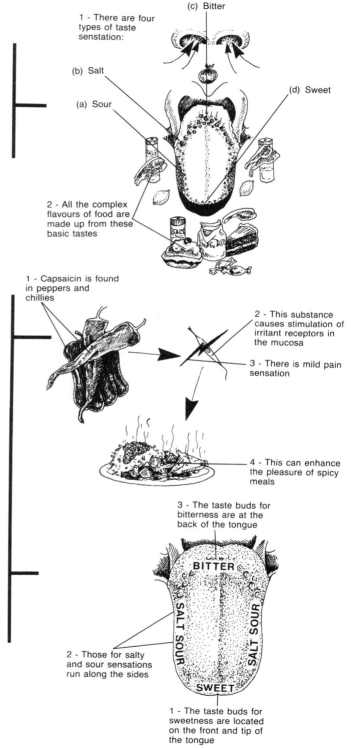

1 - There are four types of taste sensation:

(c) Bitter

(b) Salt

(a) Sour

(d) Sweet

2 - All the complex flavours of food are made up from these basic tastes

1 - Capsaicin is found in peppers and chillies

2 - This substance causes stimulation of irritant receptors in the mucosa

3 - There is mild pain sensation

4 - This can enhance the pleasure of spicy meals

3 - The taste buds for bitterness are at the back of the tongue

BITTER

SALT SOUR

SALT SOUR

SWEET

2 - Those for salty and sour sensations run along the sides

1 - The taste buds for sweetness are located on the front and tip of the tongue

Stimulation of taste buds with the appropriate chemical causes a generator potential which initiates the discharge of action potentials in the primary sensory axons. These run first in the fifth cranial nerve (trigeminal) then pass via the **chorda tympani** nerve (near the eardrum) to the seventh (facial) cranial nerve, and to the **tractus solitarius** in the brain stem. Axons from the circumvallate papillae and the pharynx pass via the vagus (tenth) or glossopharyngeal (ninth) nerves to the tractus solitarius. Here they all relay with the secondary sensory neurones which pass to the thalamus, where the tertiary neurones originate and project to a special taste area of the cerebral cortex.

Some of the taste fibres participate in the reflex control of secretion of saliva; fibres from the tractus solitarius pass to the salivatory nuclei.

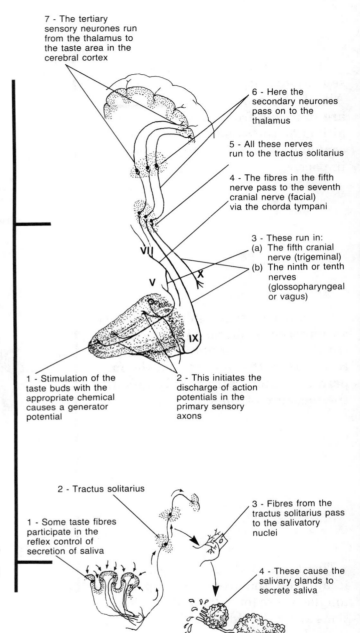

7 - The tertiary sensory neurones run from the thalamus to the taste area in the cerebral cortex

6 - Here the secondary neurones pass on to the thalamus

5 - All these nerves run to the tractus solitarius

4 - The fibres in the fifth nerve pass to the seventh cranial nerve (facial) via the chorda tympani

3 - These run in:
(a) The fifth cranial nerve (trigeminal)
(b) The ninth or tenth nerves (glossopharyngeal or vagus)

VII

V

X

IX

1 - Stimulation of the taste buds with the appropriate chemical causes a generator potential

2 - This initiates the discharge of action potentials in the primary sensory axons

2 - Tractus solitarius

1 - Some taste fibres participate in the reflex control of secretion of saliva

3 - Fibres from the tractus solitarius pass to the salivatory nuclei

4 - These cause the salivary glands to secrete saliva

SPECIAL SENSES: HEARING AND BALANCE

The special senses of hearing and balance are closely connected, and reside in the ear. There are several complicated accessory structures in both systems before the actual sensory cells are activated.

The outermost, visible part is known as the **outer ear**; the **middle ear**, beyond the eardrum, is an air-filled cavity containing structures for the efficient transfer of sound energy to the **inner ear**, which is where the actual sound receptors are located. The receptors for balance and equilibrium are also found in the inner ear.

The organs of hearing and balance use a common type of sensor, the **hair cell**, which is a tall cell, standing upon a basement membrane, with a series of deformable hairs, the **kinocilia** and **stereocilia** at its tip. These hairs are embedded in a gelatinous matrix or **cupula**, and mechanical deformation of the cupula causes hairs to bend and excite the cell.

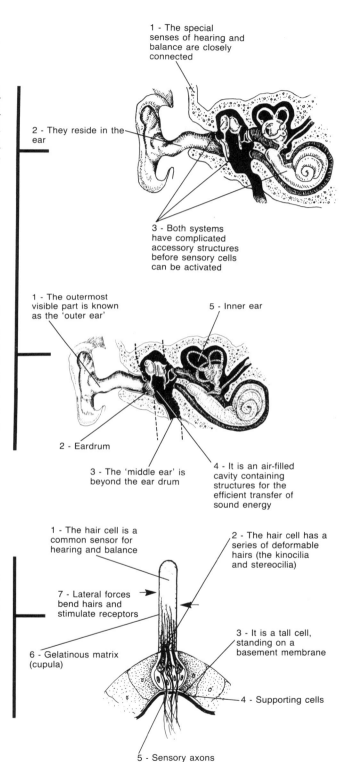

1 - The special senses of hearing and balance are closely connected

2 - They reside in the ear

3 - Both systems have complicated accessory structures before sensory cells can be activated

1 - The outermost visible part is known as the 'outer ear'

5 - Inner ear

2 - Eardrum

3 - The 'middle ear' is beyond the ear drum

4 - It is an air-filled cavity containing structures for the efficient transfer of sound energy

1 - The hair cell is a common sensor for hearing and balance

2 - The hair cell has a series of deformable hairs (the kinocilia and stereocilia)

7 - Lateral forces bend hairs and stimulate receptors

3 - It is a tall cell, standing on a basement membrane

6 - Gelatinous matrix (cupula)

4 - Supporting cells

5 - Sensory axons

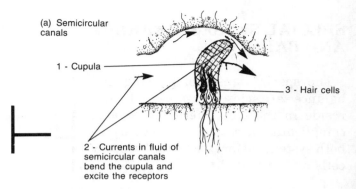

(a) Semicircular canals

1 - Cupula

3 - Hair cells

2 - Currents in fluid of semicircular canals bend the cupula and excite the receptors

The differences between the various organs lie chiefly in the arrangement of the cupula.

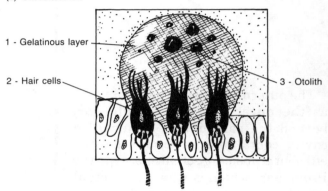

(b) Saccule/utricle

1 - Gelatinous layer

2 - Hair cells

3 - Otolith

Modifications of the organ

Physiology of the accessory organs

The accessory organs for hearing consist first of the **pinna** or external ear, which is fixed in position in man but can be moved around to various positions by muscular control in other animals such as dogs or donkeys, so that the best direction for hearing can be achieved.

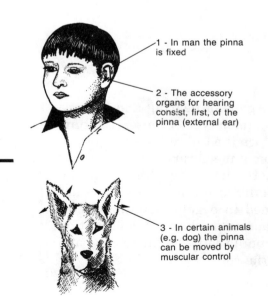

1 - In man the pinna is fixed

2 - The accessory organs for hearing consist, first, of the pinna (external ear)

3 - In certain animals (e.g. dog) the pinna can be moved by muscular control

The pinna leads into the skin-lined **external auditory meatus**, which is terminated by the **tympanic membrane** or eardrum. This, too, is covered on its outer surface by skin and on its inner surface by the mucous membrane of the middle ear, which is in turn continuous with the lining of the throat, nose and mouth.

1 - Pinna

2 - External auditory meatus

3 - Tympanic membrane (eardrum)

4 - The eardrum is covered by skin and inside the surface is covered with mucous membrane

External ear

The tympanic membrane is connected to the **malleus** (hammer), the first of three small bones or **ossicles** in the middle ear; the other two are the **incus** (anvil) and **stapes** (stirrup); these bones articulate together to form a lever system which bridges the middle ear cavity to transmit sound vibrations to the inner ear on the medial side of the middle ear.

1 - Tympanic membrane

2 - Malleus (hammer) (1st of three small bones or ossicles)

3 - Incus (anvil) (2nd small bone)

4 - Stapes (stirrup) (3rd small bone)

5 - These bones articulate together to form a lever system. This bridges the middle ear cavity, transmitting sound vibrations to the inner ear

6 - Middle ear cavity

Middle ear

The eardrum and ossicle system convert the incident sound waves arriving through the air, having large amplitude but little pressure, into movements with small amplitude but large pressure. These movements occur at the foot of the stapes where it transfers its vibratory energy to the fluid of the inner ear through the oval window.

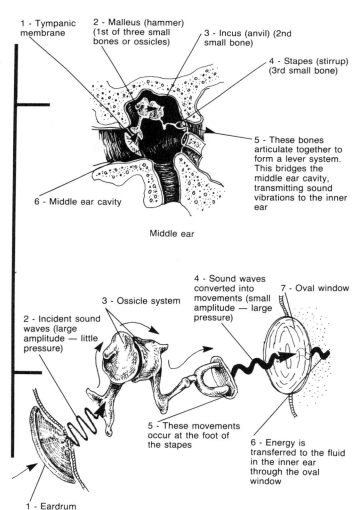

2 - Incident sound waves (large amplitude — little pressure)

3 - Ossicle system

4 - Sound waves converted into movements (small amplitude — large pressure)

7 - Oval window

5 - These movements occur at the foot of the stapes

6 - Energy is transferred to the fluid in the inner ear through the oval window

1 - Eardrum

If the eardrum or ossicles become damaged, some conduction of sound can still occur through the temporal bone, but this **bone conduction** is never as efficient as the so-called **air conduction**.

1 - Normal conduction of sound waves (air conduction)

2 - Damaged eardrum or ossicles

4 - This is not as effective

3 - Conduction of sound through temporal bone

The tightness of the eardrum is controlled by a small muscle called the **tensor tympani**, and another small muscle, the **stapedius**, controls the stiffness in the chain of ossicles. If a very loud noise is detected by the ear, these voluntary muscles contract reflexly in an attempt to protect the middle and inner ear structures from excessive vibration.

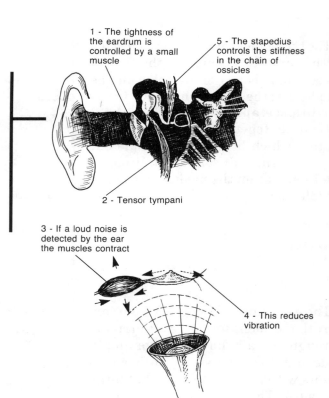

1 - The tightness of the eardrum is controlled by a small muscle

5 - The stapedius controls the stiffness in the chain of ossicles

2 - Tensor tympani

3 - If a loud noise is detected by the ear the muscles contract

4 - This reduces vibration

The middle ear cavity is filled with air, and can communicate with the pharynx through the **Eustachian tube**, which remains closed for most of the time, but may be opened by the acts of yawning, sneezing, swallowing or pinching the nostrils while attempting to exhale.

These manoeuvres allow the pressures in the middle ear and pharynx to be equalized, which may be important in flying and underwater swimming; they allow any secretions in the middle ear to drain into the pharynx and, of course, they also allow infection present in the pharynx to ascend into the middle ear.

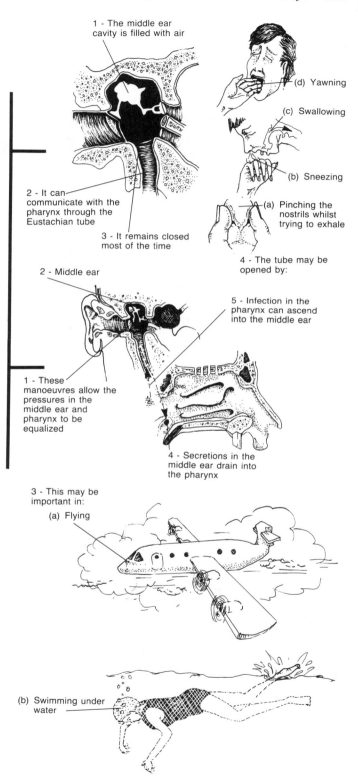

1 - The middle ear cavity is filled with air

2 - It can communicate with the pharynx through the Eustachian tube

3 - It remains closed most of the time

(d) Yawning

(c) Swallowing

(b) Sneezing

(a) Pinching the nostrils whilst trying to exhale

4 - The tube may be opened by:

2 - Middle ear

5 - Infection in the pharynx can ascend into the middle ear

1 - These manoeuvres allow the pressures in the middle ear and pharynx to be equalized

4 - Secretions in the middle ear drain into the pharynx

3 - This may be important in:

(a) Flying

(b) Swimming under water

Function of the cochlea

The sound transducer in the inner ear is known as the **cochlea**, and is a complex spiral organ.

If it were straightened out, it could be seen to consist of a tube filled with **perilymph** and folded back upon itself, with another tube containing **endolymph** in the space between.

The various tubular elements are separated by two membranes, the **basilar membrane** and **Reissner's membrane**. The basilar membrane is a fairly stiff structure which supports the sensitive **hair cells**, but Reissner's membrane is a relatively slack, thin layer which simply acts as a barrier between endolymph and perilymph but offers almost no resistance to the passage of acoustic energy. From the point of view of the sound waves, the scala vestibuli and the scala media form a single functional unit.

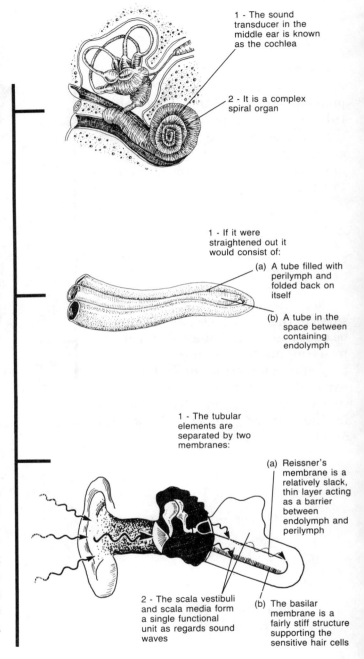

1 - The sound transducer in the middle ear is known as the cochlea

2 - It is a complex spiral organ

1 - If it were straightened out it would consist of:
(a) A tube filled with perilymph and folded back on itself
(b) A tube in the space between containing endolymph

1 - The tubular elements are separated by two membranes:
(a) Reissner's membrane is a relatively slack, thin layer acting as a barrier between endolymph and perilymph
2 - The scala vestibuli and scala media form a single functional unit as regards sound waves
(b) The basilar membrane is a fairly stiff structure supporting the sensitive hair cells

The hair cells of the cochlea lie upon the basilar membrane, and their hairs are embedded in the **tectorial membrane**, which is the cochlea's version of the cupula and constitutes a single gelatinous structure.

Sound waves cause vibration of the eardrum and ossicles, and these vibrations are transmitted via the foot of the stapes to the **oval window**, which in turn transmits them to the perilymph of the scala vestibuli.

The vibrations make the basilar membrane move up and down while the tectorial membrane remains stationary; this deforms the sensory hairs and produces generator or receptor potentials in the hair cells.

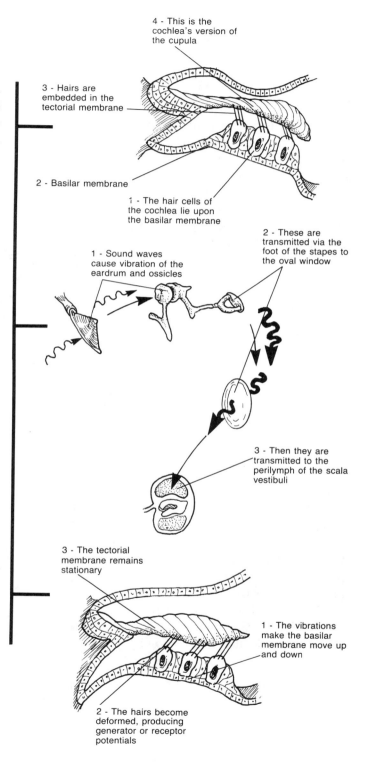

4 - This is the cochlea's version of the cupula

3 - Hairs are embedded in the tectorial membrane

2 - Basilar membrane

1 - The hair cells of the cochlea lie upon the basilar membrane

1 - Sound waves cause vibration of the eardrum and ossicles

2 - These are transmitted via the foot of the stapes to the oval window

3 - Then they are transmitted to the perilymph of the scala vestibuli

3 - The tectorial membrane remains stationary

1 - The vibrations make the basilar membrane move up and down

2 - The hairs become deformed, producing generator or receptor potentials

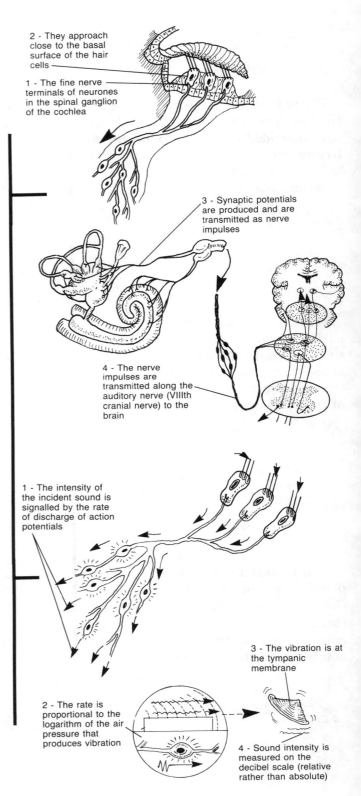

2 - They approach close to the basal surface of the hair cells

1 - The fine nerve terminals of neurones in the spinal ganglion of the cochlea

The fine nerve terminals of neurones in the spiral ganglion of the cochlea approach close to the basal surface of the hair cells, and the receptor potentials produce synaptic potentials in these terminals and the transmission of nerve impulses along the **auditory nerve** (VIIIth cranial nerve) to the brain.

3 - Synaptic potentials are produced and are transmitted as nerve impulses

4 - The nerve impulses are transmitted along the auditory nerve (VIIIth cranial nerve) to the brain

1 - The intensity of the incident sound is signalled by the rate of discharge of action potentials

The **intensity** of the incident sound is signalled to the brain by the rate of discharge of action potentials along each neurone; the rate is proportional to the **logarithm** of the air pressure producing the vibration at the tympanic membrane. Sound intensity is measured on the **decibel** scale: this is a relative rather than an absolute scale, and a decibel is a **ratio** of powers such that:

Difference in power (dB) =
   $10 \log_{10} \times$ ratio of powers

3 - The vibration is at the tympanic membrane

2 - The rate is proportional to the logarithm of the air pressure that produces vibration

4 - Sound intensity is measured on the decibel scale (relative rather than absolute)

The **pitch** of the sound is signalled in a more complex way, and depends upon the stiffness of the basilar membrane. If waves of low frequency or long wavelength arrive at the oval window, they can transmit their energy to almost the whole length of the fluid column in the scala vestibuli, and cause vibration of almost the whole length of the basilar membrane.

If the waves have a higher frequency or shorter wavelength, they transmit most of their energy to the most proximal part of the basilar membrane, but because of the stiffness of this structure the wave becomes attenuated over a relatively short distance.

Consequently, high-pitched sounds excite only the most proximal groups of hair cells, whereas low-pitched sounds excite hair cells along most of the length of the basilar membrane. The brain learns to recognize this essentially **spatial** information as signalling the pitch of the sounds.

Since there are two ears, on opposite sides of the head, the sound waves from a laterally placed source will arrive slightly earlier at one ear than at the other. The brain can interpret these slight differences in timing and detect the direction of the sound source, allowing the appreciation of **stereophonic** sound.

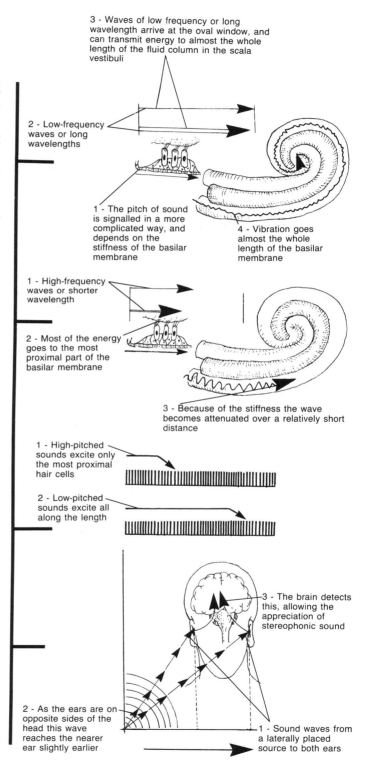

3 - Waves of low frequency or long wavelength arrive at the oval window, and can transmit energy to almost the whole length of the fluid column in the scala vestibuli

2 - Low-frequency waves or long wavelengths

1 - The pitch of sound is signalled in a more complicated way, and depends on the stiffness of the basilar membrane

4 - Vibration goes almost the whole length of the basilar membrane

1 - High-frequency waves or shorter wavelength

2 - Most of the energy goes to the most proximal part of the basilar membrane

3 - Because of the stiffness the wave becomes attenuated over a relatively short distance

1 - High-pitched sounds excite only the most proximal hair cells

2 - Low-pitched sounds excite all along the length

3 - The brain detects this, allowing the appreciation of stereophonic sound

2 - As the ears are on opposite sides of the head this wave reaches the nearer ear slightly earlier

1 - Sound waves from a laterally placed source to both ears

The auditory pathway

The auditory nerve on each side passes into the cranial cavity and enters the brain stem in the pons. In the **dorsal and ventral cochlear nuclei** the fibres synapse, and some second-order neurones cross the midline to run to the opposite olivary nucleus or the nuclei of the lateral lemniscus; others run on the same side to the olivary or lemniscal nuclei or the inferior colliculus. All of the fibres eventually reach the **medial geniculate body**, a major relay station from which neurones project to the **auditory cortex** in the temporal lobe of the cerebrum.

Unlike most other sensory pathways where there are exactly three neurones between primary sensory neurone and cortex, the auditory pathway may have as many as six neurones.

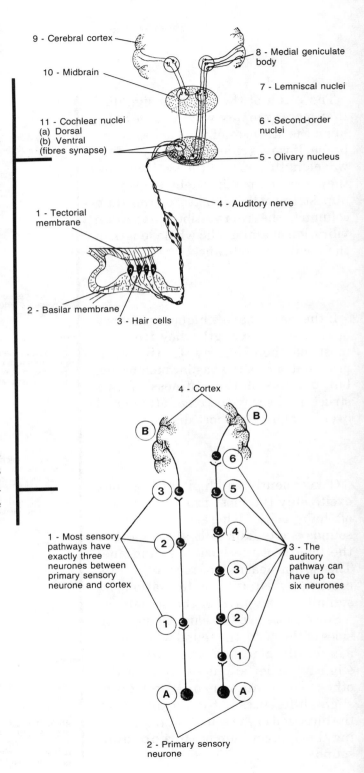

9 - Cerebral cortex

8 - Medial geniculate body

10 - Midbrain

7 - Lemniscal nuclei

11 - Cochlear nuclei
(a) Dorsal
(b) Ventral
(fibres synapse)

6 - Second-order nuclei

5 - Olivary nucleus

4 - Auditory nerve

1 - Tectorial membrane

2 - Basilar membrane

3 - Hair cells

4 - Cortex

1 - Most sensory pathways have exactly three neurones between primary sensory neurone and cortex

3 - The auditory pathway can have up to six neurones

2 - Primary sensory neurone

The auditory cortex has connections with the **speech area**; there is also an **auditory association area** for the processing, recall and recognition of complex sound experiences.

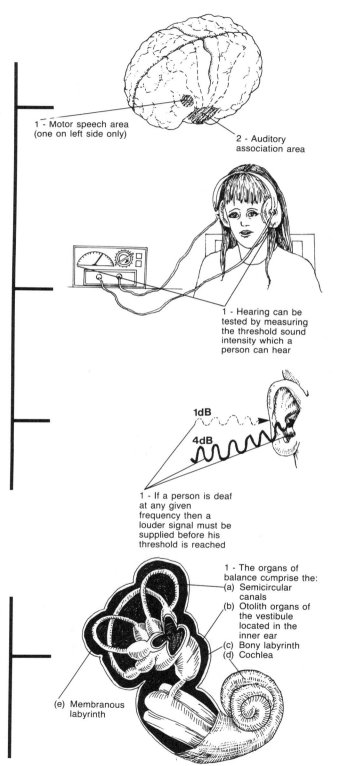

1 - Motor speech area (one on left side only)

2 - Auditory association area

Hearing can be tested by measuring the **threshold** sound intensity which a person can hear. The absolute magnitude of the threshold varies considerably with frequency, even in normal people, so the **audiometers** which are used to test hearing produce pure tones over a wide range of frequencies. They are calibrated on a decibel scale, so that the zero level at any given frequency is equal to the threshold value for the average normal person. If a person is deaf at any given frequency, then a louder signal must be supplied before his threshold is reached; this is recorded as a hearing **loss**, so that if a person needs a signal 3 dB louder than normal before he can hear it, he has a hearing loss of -3 dB.

1 - Hearing can be tested by measuring the threshold sound intensity which a person can hear

1dB

4dB

1 - If a person is deaf at any given frequency then a louder signal must be supplied before his threshold is reached

The vestibular apparatus

The organs of balance comprise the **semicircular canals** and the **otolith organs** of the **vestibule**. They are located in the inner ear, within a series of hollows (containing perilymph) in the temporal bone called the **bony labyrinth**; they consist of a set of tubes (containing endolymph) which together with the cochlea comprise the **membranous labyrinth**.

1 - The organs of balance comprise the:
(a) Semicircular canals
(b) Otolith organs of the vestibule located in the inner ear
(c) Bony labyrinth
(d) Cochlea
(e) Membranous labyrinth

The semicircular canals are a set of three tubes (on each side) placed at right angles to one another in three planes, in order to detect movement of the head in any direction. The otolith organs are located in the **utricle** and **saccule** of the vestibule — tubes connected to the semicircular canals.

The otolith organs each have a **macula** consisting of a number of hair cells whose hair tufts are embedded in a gelatinous mass (this organ's version of the cupula) which contains large quantities of calcium carbonate crystals, the **otoconia**.

Under the influence of gravity the otoconia bend the cupula and hence the hair cells in one or the other direction; since the maculae of the otolith organs are oriented in different directions, there will always be one or more organs whose receptors are being intensely activated, and the brain can integrate the information reaching it to work out the position of the head in space.

Another set of receptors senses rotary movement of the head; if one starts to rotate about the midline, one experiences a sensation of dizziness which soon passes off during rotation at constant velocity, but when one stops rotating the dizziness returns, and one feels as if rotation is now occurring in the opposite direction. These sensations are registered by the semicircular canals.

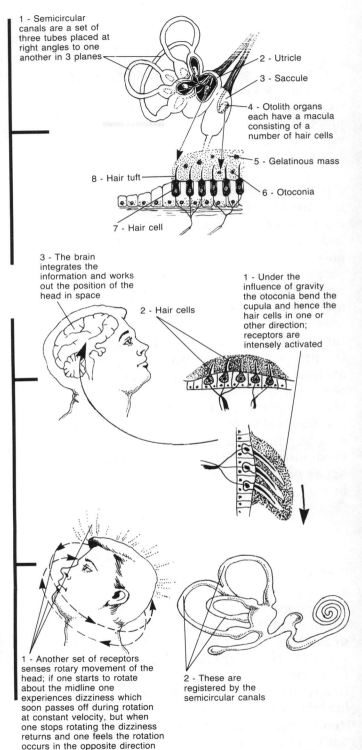

1 - Semicircular canals are a set of three tubes placed at right angles to one another in 3 planes

2 - Utricle

3 - Saccule

4 - Otolith organs each have a macula consisting of a number of hair cells

5 - Gelatinous mass

8 - Hair tuft

6 - Otoconia

7 - Hair cell

3 - The brain integrates the information and works out the position of the head in space

2 - Hair cells

1 - Under the influence of gravity the otoconia bend the cupula and hence the hair cells in one or other direction; receptors are intensely activated

1 - Another set of receptors senses rotary movement of the head; if one starts to rotate about the midline one experiences dizziness which soon passes off during rotation at constant velocity, but when one stops rotating the dizziness returns and one feels the rotation occurs in the opposite direction

2 - These are registered by the semicircular canals

The maculae of the semicircular canals are found in the **ampullae**, which are dilatations at one end of each canal. The hairs of the sensory cells are embedded in the cupula, which extends most of the way across the ampulla, and can be bent by movement of the endolymph fluid within the semicircular canal. If the head begins to rotate in the plane of one pair of canals, the inertia of the fluid within will cause the cupula to bend, exciting one group of hair cells.

If the head rotates with constant velocity, the fluid eventually reaches the same speed as the walls of the canal and the cupula is no longer deformed, so the discharge of the hair cells ceases. If the head is now slowed down and stopped, the fluid in the canals will continue to rotate faster than the walls of the canal, and will deflect the cupula in the opposite direction; eventually the fluid stops moving and the cupula is no longer deflected. Thus the maculae of the semicircular canals are rapidly adapting receptors; they respond to **changes** in angular velocity or to accelerations and decelerations.

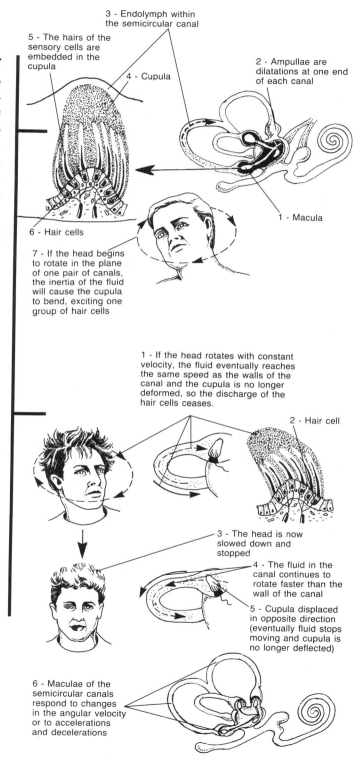

3 - Endolymph within the semicircular canal

5 - The hairs of the sensory cells are embedded in the cupula

4 - Cupula

2 - Ampullae are dilatations at one end of each canal

1 - Macula

6 - Hair cells

7 - If the head begins to rotate in the plane of one pair of canals, the inertia of the fluid will cause the cupula to bend, exciting one group of hair cells

1 - If the head rotates with constant velocity, the fluid eventually reaches the same speed as the walls of the canal and the cupula is no longer deformed, so the discharge of the hair cells ceases.

2 - Hair cell

3 - The head is now slowed down and stopped

4 - The fluid in the canal continues to rotate faster than the wall of the canal

5 - Cupula displaced in opposite direction (eventually fluid stops moving and cupula is no longer deflected)

6 - Maculae of the semicircular canals respond to changes in the angular velocity or to accelerations and decelerations

Since there are three orthogonal sets of canals, almost any movement of the head can be translated into an acceleration in one or more planes, so there will be some excitation of the receptors and some signals reaching the brain to inform it about the movement of the head.

Bending of the hairs of the sensory cells causes a receptor potential, and a synaptic potential causes discharge of action potentials in the neurones of the **vestibular nerve** (part of cranial nerve **VIII**, along with the auditory nerve).

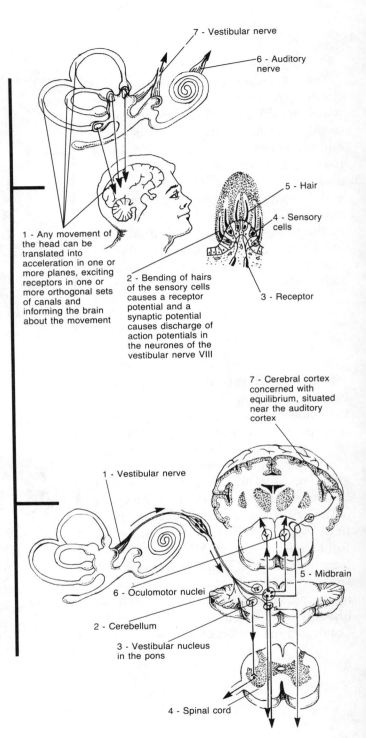

7 - Vestibular nerve

6 - Auditory nerve

5 - Hair

4 - Sensory cells

1 - Any movement of the head can be translated into acceleration in one or more planes, exciting receptors in one or more orthogonal sets of canals and informing the brain about the movement

2 - Bending of hairs of the sensory cells causes a receptor potential and a synaptic potential causes discharge of action potentials in the neurones of the vestibular nerve VIII

3 - Receptor

The vestibular nerve relays in the **vestibular nucleus** in the pons; this nucleus has connections with the cerebellum (which is concerned with balance and coordination of motor activity), with the spinal cord (whence it modifies motor activity of muscles at several levels in the body), with the oculomotor nuclei (producing movements of the eyes in an attempt to fix on objects as the head rotates), and with an area of the cerebral cortex concerned with equilibrium, situated near to the auditory cortex.

7 - Cerebral cortex concerned with equilibrium, situated near the auditory cortex

1 - Vestibular nerve

5 - Midbrain

6 - Oculomotor nuclei

2 - Cerebellum

3 - Vestibular nucleus in the pons

4 - Spinal cord

The semicircular canals can be stimulated artificially in a clinical test by instilling warm or cold water into the ears. This sets up convection currents in the endolymph of the canals, causing deformation of the cupula and producing the sensation of rotation.

Stimulation of the semicircular canals causes characteristic repetitive eye movements known as **nystagmus**, where the eyes move from one side to the other relatively slowly and then flick back rapidly to the original position.

If arrangements are made to record the eye movements (by electromyography or 'nystagmography') then the duration of the nystagmus can be assessed, and any deviation from normal is noted. This **caloric** test is considerably easier to perform than rotating the subject on a swivelling chair; it is also much easier to record nystagmus from a stationary subject.

Nystagmus represents the attempt by the brain to fix the eyes on some point of reference while the head rotates, and during actual rotation is very useful in assisting the individual to appreciate where he is in space. Of course, when warm water is poured into the ears the nystagmus has no true orienting function.

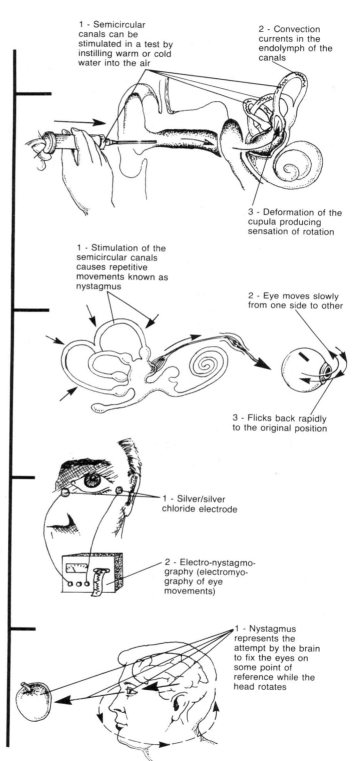

1 - Semicircular canals can be stimulated in a test by instilling warm or cold water into the air

2 - Convection currents in the endolymph of the canals

3 - Deformation of the cupula producing sensation of rotation

1 - Stimulation of the semicircular canals causes repetitive movements known as nystagmus

2 - Eye moves slowly from one side to other

3 - Flicks back rapidly to the original position

1 - Silver/silver chloride electrode

2 - Electro-nystagmography (electromyography of eye movements)

1 - Nystagmus represents the attempt by the brain to fix the eyes on some point of reference while the head rotates

SPECIAL SENSES: THE EYE

The eye is the most complex of all the sensory organs: this applies both to the sensory process itself and to the arrangement of the accessory structures. The ultimate function of all of the accessory structures is to allow the retina, the light-sensitive part of the eye, to receive the best possible image of the external world.

Overview of accessory structures

A pair of skin flaps, the **eyelids**, forms a protective retractable cover for the eyes; the **lacrimal glands** produce a watery secretion, the tears, to clean and lubricate the front surface of the eye in the **conjunctival sac**. The eyeball itself has a fibrous outer sheath, the **sclera**, the front part of which is very transparent, forming the **cornea**, the first and perhaps the most important part of the optical pathway to the retina.

The **extrinsic ocular muscles**, which move the whole eyeball, are attached to the sclera. Each eye has six muscles, the four **recti** and two **obliques**, which execute very complex and well-coordinated movements to point the eyes in the appropriate direction and ensure that both eyes receive the same image on corresponding parts of the retina.

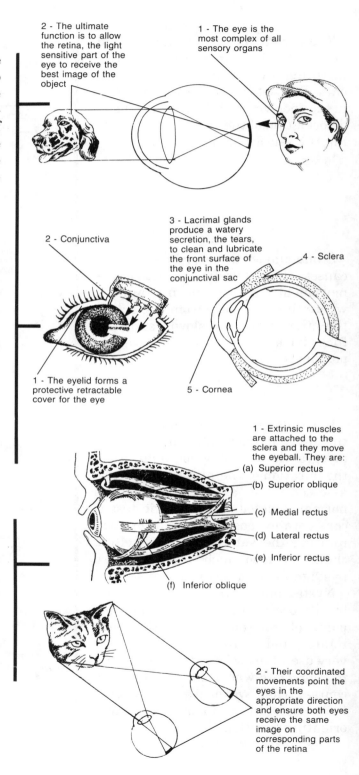

2 - The ultimate function is to allow the retina, the light sensitive part of the eye to receive the best image of the object

1 - The eye is the most complex of all sensory organs

2 - Conjunctiva

3 - Lacrimal glands produce a watery secretion, the tears, to clean and lubricate the front surface of the eye in the conjunctival sac

4 - Sclera

1 - The eyelid forms a protective retractable cover for the eye

5 - Cornea

1 - Extrinsic muscles are attached to the sclera and they move the eyeball. They are:
(a) Superior rectus
(b) Superior oblique
(c) Medial rectus
(d) Lateral rectus
(e) Inferior rectus
(f) Inferior oblique

2 - Their coordinated movements point the eyes in the appropriate direction and ensure both eyes receive the same image on corresponding parts of the retina

So important are the movements of these tiny voluntary muscles that three separate cranial nerves on each side are allocated the task of controlling them, and the motor units of these muscles contain only six to a dozen muscle fibres each (in contrast to some of the leg muscles which may have motor units of several hundred muscle fibres).

Behind the cornea is the **anterior chamber** of the eye, filled with a watery fluid or **aqueous humour**. Next comes the pigmented **iris**, which has a central aperture or **pupil** whose size may be increased or decreased (by muscular action) to allow more or less light to pass along the optical pathway. Behind the pupil is the **lens**, whose thickness is controlled by the **ciliary muscle**, producing changes in the total refractive power of the eye and hence bringing near or distant objects to a focus on the retina.

The main central part of the eyeball is filled with a thick, transparent jelly, the **vitreous humour**. At the back of the eye, covering almost the whole of the inner surface, is the **retina**, which houses the light-sensitive receptors. Just in front of the receptors are the retinal blood vessels, but being very fine and transparent they do not affect the transmission of light to the receptors.

The layer just outside the retina, and separating it from the sclera, is the **choroid**, which is a fibrous layer containing many blood vessels; its anterior part is specialized to form the ciliary body and iris.

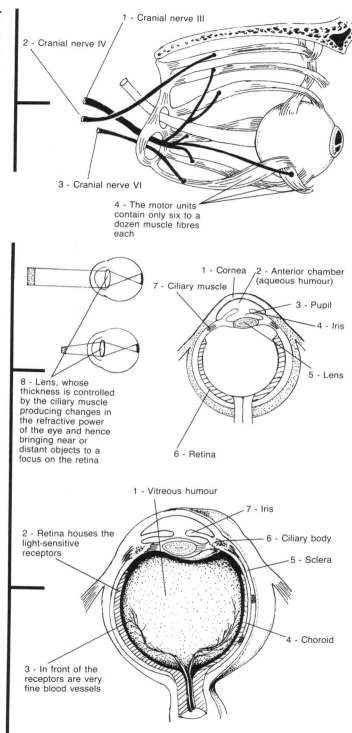

1 - Cranial nerve III

2 - Cranial nerve IV

3 - Cranial nerve VI

4 - The motor units contain only six to a dozen muscle fibres each

1 - Cornea 2 - Anterior chamber (aqueous humour)

7 - Ciliary muscle

3 - Pupil

4 - Iris

5 - Lens

6 - Retina

8 - Lens, whose thickness is controlled by the ciliary muscle producing changes in the refractive power of the eye and hence bringing near or distant objects to a focus on the retina

1 - Vitreous humour

7 - Iris

2 - Retina houses the light-sensitive receptors

6 - Ciliary body

5 - Sclera

4 - Choroid

3 - In front of the receptors are very fine blood vessels

Physiology of the accessory structures

The eyelids are folds of skin whose opening and closing are controlled by voluntary muscles innervated by the facial nerve. The upper eyelid also has some smooth muscle fibres (the **levator palpebrae superioris**) which open the eye and are controlled by sympathetic nerves originating in the superior cervical ganglion.

Some animals, including the cat, have a 'third eyelid', the **nictitating membrane**, whose closure is controlled by autonomic nerves.

The closing of the eyelids (blinking) is an essentially automatic action, though the eyes can of course be closed voluntarily; the main function of blinking is to wipe tears across the corneal surface and to protect the cornea.

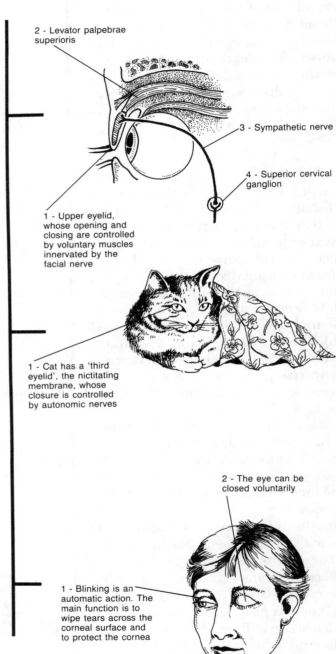

2 - Levator palpebrae superioris

3 - Sympathetic nerve

4 - Superior cervical ganglion

1 - Upper eyelid, whose opening and closing are controlled by voluntary muscles innervated by the facial nerve

1 - Cat has a 'third eyelid', the nictitating membrane, whose closure is controlled by autonomic nerves

2 - The eye can be closed voluntarily

1 - Blinking is an automatic action. The main function is to wipe tears across the corneal surface and to protect the cornea

Each **lacrimal gland** is found at the upper outer aspect of the orbit and its duct discharges into the conjunctival sac. The fluid is a watery secretion containing some electrolytes and the non-specific antibacterial enzyme **lysozyme**. Its secretion is under the control of the parasympathetic nervous system via the oculomotor nerve, and is stimulated by irritation of the eye, particularly the cornea, and of course by excessive emotion. If tears are secreted at a rate greater than their removal by evaporation, the excess fluid passes into the nasal cavity through the **nasolacrimal duct** or occasionally tumbles down the cheeks.

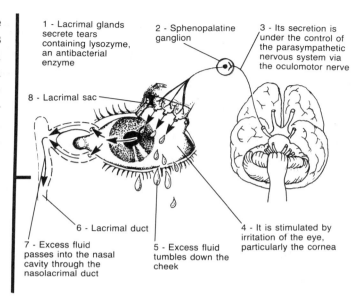

1 - Lacrimal glands secrete tears containing lysozyme, an antibacterial enzyme

2 - Sphenopalatine ganglion

3 - Its secretion is under the control of the parasympathetic nervous system via the oculomotor nerve

8 - Lacrimal sac

6 - Lacrimal duct

7 - Excess fluid passes into the nasal cavity through the nasolacrimal duct

5 - Excess fluid tumbles down the cheek

4 - It is stimulated by irritation of the eye, particularly the cornea

The optical path

The most important component in the refraction of light and the production of a focused image is the interface between the air and the cornea. This is the point with the highest difference in refractive indices: the transition from air to fluid. The curvature of the cornea is thus the primary focusing element, much more important than the lens, whose refractive index differs only slightly from that of its surroundings; the lens merely produces fine adjustments in the total refractive power of the eye.

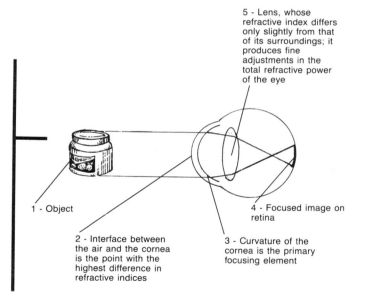

5 - Lens, whose refractive index differs only slightly from that of its surroundings; it produces fine adjustments in the total refractive power of the eye

1 - Object

2 - Interface between the air and the cornea is the point with the highest difference in refractive indices

3 - Curvature of the cornea is the primary focusing element

4 - Focused image on retina

The cornea is an unusually transparent epithelial layer. Its outer surface is anatomically continuous with the lining of the conjunctival sac and is derived from skin; the inner layer is mesodermal in origin, and is a single layer of cells. The region between the two epithelia is filled with a very thin layer of collagen. The cornea contains no blood vessels (as their presence would affect the transparency and purity of the optical properties at such a critical interface) so it must obtain its oxygen by diffusion from the atmosphere and its nutrients like glucose by diffusion from the aqueous humour bathing its inner surface, or from the tears.

The cornea does, however, contain a very high density of sensory nerve fibres, and is extremely sensitive to pain or irritation; the corneal blink reaction is a very powerful protective reflex and is one of the last to disappear during anaesthesia or coma.

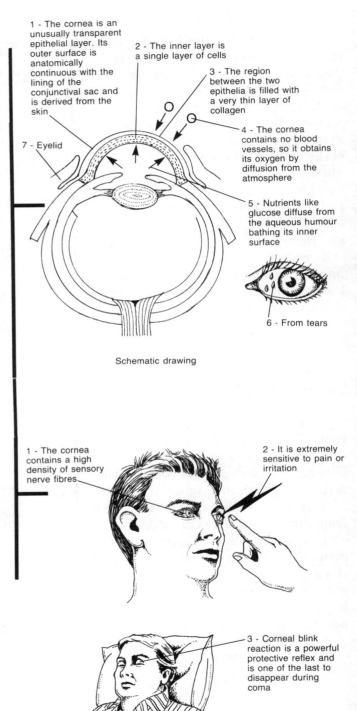

1 - The cornea is an unusually transparent epithelial layer. Its outer surface is anatomically continuous with the lining of the conjunctival sac and is derived from the skin

2 - The inner layer is a single layer of cells

3 - The region between the two epithelia is filled with a very thin layer of collagen

4 - The cornea contains no blood vessels, so it obtains its oxygen by diffusion from the atmosphere

5 - Nutrients like glucose diffuse from the aqueous humour bathing its inner surface

6 - From tears

7 - Eyelid

Schematic drawing

1 - The cornea contains a high density of sensory nerve fibres

2 - It is extremely sensitive to pain or irritation

3 - Corneal blink reaction is a powerful protective reflex and is one of the last to disappear during coma

Behind the cornea is the aqueous humour. This transparent fluid is secreted by the **ciliary glands** in the ciliary body just behind the iris, passes forward through the pupil, and is reabsorbed into the circulation by the **canal of Schlemm**, which runs around the circumference of the cornea. It is essential that the rate of formation of the aqueous humour just balances its reabsorption, in order to maintain a constant intra-ocular pressure; any increase in pressure (**glaucoma**) can occlude the retinal and choroidal blood vessels, which can cause blindness.

The aqueous humour has a composition very similar to an ultrafiltrate of plasma, but the mechanism is probably more complex than simple ultrafiltration, as drugs which block carbonic anhydrase can reduce the rate of aqueous humour formation. The rate of production is normally such that about 1% of the volume is replaced each minute.

The **lens** is composed of an elastic capsule filled with viscous protein fibres which are quite transparent. It is supported by a **suspensory ligament** attached to the ciliary muscle. Contraction of this muscle does not stretch the lens, as might be expected, but causes the support of the suspensory ligament to move forwards on the eyeball, thus reducing the tension in the ligament and allowing the lens to assume and thicker, fatter shape and hence produce a greater refractive effect. This process is called **accommodation**.

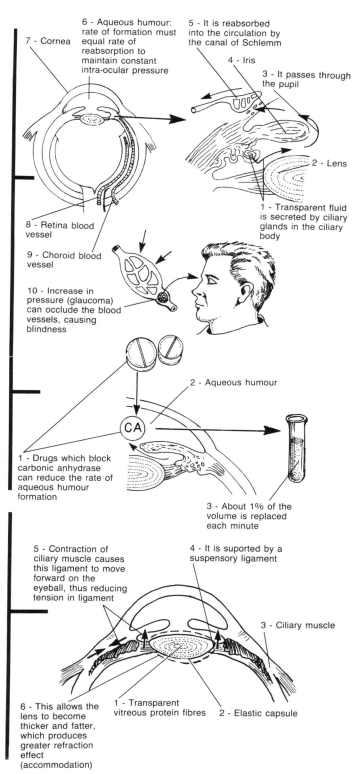

7 - Cornea

6 - Aqueous humour: rate of formation must equal rate of reabsorption to maintain constant intra-ocular pressure

5 - It is reabsorbed into the circulation by the canal of Schlemm

4 - Iris

3 - It passes through the pupil

2 - Lens

1 - Transparent fluid is secreted by ciliary glands in the ciliary body

8 - Retina blood vessel

9 - Choroid blood vessel

10 - Increase in pressure (glaucoma) can occlude the blood vessels, causing blindness

2 - Aqueous humour

CA

1 - Drugs which block carbonic anhydrase can reduce the rate of aqueous humour formation

3 - About 1% of the volume is replaced each minute

5 - Contraction of ciliary muscle causes this ligament to move forward on the eyeball, thus reducing tension in ligament

4 - It is suported by a suspensory ligament

3 - Ciliary muscle

6 - This allows the lens to become thicker and fatter, which produces greater refraction effect (accommodation)

1 - Transparent vitreous protein fibres

2 - Elastic capsule

Contraction of the ciliary muscle causes the lens to throw near objects into focus on the retina; relaxation of the muscle allows distant objects (at infinity) to come into focus by increasing the eye's focal length.

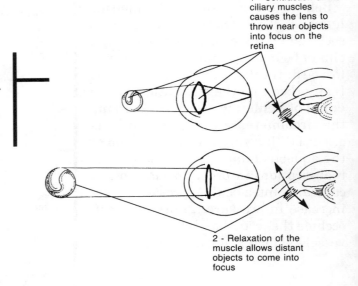

1 - Contraction of the ciliary muscles causes the lens to throw near objects into focus on the retina

2 - Relaxation of the muscle allows distant objects to come into focus

The ciliary muscle is under the control of parasympathetic nerve fibres originating in the Edinger—Westphal nucleus (see below), running in the oculomotor nerve (cranial nerve **III**) and relaying in the ciliary ganglion.

1 - Edinger—Westphal nucleus

4 - Ciliary muscle is under the control of parasympathetic nerve fibres

2 - Cranial nerve III

3 - Ciliary ganglion

The optical system consisting of cornea, aqueous humour, lens and vitreous humour projects an inverted image of the outside world upon the retina. The brain automatically interprets this as representing right-side-up reality.

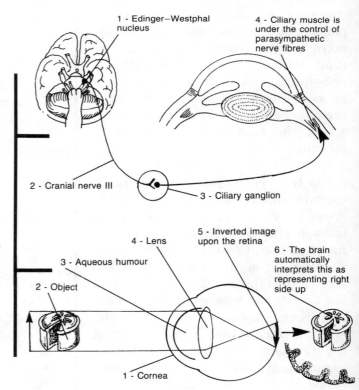

5 - Inverted image upon the retina

6 - The brain automatically interprets this as representing right side up

4 - Lens

3 - Aqueous humour

2 - Object

1 - Cornea

In fact in experiments in which volunteers wore special glasses which threw an erect image on to the retina, the brain became hopelessly confused. Within a few days, however, the subjects had learned to interpret their new view of the world, and when the glasses were taken off they once again went through a period of intense confusion.

1 - In an experiment volunteers wore special glasses which threw an erect image on the retina; the brain became confused, but within a few days the subjects had learned to interpret their new view of the world

2 - When the glasses were taken off they once again went through confusion

The **iris** acts as a curtain, controlling the amount of light passing through the eye to the retina. In very bright light the pupil may become constricted almost to the size of a pin-hole, and in darkness the pupil dilates widely. The effect of such constriction or dilatation is not simply to protect the eye; it means that the eye can respond to images over a very wide range of illumination. For instance, in the dark the widely dilated pupil allows the maximum amount of light to reach the retina, but in bright light the constricted pupil reduces the light reaching the retina, while still allowing for a wide range of intensity between the brightest object seen and the dimmest.

3 - Iris acts as a curtain controlling the amount of light passing through the eye to the retina

1 - Iris

2 - Pupil

4 - In darkness the pupil dilates widely, allowing the maximum amount of light to reach the retina

5 - In bright light the constricted pupil reduces the light reaching the retina, while still allowing for a wide range of intensity between the brightest object seen and the dimmest

The iris has two separate layers of smooth muscle: the anterior **sphincter pupillae** composed of circularly oriented fibres, and a more posterior **dilator pupillae** with radially arranged fibres. The sphincter is controlled by parasympathetic nerves whose presynaptic fibres arise in the **Edinger—Westphal nucleus**, part of the nucleus of the oculomotor nerve (cranial nerve **III**) in the midbrain. This nucleus receives fibres from the optic tract, informing it when a bright light shines on the retina. The parasympathetic fibres run in the oculomotor nerve, relaying in the ciliary ganglion. The dilator pupillae is controlled by sympathetic nerves from the upper thoracic levels relaying in the superior cervical ganglion.

The size of the pupillary aperture not only determines the level of illumination of the retina, but also affects the depth of field of the optical system. Just as in a camera, the presence of a very small pupil means that images from both near and far can be simultaneously brought to a focus on the retina.

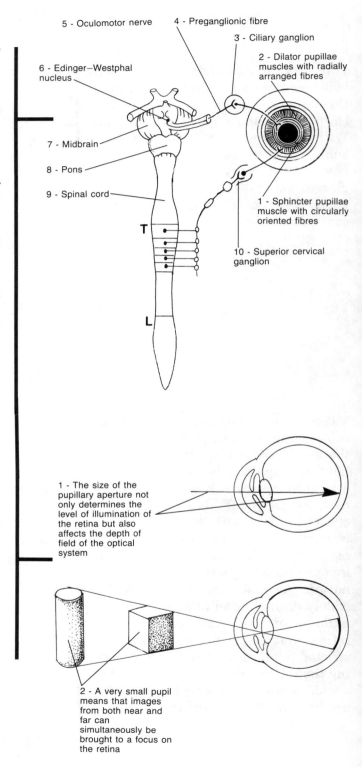

5 - Oculomotor nerve

4 - Preganglionic fibre

3 - Ciliary ganglion

2 - Dilator pupillae muscles with radially arranged fibres

6 - Edinger—Westphal nucleus

7 - Midbrain

8 - Pons

9 - Spinal cord

1 - Sphincter pupillae muscle with circularly oriented fibres

10 - Superior cervical ganglion

1 - The size of the pupillary aperture not only determines the level of illumination of the retina but also affects the depth of field of the optical system

2 - A very small pupil means that images from both near and far can simultaneously be brought to a focus on the retina

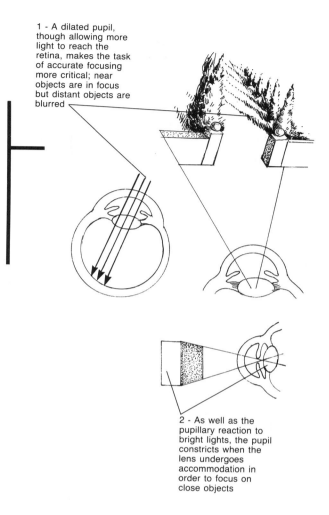

A dilated pupil, though allowing more light to reach the retina, makes the task of accurate focusing more critical, so that if near objects are well in focus then distant objects appear blurred. As well as the pupillary reaction to bright lights, there is another reaction whereby the pupil constricts when the lens undergoes accommodation in order to focus on close objects.

1 - A dilated pupil, though allowing more light to reach the retina, makes the task of accurate focusing more critical; near objects are in focus but distant objects are blurred

The pigment deposited in the iris helps it to exclude light; it also gives the eye its characteristic colour, which makes an important contribution to an individual's appearance. Persons with blue or grey eyes have relatively little pigment and may be rather intolerant of bright sunlight; persons with darkly pigmented irises are better equipped to deal with very strong sunshine.

2 - As well as the pupillary reaction to bright lights, the pupil constricts when the lens undergoes accommodation in order to focus on close objects

The retina

The light-sensitive retina is the most important part of the eye; without it all of the accessory structures would be pointless. The arrangement of cells within the retina appears odd and perhaps illogical; the photoreceptor cells are in the most posterior layer, and light has to pass through various layers of nerve fibres and nerve cells before reaching the receptors. There are two types of receptor: rods and cones (so called because of their shape).

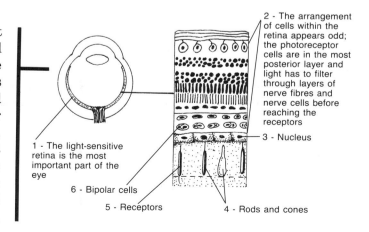

2 - The arrangement of cells within the retina appears odd; the photoreceptor cells are in the most posterior layer and light has to filter through layers of nerve fibres and nerve cells before reaching the receptors

3 - Nucleus

1 - The light-sensitive retina is the most important part of the eye

6 - Bipolar cells

5 - Receptors

4 - Rods and cones

The rods are much more sensitive to light than the cones but can only respond to the presence or absence of light — to light and dark; they are for monochrome vision. The cones, though less sensitive, can respond to different colours of light, and are also capable of resolving much smaller areas and so allow a much finer image to be perceived. The cones are found in high density at the centre of the retina, in an area known as the **fovea** or yellow spot; the rods are found in highest numbers around the periphery of the eye.

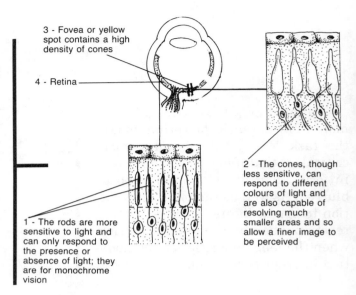

3 - Fovea or yellow spot contains a high density of cones

4 - Retina

2 - The cones, though less sensitive, can respond to different colours of light and are also capable of resolving much smaller areas and so allow a finer image to be perceived

1 - The rods are more sensitive to light and can only respond to the presence or absence of light; they are for monochrome vision

In front of the layer of rods and cones come the **bipolar cells**, which are the equivalent of interneurones in the central nervous system. In front of these are the **ganglion cells**, whose axons run across the surface of the retina and are gathered together to form the **optic nerve**, which penetrates the retina at the back and runs through the orbit towards the brain. The point at which the optic nerve penetrates the retina has no photoreceptors present and constitutes a **blind spot**, which is situated slightly medial to the fovea.

As well as the bipolar cells, the intermediate part of the retina contains a number of other types of interneurones whose function is to integrate the information coming from adjacent parts of the retina. These are known as horizontal cells, amacrine cells and the fibres of Muller.

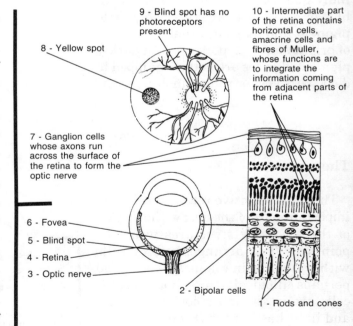

9 - Blind spot has no photoreceptors present

10 - Intermediate part of the retina contains horizontal cells, amacrine cells and fibres of Muller, whose functions are to integrate the information coming from adjacent parts of the retina

8 - Yellow spot

7 - Ganglion cells whose axons run across the surface of the retina to form the optic nerve

6 - Fovea
5 - Blind spot
4 - Retina
3 - Optic nerve

2 - Bipolar cells

1 - Rods and cones

Behind the retina is a pigment layer containing large quantities of **melanin**, which absorbs any light penetrating through the sensitive layer, preventing it from being scattered and exciting inappropriate cells in the retina. The pigment layer also stores vitamin **A**, which is important in the generation of the photopigments.

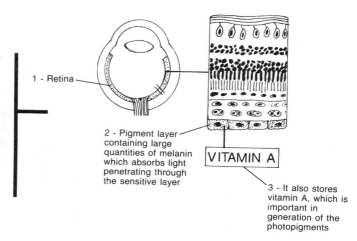

1 - Retina

2 - Pigment layer containing large quantities of melanin which absorbs light penetrating through the sensitive layer

VITAMIN A

3 - It also stores vitamin A, which is important in generation of the photopigments

Structure of rods and cones

The part of the rod or cone nearest the pigment layer has its membrane thrown into a large number of folds or shelves and is known as the outer segment. The shelves are lined with the visual pigments which constitute the actual light-sensing element. The inner segment is a tubular region which is packed with mitochondria; this is the region where the photopigments are synthesized. Next there is a region containing the nucleus, and finally a synaptic body which makes contact with the bipolar cells, the next component in the chain of the visual pathway to the brain.

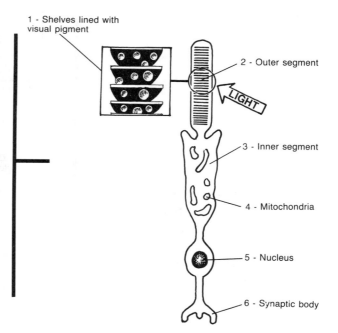

1 - Shelves lined with visual pigment

2 - Outer segment

LIGHT

3 - Inner segment

4 - Mitochondria

5 - Nucleus

6 - Synaptic body

The visual process

The photopigment found in the rods is called **rhodopsin** or **visual purple**. It is manufactured in the retina from dietary vitamin A, and is capable of being transformed by the action of light. Vitamin A occurs in a *cis* and a *trans* form, and can be converted enzymatically into cis- or trans-retinene; these two forms may be transformed one into the other by the enzyme **retinene isomerase**. Retinene can be converted into rhodopsin, the actual purple-coloured pigment.

Light falling upon rhodopsin bleaches it, converting it into **prelumirhodopsin** and then via **lumirhodopsin** into **metarhodopsin**; these can either be converted into retinene, or via an intermediate substance **scotopsin** back into rhodopsin.

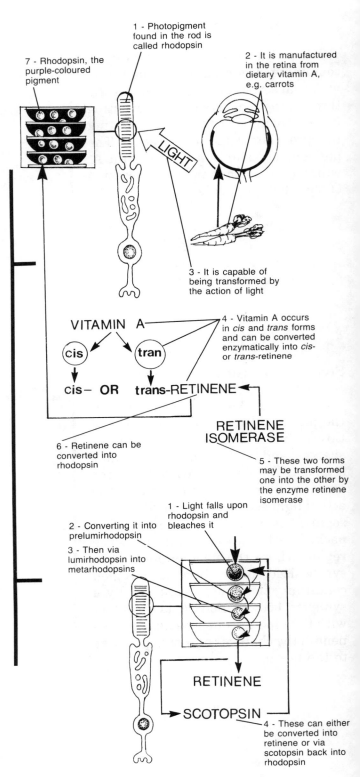

7 - Rhodopsin, the purple-coloured pigment

1 - Photopigment found in the rod is called rhodopsin

2 - It is manufactured in the retina from dietary vitamin A, e.g. carrots

3 - It is capable of being transformed by the action of light

VITAMIN A

cis   tran

cis— OR trans-RETINENE

RETINENE ISOMERASE

4 - Vitamin A occurs in *cis* and *trans* forms and can be converted enzymatically into *cis*- or *trans*-retinene

6 - Retinene can be converted into rhodopsin

5 - These two forms may be transformed one into the other by the enzyme retinene isomerase

1 - Light falls upon rhodopsin and bleaches it

2 - Converting it into prelumirhodopsin

3 - Then via lumirhodopsin into metarhodopsins

RETINENE

SCOTOPSIN

4 - These can either be converted into retinene or via scotopsin back into rhodopsin

If a person goes into bright light, all of his rhodopsin rapidly becomes bleached, and if he then goes into the dark he cannot see very well at all. After some time he undergoes **dark adaptation** as his retina regenerates rhodopsin, and gradually the sensitivity of his eyes to dim light increases. It may take from 10 to 60 minutes for full light sensitivity to be regained on going into the dark.

Rhodopsin is the pigment found in the rods; it is very sensitive to small amounts of light, and a single dark-adapted rod can respond to a single quantum of light energy, causing a flash to be perceived by the brain. Rods are only sensitive to the presence or absence of light, and are of no use in colour vision.

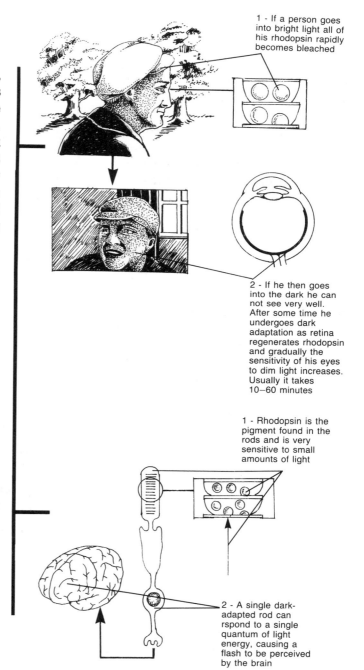

1 - If a person goes into bright light all of his rhodopsin rapidly becomes bleached

2 - If he then goes into the dark he can not see very well. After some time he undergoes dark adaptation as retina regenerates rhodopsin and gradually the sensitivity of his eyes to dim light increases. Usually it takes 10–60 minutes

1 - Rhodopsin is the pigment found in the rods and is very sensitive to small amounts of light

2 - A single dark-adapted rod can rspond to a single quantum of light energy, causing a flash to be perceived by the brain

The cones are the receptors responsible for colour vision. They have three different types of pigments, which are maximally sensitive in different parts of the visual spectrum, corresponding to blue, green and red; each cone contains only one type of pigment, so that light of different colours will produce excitation of different populations of cones.

Any given colour or hue of light will produce a characteristic pattern of excitation of cones, so that the brain will be able to recognize a particular pattern of discharge as being due to a unique colour. The absolute sensitivity of the cones to light is much less than that of the rods, so that colour vision can only take place in fairly well-lit surroundings.

Congenital absence of one or more pigments for colour vision causes **colour blindness**, which is inherited as a recessive sex-linked character.

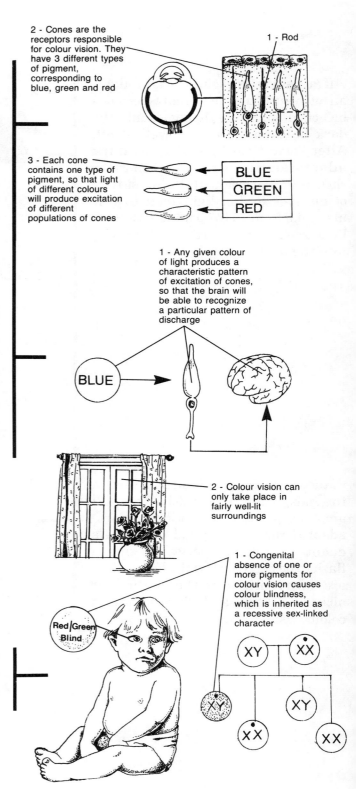

2 - Cones are the receptors responsible for colour vision. They have 3 different types of pigment, corresponding to blue, green and red

1 - Rod

3 - Each cone contains one type of pigment, so that light of different colours will produce excitation of different populations of cones

BLUE
GREEN
RED

1 - Any given colour of light produces a characteristic pattern of excitation of cones, so that the brain will be able to recognize a particular pattern of discharge

BLUE

2 - Colour vision can only take place in fairly well-lit surroundings

1 - Congenital absence of one or more pigments for colour vision causes colour blindness, which is inherited as a recessive sex-linked character

Red/Green Blind

When a dark-adapted rod or cone is stimulated by a brief flash of light, the chemical change in the photopigment produces a change in the membrane potential which can be recorded with a microelectrode. This change is a **hyperpolarization** rather than a depolarization (which is what might have been expected). The receptor potential causes synaptic transmission to a bipolar cell, which also becomes hyperpolarized; the bipolar cells in turn make synaptic connections to ganglion cells, whose long axon processes form the fibres of the optic nerve. It is not completely clear how the hyperpolarizations of the receptor cells eventually cause depolarization and action potentials in the ganglion cells, but it appears that some of the cells in the retina (bipolar and horizontal cells) exercise a tonic inhibitory discharge; hyperpolarization of these cells might turn off inhibition and allow the bipolar cells to become depolarized.

The interactions between cells in the retina are quite complex; if a particular photoreceptor is excited with a spot of light, the area of retina immediately around it is profoundly depressed (lateral inhibition). This has the useful effect of making the outline of the spot sharper by exaggerating the contrast between light and dark.

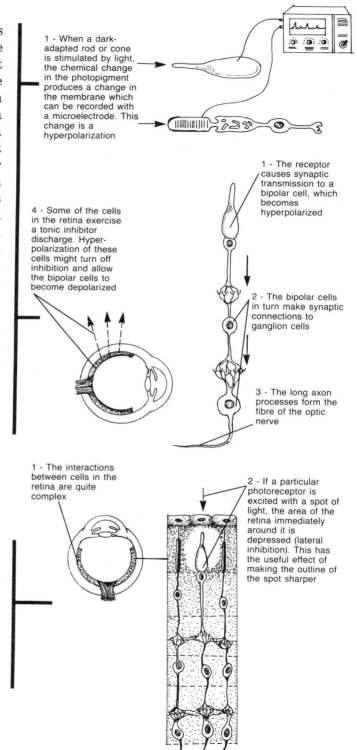

1 - When a dark-adapted rod or cone is stimulated by light, the chemical change in the photopigment produces a change in the membrane which can be recorded with a microelectrode. This change is a hyperpolarization

1 - The receptor causes synaptic transmission to a bipolar cell, which becomes hyperpolarized

4 - Some of the cells in the retina exercise a tonic inhibitor discharge. Hyperpolarization of these cells might turn off inhibition and allow the bipolar cells to become depolarized

2 - The bipolar cells in turn make synaptic connections to ganglion cells

3 - The long axon processes form the fibre of the optic nerve

1 - The interactions between cells in the retina are quite complex

2 - If a particular photoreceptor is excited with a spot of light, the area of the retina immediately around it is depressed (lateral inhibition). This has the useful effect of making the outline of the spot sharper

The visual pathway

The optic nerve runs backward through the orbit and enters the cranial cavity, lying underneath the cerebral hemispheres. The two optic nerves come together in the **optic chiasma** at the base of the brain between the hypothalamus and the pituitary gland, and some of the nerve fibres from the left eye cross over to run in the right optic nerve and vice versa.

The consequence is that the left half of the visual field of each eye (as seen by the right half of the retina, since the image on the retina is inverted) is represented in the right optic nerve, and eventually reaches the right visual cortex; the right half of the visual field (seen by the left half of the retina) is represented in the left optic nerve and arrives at the left visual cortex. The fibres in the optic nerve from the foveal region are represented in both optic nerves (some crossing and some remaining uncrossed) so that both sides of the visual cortex receive information from the foveae.

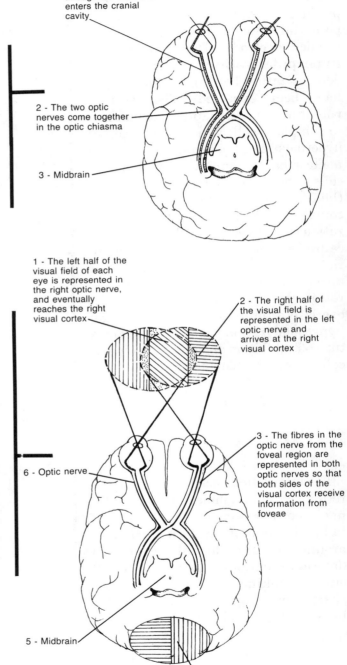

1 - The optic nerve runs backward through the orbit and enters the cranial cavity

2 - The two optic nerves come together in the optic chiasma

3 - Midbrain

1 - The left half of the visual field of each eye is represented in the right optic nerve, and eventually reaches the right visual cortex

2 - The right half of the visual field is represented in the left optic nerve and arrives at the right visual cortex

3 - The fibres in the optic nerve from the foveal region are represented in both optic nerves so that both sides of the visual cortex receive information from foveae

6 - Optic nerve

5 - Midbrain

4 - Visual cortex

From the optic chiasma the optic nerves run backwards to the **lateral geniculate bodies**, which fulfil the same function for vision as does the thalamus for somatic sensation; they are major relay centres, but also perform some information processing, and the **optic tracts** radiate back from the lateral geniculate bodies to the **visual cortex** in the **occipital lobe** of the cerebral hemispheres. Each point on the retina can be mapped on to an area of the visual cortex; a disproportionately large area is devoted to the fovea, as this is the region of the retina with the greatest acuity, where most of the fine detail of the incident image is resolved.

There is some complex signal processing in the visual cortex. Individual neurones in the cortex do not respond to single flashes of light; rather they respond to patterns and in particular to movement.

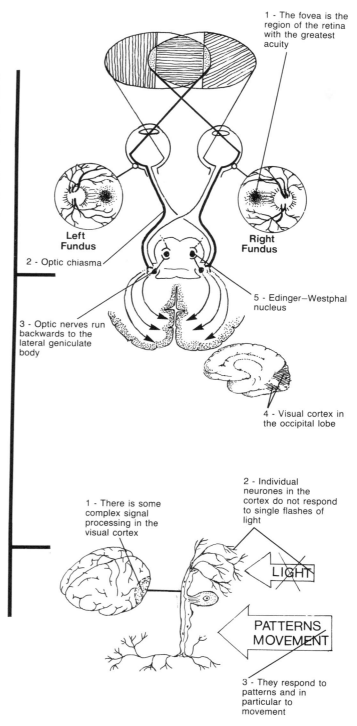

1 - The fovea is the region of the retina with the greatest acuity

Left Fundus

Right Fundus

2 - Optic chiasma

3 - Optic nerves run backwards to the lateral geniculate body

5 - Edinger–Westphal nucleus

4 - Visual cortex in the occipital lobe

1 - There is some complex signal processing in the visual cortex

2 - Individual neurones in the cortex do not respond to single flashes of light

LIGHT

PATTERNS MOVEMENT

3 - They respond to patterns and in particular to movement

If the impulse discharge of a particular neurone is monitored, it is found that it responds maximally when a rectangular bar of light is moved across the corresponding area of the retina in a particular orientation and direction; another neurone will have a different characteristic orientation and direction of movement to which it is sensitive.

There are columns of cells arranged between the surface and depth of the visual cortex, all of which respond to the same orientation of movement.

The **visual association area**, just anterior to the main visual cortex, is concerned with still more complex interpretation, recognizing shapes, visual textures and hues, and assisting in the identification of objects by comparison with images from one's previous visual experience.

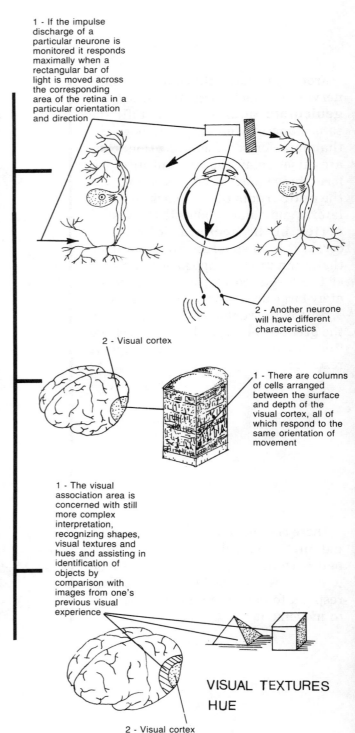

1 - If the impulse discharge of a particular neurone is monitored it responds maximally when a rectangular bar of light is moved across the corresponding area of the retina in a particular orientation and direction

2 - Another neurone will have different characteristics

2 - Visual cortex

1 - There are columns of cells arranged between the surface and depth of the visual cortex, all of which respond to the same orientation of movement

1 - The visual association area is concerned with still more complex interpretation, recognizing shapes, visual textures and hues and assisting in identification of objects by comparison with images from one's previous visual experience

VISUAL TEXTURES
HUE

2 - Visual cortex

There are two eyes, and the images falling upon the two retinae are slightly different. The brain can control the extrinsic ocular muscles to move the eyes in such a way that the retinal images are almost identical, but any small differences in the two images are interpreted as clues to the distance of an object away from the observer. This phenomenon of **binocular vision** is very useful for creating an impression of depth or of solidity in nearby objects, but only works over distances of a few metres.

Depth perception over larger distances depends on the brain's interpretation of other cues such as perspective or the rate of change in size. For instance, binocular vision is of almost no use in warning of an approaching car; rather it is the rapid increase in the **size** of the retinal image which informs the brain that the object is coming nearer.

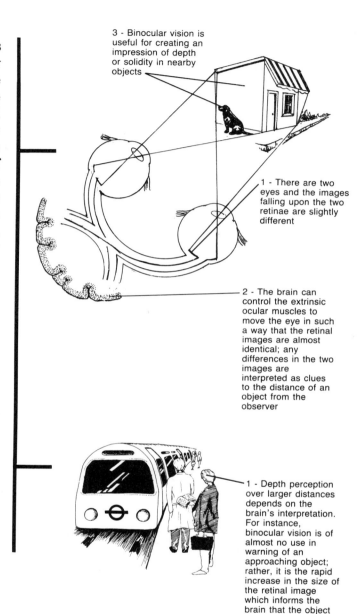

3 - Binocular vision is useful for creating an impression of depth or solidity in nearby objects

1 - There are two eyes and the images falling upon the two retinae are slightly different

2 - The brain can control the extrinsic ocular muscles to move the eye in such a way that the retinal images are almost identical; any differences in the two images are interpreted as clues to the distance of an object from the observer

1 - Depth perception over larger distances depends on the brain's interpretation. For instance, binocular vision is of almost no use in warning of an approaching object; rather, it is the rapid increase in the size of the retinal image which informs the brain that the object is coming

The Autonomic Nervous System

The autonomic nervous system is that part of the motor system which has the cell bodies of its most distal neurones outside the central nervous system. It is chiefly concerned with the rather undramatic visceral or vegetative functions of the body such as the regulation of the circulation or digestion, though its effects can sometimes be very dramatic, when the organism is highly aroused and is about to attack or defend itself.

The system carries out the automatic control of most involuntary functions (although respiration, a largely automatic function, is not controlled by the autonomic nervous system; conversely, it is possible to exercise some voluntary control over several autonomic functions such as micturition and defecation).

Several of the body's autonomic functions are regulated by the brain: the autonomic functions of the eye are controlled by nuclei in the brain stem; parts of the **hypothalamus** affect the circulation, or take part in thermoregulation; many circulatory and respiratory functions are controlled in the medulla oblongata. However, many other autonomic functions are controlled by spinal reflexes, and many are even regulated locally outside the central nervous system, by means of the often extensive networks or **plexuses** of nerves in the walls of the viscera.

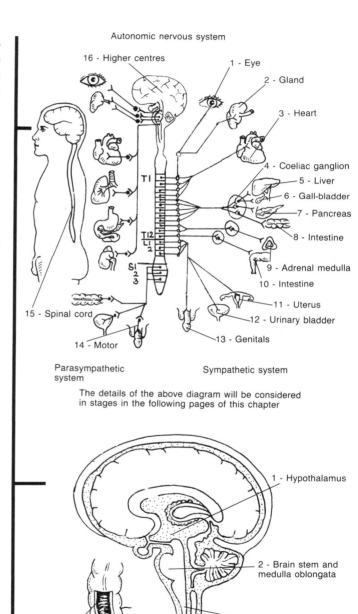

Autonomic nervous system

16 - Higher centres

1 - Eye
2 - Gland
3 - Heart
4 - Coeliac ganglion
5 - Liver
6 - Gall-bladder
7 - Pancreas
8 - Intestine
9 - Adrenal medulla
10 - Intestine
11 - Uterus
12 - Urinary bladder
13 - Genitals

T1
T12
L1
2
S1
2
3

15 - Spinal cord

14 - Motor

Parasympathetic system

Sympathetic system

The details of the above diagram will be considered in stages in the following pages of this chapter

1 - Hypothalamus

2 - Brain stem and medulla oblongata

3 - Spinal cord

4 - Local reflexes in nerve plexuses in the walls of the gut

THE HYPOTHALAMUS AND LIMBIC SYSTEM

Although the hypothalamus is a major centre of autonomic integration, it also has effects on a number of other systems in the body, including the endocrine glands and some skeletal muscular systems as well as certain aspects of behaviour.

It has centres for the regulation of temperature, and these not only affect vasoconstriction and sweating (autonomic functions) but also shivering (skeletal muscles). There are centres for regulation of the gut (autonomic) and also of the appetite (behavioural); for regulation of the kidney (endocrine) and also for thirst (behavioural). There are centres for regulating the endocrine system and reproduction.

There is a centre which produces an arousal state with dilated pupils and vasodilated muscles, vasoconstricted skin and a raised blood pressure (autonomic effects), together with facial grimacing and the adoption of a threatening posture (motor functions such as arching the back and waving the tail in cats, or growling in dogs).

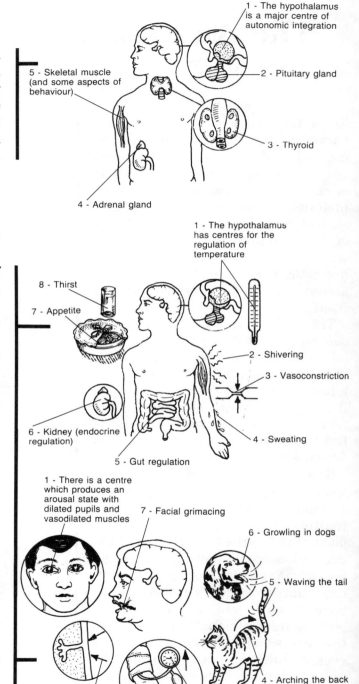

1 - The hypothalamus is a major centre of autonomic integration
2 - Pituitary gland
3 - Thyroid
4 - Adrenal gland
5 - Skeletal muscle (and some aspects of behaviour)

1 - The hypothalamus has centres for the regulation of temperature
2 - Shivering
3 - Vasoconstriction
4 - Sweating
5 - Gut regulation
6 - Kidney (endocrine regulation)
7 - Appetite
8 - Thirst

1 - There is a centre which produces an arousal state with dilated pupils and vasodilated muscles
2 - Vasoconstricted skin
3 - Raised blood pressure
4 - Arching the back
5 - Waving the tail
6 - Growling in dogs
7 - Facial grimacing

The hypothalamus is anatomically and functionally related to a number of rather primitive parts of the cerebral cortex including the amygdala, the hippocampus, the uncus and pyriform area, the cingulate gyrus and the insula. These centres together constitute the **limbic system**, whose functions are still poorly understood, but contribute to the control of appetite, aggression, sexual behaviour, as well as some of the more vegetative autonomic functions. They seem to constitute a route whereby emotional influences can produce autonomic or endocrine changes, and may be part of the pathway in producing psychosomatic illness.

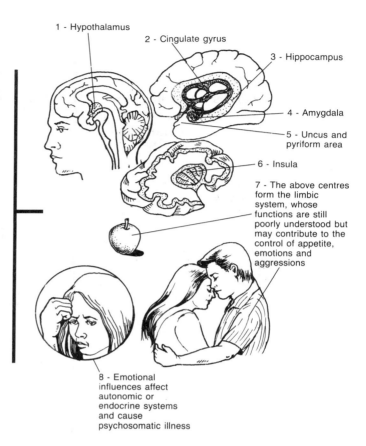

1 - Hypothalamus

2 - Cingulate gyrus

3 - Hippocampus

4 - Amygdala

5 - Uncus and pyriform area

6 - Insula

7 - The above centres form the limbic system, whose functions are still poorly understood but may contribute to the control of appetite, emotions and aggressions

8 - Emotional influences affect autonomic or endocrine systems and cause psychosomatic illness

DIVISIONS OF THE AUTONOMIC SYSTEM

The autonomic system is divided into a **sympathetic** part, whose nerves leave the spinal cord in the thoracic and lumbar segments (thoracolumbar outflow), and a **parasympathetic** part, whose nerve axons leave the brain stem or the sacral part of the spinal cord (craniosacral outflow). Both of these divisions have **ganglia** or synaptic relay stations outside the central nervous system; the motor nerves leaving the brain or spinal cord are called **preganglionic** nerves, and those leaving the ganglia after the synapse are known as **postganglionic** nerves.

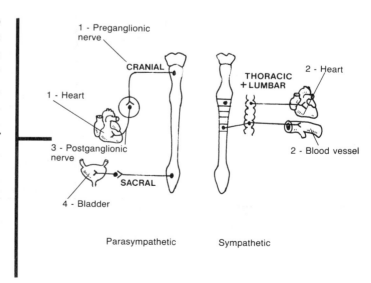

1 - Preganglionic nerve

CRANIAL

1 - Heart

3 - Postganglionic nerve

SACRAL

4 - Bladder

THORACIC + LUMBAR

2 - Heart

2 - Blood vessel

Parasympathetic   Sympathetic

Many of the organs innervated by the autonomic system are supplied by nerves of both divisions, and often the two types of nerves have opposite or contrasting effects. For instance, in some parts of the gut the parasympathetic nerves stimulate motility while the sympathetic nerves inhibit it. The pupil of the eye is constricted by parasympathetic nerves but is dilated by the sympathetic. The parasympathetic nerves cause erection of the penis while the sympathetic nerves cause ejaculation and flaccidity. The parasympathetic nerves slow the heart, while the sympathetic nerves accelerate it and make it beat more forcefully.

In some cases the two divisions of the autonomic system achieve their antagonistic effects by separately innervating different though related structures; for instance, in the eye the parasympathetic nerves innervate the sphincter pupillae while the sympathetic nerves innervate the separate dilator muscle.

In other cases they achieve their separate effects by using different and antagonistic neurotransmitters; in the heart the vagus (parasympathetic) nerve secretes acetylcholine, which slows the heart, while the sympathetic nerves secrete noradrenaline, which increases the heart rate.

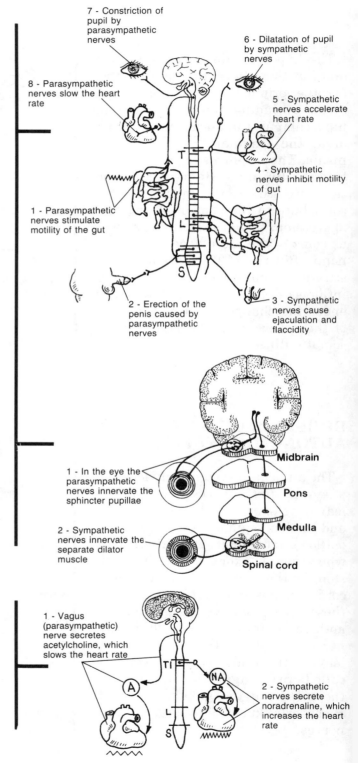

7 - Constriction of pupil by parasympathetic nerves

6 - Dilatation of pupil by sympathetic nerves

8 - Parasympathetic nerves slow the heart rate

5 - Sympathetic nerves accelerate heart rate

4 - Sympathetic nerves inhibit motility of gut

1 - Parasympathetic nerves stimulate motility of the gut

2 - Erection of the penis caused by parasympathetic nerves

3 - Sympathetic nerves cause ejaculation and flaccidity

1 - In the eye the parasympathetic nerves innervate the sphincter pupillae

2 - Sympathetic nerves innervate the separate dilator muscle

Midbrain

Pons

Medulla

Spinal cord

1 - Vagus (parasympathetic) nerve secretes acetylcholine, which slows the heart rate

2 - Sympathetic nerves secrete noradrenaline, which increases the heart rate

The position of the ganglia and their synapses is different in the two divisions. In the parasympathetic system there is a long preganglionic nerve and the ganglia are very close to the target organ — perhaps in the walls of the organ itself — with a very short postganglionic nerve. In the sympathetic system there is a relatively short preganglionic nerve, the ganglia are quite close to the spinal cord, and the postganglionic nerve going out to the target organ is relatively long.

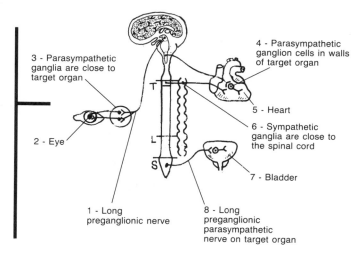

3 - Parasympathetic ganglia are close to target organ

4 - Parasympathetic ganglion cells in walls of target organ

5 - Heart

6 - Sympathetic ganglia are close to the spinal cord

2 - Eye

7 - Bladder

1 - Long preganglionic nerve

8 - Long preganglionic parasympathetic nerve on target organ

Parasympathetic division

The parasympathetic nerves leave the central nervous system in several of the cranial nerves: the oculomotor (III — controlling the iris and ciliary body), the facial (VII — controlling lacrimation and salivary secretion), the glossopharyngeal (IX — controlling salivation) and the vagus (X — controlling bronchi, the heart and the upper half of the alimentary canal). The lower part of the parasympathetic outflow is from the sacral part of the spinal cord — the **nervi erigentes**, so called because one of their prime actions is to cause erection of the penis, though they also control the whole of the lower gut and the urinary tract.

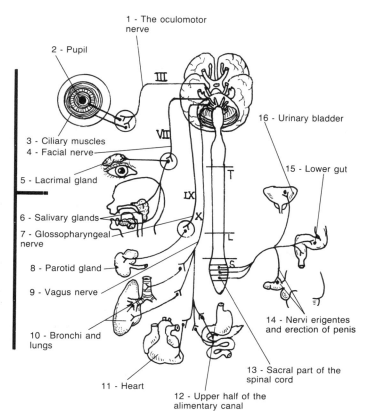

1 - The oculomotor nerve

2 - Pupil

3 - Ciliary muscles

4 - Facial nerve

5 - Lacrimal gland

6 - Salivary glands

7 - Glossopharyngeal nerve

8 - Parotid gland

9 - Vagus nerve

10 - Bronchi and lungs

11 - Heart

16 - Urinary bladder

15 - Lower gut

14 - Nervi erigentes and erection of penis

13 - Sacral part of the spinal cord

12 - Upper half of the alimentary canal

Parasympathetic transmitters

In each parasympathetic nerve the cell body lies in the grey matter of the brain stem or cord — in specific nuclei of the brain stem or in the intermediolateral cell column of the spinal grey matter. The long preganglionic nerves run in major trunks to the target organ, where they relay with the short non-myelinated postganglionic nerves. The synapse at these distributed ganglia is cholinergic, and the postganglionic fibres almost all secrete acetylcholine at their junction with the target smooth muscle or gland.

Although both of these synapses use acetylcholine as their transmitter, the nature of the synapses is different: the ganglionic synapse resembles the skeletal neuromuscular junction in being blocked by curare and being mimicked by nicotine (hence 'nicotinic' synapse), while the nerve—muscle or nerve—gland synapse is blocked by atropine and mimicked by muscarine (hence 'muscarinic' synapse). There must be differences in the shape of the receptor molecule which binds to the acetylcholine molecule; possibly the two types of receptor bind to different parts of the acetylcholine molecule.

Sympathetic division

The sympathetic nerve axons arise from cell bodies in the intermediolateral column of the spinal grey matter in the thoracic and lumbar parts of the spinal cord. The axons leave the cord in the ventral roots, join the mixed spinal nerves and then run to the **paravertebral** ganglia of the sympathetic chain in the white **rami communicantes** or communicating branches — white because the axons are myelinated.

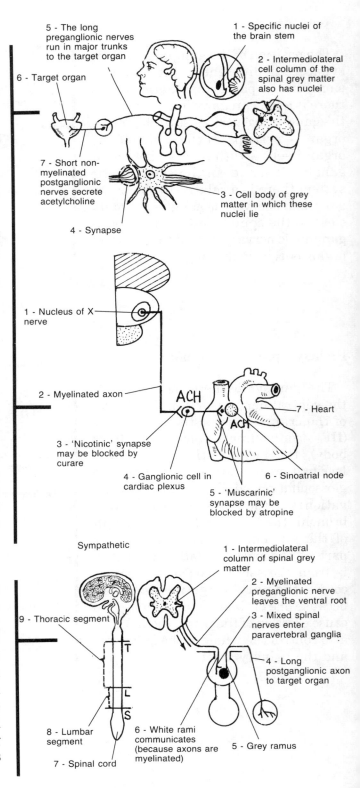

5 - The long preganglionic nerves run in major trunks to the target organ

6 - Target organ

1 - Specific nuclei of the brain stem

2 - Intermediolateral cell column of the spinal grey matter also has nuclei

7 - Short non-myelinated postganglionic nerves secrete acetylcholine

3 - Cell body of grey matter in which these nuclei lie

4 - Synapse

1 - Nucleus of X nerve

2 - Myelinated axon

ACH

3 - 'Nicotinic' synapse may be blocked by curare

4 - Ganglionic cell in cardiac plexus

5 - 'Muscarinic' synapse may be blocked by atropine

6 - Sinoatrial node

7 - Heart

Sympathetic

9 - Thoracic segment

8 - Lumbar segment

7 - Spinal cord

6 - White rami communicates (because axons are myelinated)

5 - Grey ramus

1 - Intermediolateral column of spinal grey matter

2 - Myelinated preganglionic nerve leaves the ventral root

3 - Mixed spinal nerves enter paravertebral ganglia

4 - Long postganglionic axon to target organ

Once they reach the sympathetic chain, the axons may synapse in the ganglion of the same segment, may run up or down the chain to synapse in the ganglion of a different segment, or may leave the chain in one of the **visceral** or **splanchnic** nerves without forming a synapse, to relay more remotely in one of the splanchnic ganglia such as the coeliac, the superior or inferior mesenteric ganglion. If the nerve relays in a sympathetic ganglion, the postganglionic fibres return to the mixed spinal nerves in the grey rami communicantes — grey because these fibres are non-myelinated.

There are about thirty times as many postganglionic fibres leaving the ganglia as preganglionic fibres arriving; in other words, each preganglionic fibre can have a very wide sphere of influence. The postganglionic nerves run to their target organs in the mixed spinal nerves, or very often in extensive nerve plexuses which run along the walls of the major blood vessels supplying the various parts.

All of the sympathetic nerves supplying the head arise from the cervical ganglia of the sympathetic chain and run along the branches of the carotid arteries; all of the sympathetic fibres supplying the limbs run with the blood vessels (there are no parasympathetic nerves in the limbs); the sympathetic nerves supplying the viscera travel both along the blood vessels and along other pathways, including the splanchnic nerves.

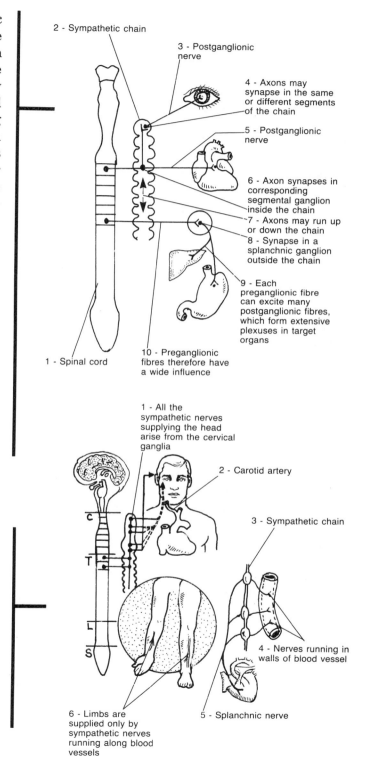

2 - Sympathetic chain

3 - Postganglionic nerve

4 - Axons may synapse in the same or different segments of the chain

5 - Postganglionic nerve

6 - Axon synapses in corresponding segmental ganglion inside the chain

7 - Axons may run up or down the chain

8 - Synapse in a splanchnic ganglion outside the chain

9 - Each preganglionic fibre can excite many postganglionic fibres, which form extensive plexuses in target organs

1 - Spinal cord

10 - Preganglionic fibres therefore have a wide influence

1 - All the sympathetic nerves supplying the head arise from the cervical ganglia

2 - Carotid artery

3 - Sympathetic chain

4 - Nerves running in walls of blood vessel

5 - Splanchnic nerve

6 - Limbs are supplied only by sympathetic nerves running along blood vessels

Sympathetic transmitters

In the sympathetic and splanchnic ganglia the synaptic neurotransmitter is again acetylcholine (nicotinic synapse), while the transmitter at the peripheral end is usually noradrenaline, though it can sometimes be adrenaline, sometimes acetylcholine and sometimes an unknown transmitter.

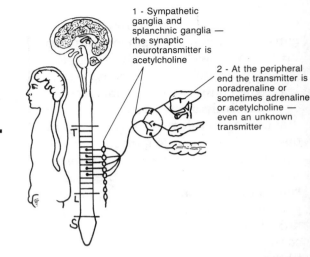

1 - Sympathetic ganglia and splanchnic ganglia — the synaptic neurotransmitter is acetylcholine

2 - At the peripheral end the transmitter is noradrenaline or sometimes adrenaline or acetylcholine — even an unknown transmitter

The most important effect of the sympathetic nerves is upon the blood vessels. In most organs the released noradrenaline causes vasoconstriction; in many cases this is the only true physiological role of the sympathetic nerves, though experimental electrical stimulation of the nerves can produce other effects such as secretion in the liver or dilatation in the bronchi. These secondary effects are often the results of overspill of neurotransmitter from the blood vessels into the main part of the innervated organ, producing effects which are only seen because the experimental stimulation results in the unnatural simultaneous activation of many nerves releasing a large quantity of transmitter. Nevertheless, in many organs the sympathetic nerves have a real and important non-vascular regulatory function.

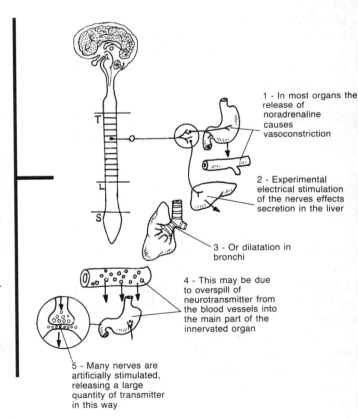

1 - In most organs the release of noradrenaline causes vasoconstriction

2 - Experimental electrical stimulation of the nerves effects secretion in the liver

3 - Or dilatation in bronchi

4 - This may be due to overspill of neurotransmitter from the blood vessels into the main part of the innervated organ

5 - Many nerves are artificially stimulated, releasing a large quantity of transmitter in this way

The effects of the sympathetic neuro-transmitters noradrenaline and adrenaline are sometimes rather different. This is because of the existence of at least two separate types of adrenergic receptor: alpha and beta. Different target organs have different proportions of the two types, and the way they respond to a particular transmitter depends both on the activity (alpha or beta) shown by the chemical and on the receptor type present.

Alpha effects include constriction of blood vessels, relaxation of the gut, dilatation of the pupil; beta effects include speeding of the heart and an increase in its contractile force, and relaxation of the bronchi, the uterus and the gut (though by a different mechanism from the alpha effect).

Noradrenaline possesses mainly alpha activity, with weak beta activity which is only manifest if a tissue has no alpha receptors or they have been blocked by alpha blockers. As the myocardium has no alpha receptors, the beta effect of noradrenaline released from the sympathetic nerves speeds the heart. Elsewhere in the circulation, the alpha constrictor effects of noradrenaline predominate.

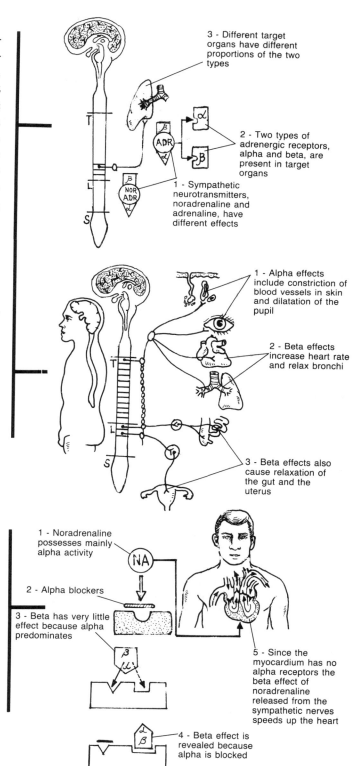

3 - Different target organs have different proportions of the two types

2 - Two types of adrenergic receptors, alpha and beta, are present in target organs

1 - Sympathetic neurotransmitters, noradrenaline and adrenaline, have different effects

1 - Alpha effects include constriction of blood vessels in skin and dilatation of the pupil

2 - Beta effects increase heart rate and relax bronchi

3 - Beta effects also cause relaxation of the gut and the uterus

1 - Noradrenaline possesses mainly alpha activity

2 - Alpha blockers

3 - Beta has very little effect because alpha predominates

4 - Beta effect is revealed because alpha is blocked

5 - Since the myocardium has no alpha receptors the beta effect of noradrenaline released from the sympathetic nerves speeds up the heart

Adrenaline has alpha and beta activity in about equal proportions, so the effects it produces depend upon the local receptor population. Some blood vessels (in the skin and the viscera) have alpha receptors and constrict in response to circulating adrenaline; others (in skeletal muscle) have beta receptors and dilate when adrenaline is present. Adrenaline can cause different effects in different vascular beds.

AUTONOMIC SUPPLY TO THE HEAD AND NECK

In the eye the parasympathetic nerves, whose ganglionic synapses are in the ciliary ganglion, cause constriction of the pupil by stimulation of the sphincter pupillae, and accommodation of the lens for near vision by stimulation of the ciliary muscle; they also cause secretion from the lacrimal gland (via a relay in the sphenopalatine ganglion).

The sympathetic nerves, arising from the upper thoracic spinal segments, synapsing in the superior and middle cervical ganglia and running in the walls of the carotid arteries, cause dilatation of the pupil by stimulating the radial fibres of the dilator pupillae, and further increase the light reaching the eye by stimulating the smooth muscle of the levator palpebrae superioris, a part of the upper eyelid. Sympathetic nerves also control the retinal and choroidal blood vessels by releasing noradrenaline to cause constriction; they cause dilatation by simply ceasing to fire.

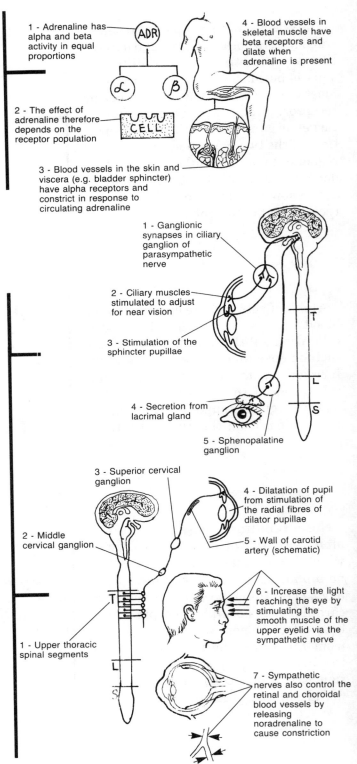

1 - Adrenaline has alpha and beta activity in equal proportions

2 - The effect of adrenaline therefore depends on the receptor population

3 - Blood vessels in the skin and viscera (e.g. bladder sphincter) have alpha receptors and constrict in response to circulating adrenaline

4 - Blood vessels in skeletal muscle have beta receptors and dilate when adrenaline is present

1 - Ganglionic synapses in ciliary ganglion of parasympathetic nerve

2 - Ciliary muscles stimulated to adjust for near vision

3 - Stimulation of the sphincter pupillae

4 - Secretion from lacrimal gland

5 - Sphenopalatine ganglion

3 - Superior cervical ganglion

2 - Middle cervical ganglion

1 - Upper thoracic spinal segments

4 - Dilatation of pupil from stimulation of the radial fibres of dilator pupillae

5 - Wall of carotid artery (schematic)

6 - Increase the light reaching the eye by stimulating the smooth muscle of the upper eyelid via the sympathetic nerve

7 - Sympathetic nerves also control the retinal and choroidal blood vessels by releasing noradrenaline to cause constriction

The salivary glands are controlled by both parasympathetic and sympathetic nerves, and the blood flow to the mucous membranes in the upper airways and all of the other vascular structures in the head and neck are controlled by the sympathetic nerves.

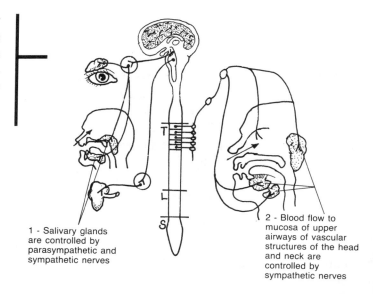

1 - Salivary glands are controlled by parasympathetic and sympathetic nerves

2 - Blood flow to mucosa of upper airways of vascular structures of the head and neck are controlled by sympathetic nerves

AUTONOMIC SUPPLY TO THE CIRCULATION

The parasympathetic innervation of the heart is by the vagus, with cholinergic fibres supplying the sinoatrial and atrioventricular nodes to slow the heart beat. The sympathetic nerves supply the nodes with adrenergic fibres and speed the heart beat; other adrenergic fibres supply the myocardium at large and increase the force of contraction.

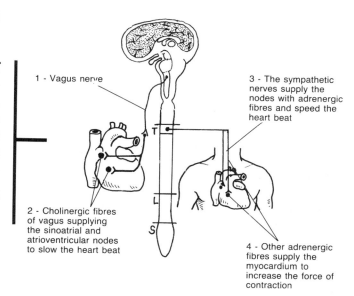

1 - Vagus nerve

3 - The sympathetic nerves supply the nodes with adrenergic fibres and speed the heart beat

2 - Cholinergic fibres of vagus supplying the sinoatrial and atrioventricular nodes to slow the heart beat

4 - Other adrenergic fibres supply the myocardium to increase the force of contraction

All areas of skin throughout the body are innervated by the sympathetic system, but receive no fibres from the parasympathetic. The sympathetic nerves control the blood vessels, causing vasoconstriction by the release of noradrenaline; vasodilatation is usually caused by cessation of vasoconstriction, but perhaps in some places by the release of acetylcholine from sympathetic nerves. The sweat glands are controlled by cholinergic fibres, and so are the small bundles of smooth muscle which cause the hairs to become erect (**arrectores pilorum**, producing piloerection or 'goose-flesh').

The blood vessels of the muscles throughout the body are controlled by the sympathetic system; there are no parasympathetic nerves to skeletal muscle. Many muscle blood vessels have beta receptors, so that adrenaline causes vasodilatation. There is also a set of cholinergic sympathetic nerves which cause intense vasodilatation in muscle during states of emotion or great distress.

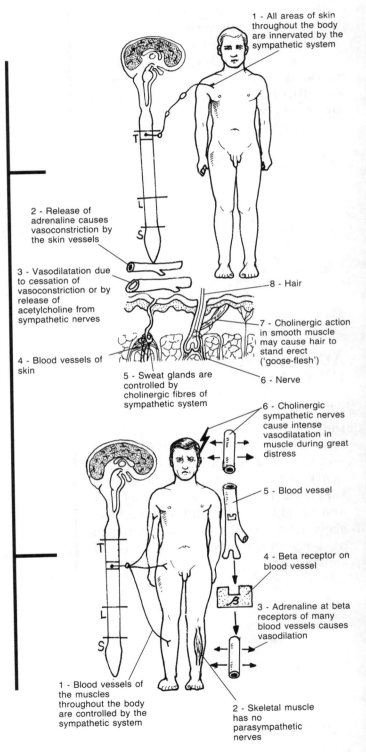

1 - All areas of skin throughout the body are innervated by the sympathetic system

2 - Release of adrenaline causes vasoconstriction by the skin vessels

3 - Vasodilatation due to cessation of vasoconstriction or by release of acetylcholine from sympathetic nerves

4 - Blood vessels of skin

5 - Sweat glands are controlled by cholinergic fibres of sympathetic system

8 - Hair

7 - Cholinergic action in smooth muscle may cause hair to stand erect ('goose-flesh')

6 - Nerve

6 - Cholinergic sympathetic nerves cause intense vasodilatation in muscle during great distress

5 - Blood vessel

4 - Beta receptor on blood vessel

3 - Adrenaline at beta receptors of many blood vessels causes vasodilation

1 - Blood vessels of the muscles throughout the body are controlled by the sympathetic system

2 - Skeletal muscle has no parasympathetic nerves

AUTONOMIC SUPPLY TO THE LUNGS

The smooth muscle in the trachea and bronchi is controlled by the vagus nerve (parasympathetic); acetylcholine causes bronchoconstriction. The role of the sympathetic nerves is more debatable; it may be that the bronchodilator effects of experimental sympathetic nerves are due to overspill from the vascular nerves, and that the true bronchodilator nerves are really parasympathetic fibres which release some other non-cholinergic transmitter such as vasoactive intestinal peptide (VIP). The sympathetic nerves undoubtedly regulate the flow of blood in both the pulmonary and the bronchial blood vessels.

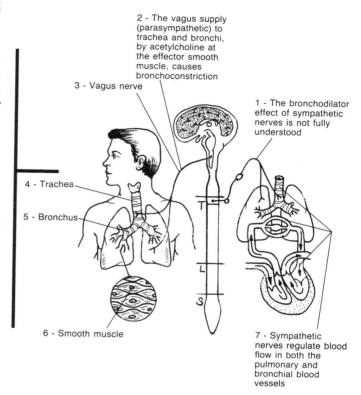

2 - The vagus supply (parasympathetic) to trachea and bronchi, by acetylcholine at the effector smooth muscle, causes bronchoconstriction

3 - Vagus nerve

1 - The bronchodilator effect of sympathetic nerves is not fully understood

4 - Trachea

5 - Bronchus

6 - Smooth muscle

7 - Sympathetic nerves regulate blood flow in both the pulmonary and bronchial blood vessels

AUTONOMIC SUPPLY TO THE GUT

The oesophagus and stomach are dually innervated by vagus and sympathetic nerves, although here again the sympathetic effects may be confined to the blood vessels. The vagus increases motility by cholinergic fibres.

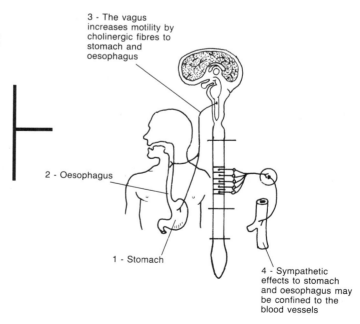

3 - The vagus increases motility by cholinergic fibres to stomach and oesophagus

2 - Oesophagus

1 - Stomach

4 - Sympathetic effects to stomach and oesophagus may be confined to the blood vessels

The lower oesophageal sphincter is relaxed by a transmitter which is probably not acetylcholine or noradrenaline, and may be VIP. The secretion of gastric acid is stimulated by acetylcholine, and may be inhibited by noradrenaline, though this may not be part of its normal physiological control. Pancreatic secretion is largely under hormonal control, but the vagus has a small role in causing secretion.

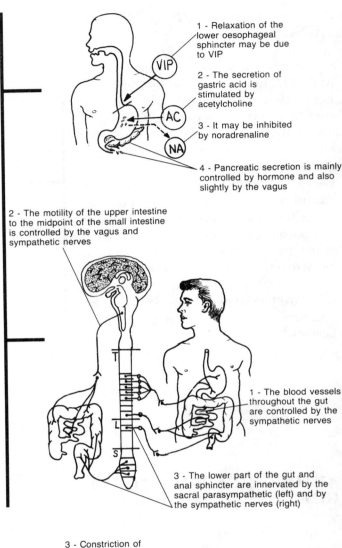

1 - Relaxation of the lower oesophageal sphincter may be due to VIP

2 - The secretion of gastric acid is stimulated by acetylcholine

3 - It may be inhibited by noradrenaline

4 - Pancreatic secretion is mainly controlled by hormone and also slightly by the vagus

2 - The motility of the upper intestine to the midpoint of the small intestine is controlled by the vagus and sympathetic nerves

The blood vessels throughout the gut are controlled by the sympathetic nerves. The motility of the upper intestine, as far as the midpoint of the small intestine, is under vagal and sympathetic control; the nerves modify the intrinsic motility of the smooth muscle cells, and modulate the activity of the myenteric nerve plexus. The lower parts of the gut, including the anal sphincter, are innervated by parasympathetic fibres from the nervi erigentes (the sacral parasympathetic) and by the sympathetic nerves.

1 - The blood vessels throughout the gut are controlled by the sympathetic nerves

3 - The lower part of the gut and anal sphincter are innervated by the sacral parasympathetic (left) and by the sympathetic nerves (right)

CONTROL OF THE BLADDER AND GENITALIA

The bladder is controlled by sacral parasympathetic fibres to the detrusor muscle which initiate micturition. It is uncertain whether the sympathetic nerves have any real role in the control of micturition, though they certainly cause constriction of the internal urethral sphincter during ejaculation, preventing reflux of semen into the bladder during sexual activity.

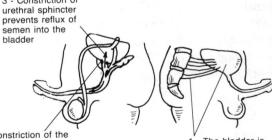

3 - Constriction of urethral sphincter prevents reflux of semen into the bladder

2 - Constriction of the internal urethral sphincter via sympathetic nerves during ejaculation (sympathetic role in micturition is uncertain)

1 - The bladder is controlled by sacral parasympathetic fibres to the detrusor muscle which initiate micturition

The parasympathetic nerves cause erection of the penis in the male and of the clitoris in the female. These effects are produced on blood vessels; this is one of the few instances where the parasympathetic nerves have a direct vascular effect. Sympathetic nerves cause ejaculation and release the erection of the penis or clitoris. They may also have a role in inhibiting uterine contractions during pregnancy.

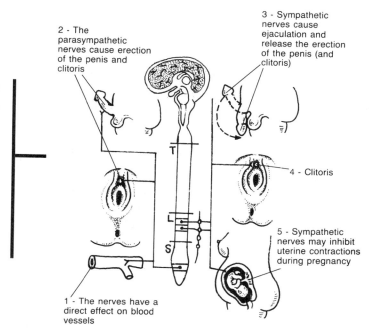

2 - The parasympathetic nerves cause erection of the penis and clitoris

3 - Sympathetic nerves cause ejaculation and release the erection of the penis (and clitoris)

4 - Clitoris

5 - Sympathetic nerves may inhibit uterine contractions during pregnancy

1 - The nerves have a direct effect on blood vessels

THE ADRENAL GLANDS

There is one place where the autonomic nervous system makes a direct input into the endocrine system. The adrenal glands are rather like modified sympathetic ganglia; they are derived from the same embryonic tissue layer, and they receive preganglionic fibres from the intermediolateral column of the spinal grey matter. Instead of sending out long axon processes to the target organs, the rounded ganglion cells secrete their neurotransmitter directly into the capillaries running past them.

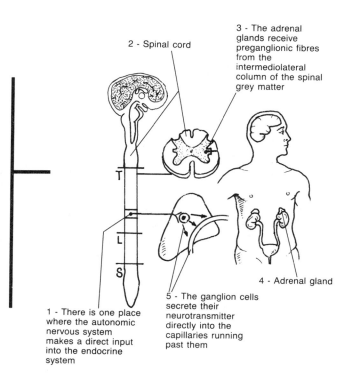

2 - Spinal cord

3 - The adrenal glands receive preganglionic fibres from the intermediolateral column of the spinal grey matter

4 - Adrenal gland

5 - The ganglion cells secrete their neurotransmitter directly into the capillaries running past them

1 - There is one place where the autonomic nervous system makes a direct input into the endocrine system

Stimulation of the preganglionic nerves results in the release of adrenaline (and a little noradrenaline) into the circulation, for carriage to all parts of the body. While most sympathetic effects can be made quite local, by the action of specific nerves supplying specific organs, the adrenal effects are felt in many organs simultaneously; the secretion of adrenaline is a good mechanism for producing widespread activation, and is important in preparing the body, and especially the circulation, for flight or fight.

As well as its effects on smooth muscle and the circulation, adrenaline has an important role in preparing the body for activity, by causing the liver to mobilize glycogen and produce glucose (a beta effect).

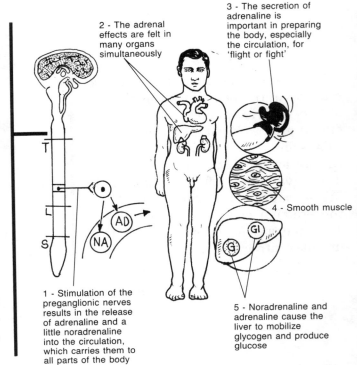

2 - The adrenal effects are felt in many organs simultaneously

3 - The secretion of adrenaline is important in preparing the body, especially the circulation, for 'flight or fight'

4 - Smooth muscle

1 - Stimulation of the preganglionic nerves results in the release of adrenaline and a little noradrenaline into the circulation, which carries them to all parts of the body

5 - Noradrenaline and adrenaline cause the liver to mobilize glycogen and produce glucose

THERMOREGULATION

The control of body temperature is one of the main actions of the autonomic nervous system; several somatic or non-autonomic effector systems are also involved.

Like other physiological systems, the thermoregulatory system requires an input from a series of sensors, a central controller which compares information from the sensors with a reference value, and a series of effector mechanisms which can modify the body temperature to return it to its correct level.

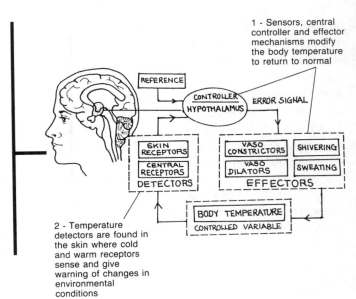

1 - Sensors, central controller and effector mechanisms modify the body temperature to return to normal

2 - Temperature detectors are found in the skin where cold and warm receptors sense and give warning of changes in environmental conditions

Temperature detectors are found in the skin, where both cold and warm receptors sense the peripheral temperature and give early warning of changes in environmental conditions. Other thermoreceptors are located in the hypothalamus — in the preoptic area and the anterior hypothalamus, in the spinal cord and in the walls of some of the viscera. The central receptors sense the temperature of the central 'core', which is the region whose temperature is maintained constant. The more peripheral parts of the body are known as the 'shell', and the temperature here varies quite considerably, being heavily influenced by the environmental temperature. If the core temperature begins to fall, some of the blood circulating to the shell is diverted to the core, maintaining heat in the core and reducing its rate of loss through the skin.

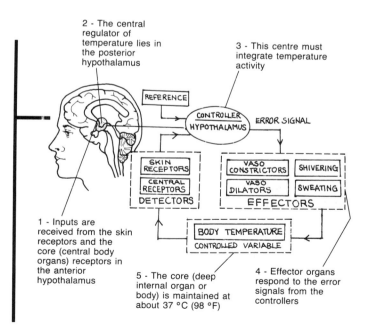

1 - Other thermoceptors are located in the preoptic area of the hypothalamus

2 - Spinal cord

3 - The walls of some viscera

4 - Core temperature of deep internal organs

5 - 'Shell', being heavily influenced by environmental temperature

6 - The core temperature may fall

7 - If so, blood circulating to the shell is then diverted to the core to maintain heat in the core and reduce the rate of heat loss through the skin

The central regulator of temperature lies in the posterior hypothalamus, which receives inputs from both the skin receptors and the core receptors in the preoptic area and anterior hypothalamus. The regulatory centre must integrate this activity, and the mechanism is not quite as simple as the control diagram might suggest, as actions can be produced in effector organs in response to signals from skin receptors, long before there is any overall change in core temperature. The central regulator attempts to maintain the core temperature (or more particularly the temperature of the hypothalamus) at around 37 °C (98.6 °F).

2 - The central regulator of temperature lies in the posterior hypothalamus

3 - This centre must integrate temperature activity

1 - Inputs are received from the skin receptors and the core (central body organs) receptors in the anterior hypothalamus

5 - The core (deep internal organ or body) is maintained at about 37 °C (98 °F)

4 - Effector organs respond to the error signals from the controllers

REFERENCE

CONTROLLER HYPOTHALAMUS   ERROR SIGNAL

SKIN RECEPTORS

CENTRAL RECEPTORS

DETECTORS

VASO CONSTRICTORS   SHIVERING

VASO DILATORS   SWEATING

EFFECTORS

BODY TEMPERATURE

CONTROLLED VARIABLE

The effector systems consist of mechanisms for generating or retaining heat, and mechanisms for eliminating heat (see previous illustration). The normal resting metabolism produces about 100 watts of heat, but in severe exercise the rate of heat production can rise to 1000–2000 watts. If the body needs to keep warm, the level of activity can be increased (and people often move about more when they feel cold); alternatively the muscles can be stimulated to undergo rhythmic purposeless alternate contraction and relaxation (shivering) to generate heat without doing external work, and this can release up to 1000 watts.

In order to conserve heat in the body, the blood vessels of the skin constrict under the influence of sympathetic nerves, and the rate of heat loss through the skin is reduced. The shell is allowed to cool towards the environmental temperature, but the heat is kept in the core.

If the core temperature rises, either due to an increase in metabolic activity (such as exercise) or because of being in a warm environment, the skin blood vessels dilate (by release of sympathetic tone) and allow blood to come near the surface; the core effectively becomes larger, at the expense of the shell. This helps the elimination of heat, but only if the environment is cooler than the skin; if air temperature exceeds about 35 °C then heat cannot be lost by conduction and convection, and the other mechanism of cooling becomes pre-eminent.

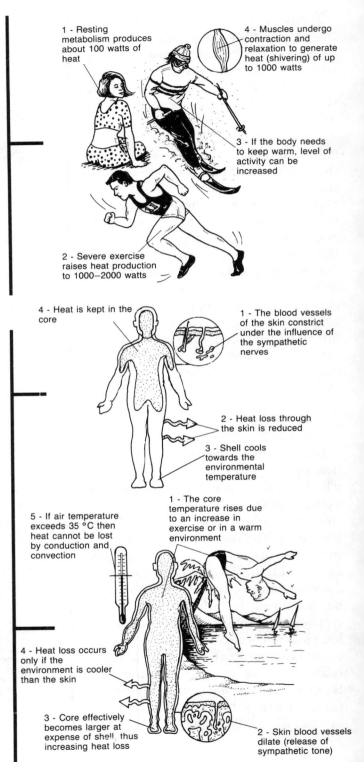

1 - Resting metabolism produces about 100 watts of heat

4 - Muscles undergo contraction and relaxation to generate heat (shivering) of up to 1000 watts

3 - If the body needs to keep warm, level of activity can be increased

2 - Severe exercise raises heat production to 1000–2000 watts

4 - Heat is kept in the core

1 - The blood vessels of the skin constrict under the influence of the sympathetic nerves

2 - Heat loss through the skin is reduced

3 - Shell cools towards the environmental temperature

1 - The core temperature rises due to an increase in exercise or in a warm environment

5 - If air temperature exceeds 35 °C then heat cannot be lost by conduction and convection

4 - Heat loss occurs only if the environment is cooler than the skin

3 - Core effectively becomes larger at expense of shell, thus increasing heat loss

2 - Skin blood vessels dilate (release of sympathetic tone)

The secretion of sweat, stimulated by cholinergic sympathetic fibres, allows heat loss by evaporation from the skin. The sweat glands can produce up to one litre per hour (though not for very long) and this can eliminate about 800 watts. Normally both vasodilatation and sweating proceed in parallel to remove heat; in fact the secretion of sweat can result in the production of bradykinin around the sweat glands, and this causes further vasodilatation.

The sweat glands produce a fluid which is essentially isosmotic with plasma, but the ducts of the glands reabsorb some of the sodium chloride, so that at low sweat rates the fluid is rather dilute. At higher rates of sweating there is not enough time for the salt to be reabsorbed, and in very hot environments the loss of both water and salt can be a very serious problem.

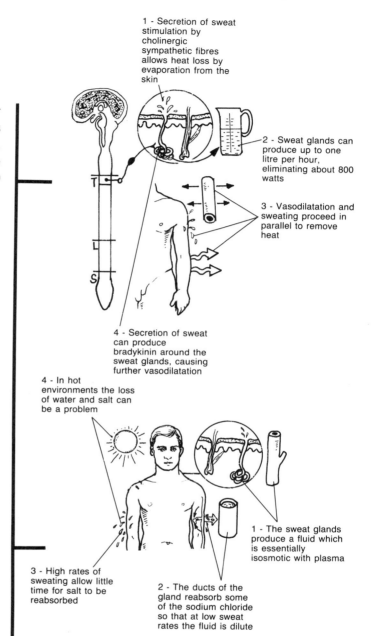

1 - Secretion of sweat stimulation by cholinergic sympathetic fibres allows heat loss by evaporation from the skin

2 - Sweat glands can produce up to one litre per hour, eliminating about 800 watts

3 - Vasodilatation and sweating proceed in parallel to remove heat

4 - Secretion of sweat can produce bradykinin around the sweat glands, causing further vasodilatation

4 - In hot environments the loss of water and salt can be a problem

1 - The sweat glands produce a fluid which is essentially isosmotic with plasma

2 - The ducts of the gland reabsorb some of the sodium chloride so that at low sweat rates the fluid is dilute

3 - High rates of sweating allow little time for salt to be reabsorbed

Functions of the Blood

Blood is the red fluid found throughout the body and contained in the blood vessels; it is pumped around the body by the heart. The main purpose of blood is **transport**; it carries oxygen to all of the tissues, takes vital foodstuffs to those organs which need them and removes waste products including gases from the tissues.

Another very important function of blood is **homeostasis**; by flowing rapidly through all of the tissues it ensures thorough mixing of the liquid elements of the body, and produces a uniformity of composition of the body fluids. Many of the body's regulatory processes control the composition of the blood and thereby ensure that the internal environment of the tissues is also kept constant.

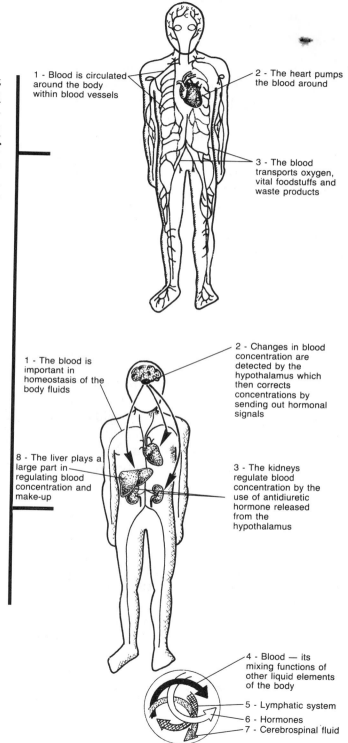

1 - Blood is circulated around the body within blood vessels

2 - The heart pumps the blood around

3 - The blood transports oxygen, vital foodstuffs and waste products

1 - The blood is important in homeostasis of the body fluids

2 - Changes in blood concentration are detected by the hypothalamus which then corrects concentrations by sending out hormonal signals

8 - The liver plays a large part in regulating blood concentration and make-up

3 - The kidneys regulate blood concentration by the use of antidiuretic hormone released from the hypothalamus

4 - Blood — its mixing functions of other liquid elements of the body

5 - Lymphatic system

6 - Hormones

7 - Cerebrospinal fluid

Temperature regulation is an example of a vital homeostatic function. If peripheral tissues become cold, the blood warmed by internal organs can deliver heat to them; alternatively the excess heat produced by active organs can be carried away by the blood and dissipated through the skin. If a person needs to conserve heat in a cold environment, the blood is diverted away from the skin and kept in the warm central body 'core'.

The blood provides a convenient **pool of nutrients** for the tissues: there are free sugars, amino acids, fatty acids and minerals in the plasma, and extra amino acids can be obtained by breaking down the plasma proteins.

There are some specific **protective functions** of the blood: if tissues or blood vessels are damaged then the **clotting** process prevents excessive blood loss; if the body is invaded by foreign materials or microorganisms then the **immune** mechanisms help to combat the invasion and destroy the invaders.

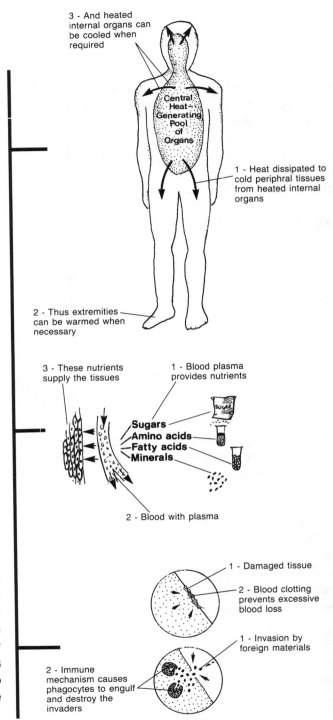

3 - And heated internal organs can be cooled when required

Central Heat - Generating Pool of Organs

1 - Heat dissipated to cold periphral tissues from heated internal organs

2 - Thus extremities can be warmed when necessary

3 - These nutrients supply the tissues

1 - Blood plasma provides nutrients

Sugars
Amino acids
Fatty acids
Minerals

2 - Blood with plasma

1 - Damaged tissue

2 - Blood clotting prevents excessive blood loss

1 - Invasion by foreign materials

2 - Immune mechanism causes phagocytes to engulf and destroy the invaders

Blood can have a **structural** or **supportive** role in some organs: for instance, the male **penis** has **erectile tissue** which is capable of being engorged with blood during sexual arousal, becoming stiff and able to enter the female genital tract.

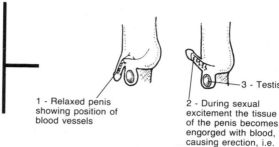

1 - Relaxed penis showing position of blood vessels

2 - During sexual excitement the tissue of the penis becomes engorged with blood, causing erection, i.e. structural function of blood

3 - Testis

COMPOSITION AND VOLUME OF BLOOD

There are two main components to blood: the fluid part or **plasma**, and the **formed elements** consisting of cells or subcellular particles suspended in the fluid medium.

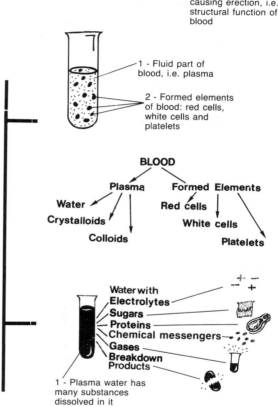

1 - Fluid part of blood, i.e. plasma

2 - Formed elements of blood: red cells, white cells and platelets

BLOOD

Plasma — Water, Crystalloids, Colloids

Formed Elements — Red cells, White cells, Platelets

Plasma consists mainly of water, in which are dissolved many electrolytes, sugars, proteins and other organic molecules, and many important chemical messengers (**hormones**) as well as trace elements, the breakdown products of cellular activity and a number of important gases.

Water with Electrolytes
Sugars
Proteins
Chemical messengers
Gases
Breakdown Products

1 - Plasma water has many substances dissolved in it

The **formed elements** are the **red cells**, whose primary purpose is to carry oxygen, the **white cells**, whose main function is the protection of the body against invaders, and the **platelets**, which are subcellular fragments important in the arrest of bleeding.

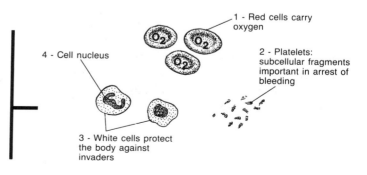

1 - Red cells carry oxygen

2 - Platelets: subcellular fragments important in arrest of bleeding

4 - Cell nucleus

3 - White cells protect the body against invaders

If a sample of blood is removed from a vein using a syringe and hypodermic needle, and the blood (after addition of a little anticoagulant) is placed in a centrifuge tube and spun at about 3000 rev/min for a few minutes, it becomes separated into its formed elements (which settle to the bottom of the tube) and the clear plasma. The machine for separating the blood is known as the **haematocrit**, and the proportion of the volume which is occupied by the formed elements is known as the **haematocrit value** or the **packed cell volume** (PCV). This is usually about 45% of the total in the normal individual.

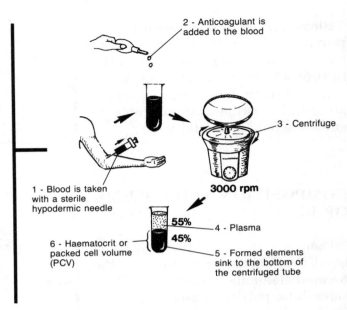

2 - Anticoagulant is added to the blood

3 - Centrifuge

1 - Blood is taken with a sterile hypodermic needle

3000 rpm

55%
45%

4 - Plasma

6 - Haematocrit or packed cell volume (PCV)

5 - Formed elements sink to the bottom of the centrifuged tube

Blood can also be separated, though much more slowly, by the influence of gravity alone. A column of blood in a narrow tube will exhibit settling of the formed elements by a few millimetres in the first hour (the **erythrocyte sedimentation rate**, ESR).

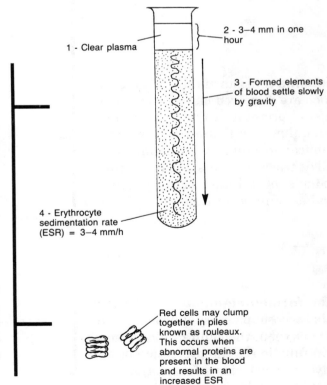

1 - Clear plasma

2 - 3–4 mm in one hour

3 - Formed elements of blood settle slowly by gravity

4 - Erythrocyte sedimentation rate (ESR) = 3–4 mm/h

This process is speeded if the red cells clump together in piles or **rouleaux**, and in many diseases where abnormal proteins which promote rouleaux formation are present in the blood there is an increased ESR.

Red cells may clump together in piles known as rouleaux. This occurs when abnormal proteins are present in the blood and results in an increased ESR

If whole blood or plasma is allowed to clot, then the clear fluid left after the clotted material has been separated off is known as **serum**; serum is plasma without the clotting factors.

It is often important to be able to measure the volume of the blood. This is usually done by an **indicator dilution** technique, which is best understood by considering a container of water whose volume is unknown. If a known mass of a dye is added, say 5 g, and thoroughly mixed with the water, then a small sample of the mixture can be taken out for measurement of the concentration of the dye. Suppose the concentration were found to be 50 mg/l; this would mean that the original 5 g had been diluted in 5000/50 or 100 litres, in other words the volume of the container was 100 litres.

Similarly, if a non-toxic dye (such as Evans Blue dye) which does not escape from the circulation and does not penetrate cells is injected into the circulation, its concentration in the plasma can be used to estimate the plasma volume. If the haematocrit value is also known, then the volume of red cells and the total blood volume can easily be calculated. A normal adult human has on average about 5 litres of blood.

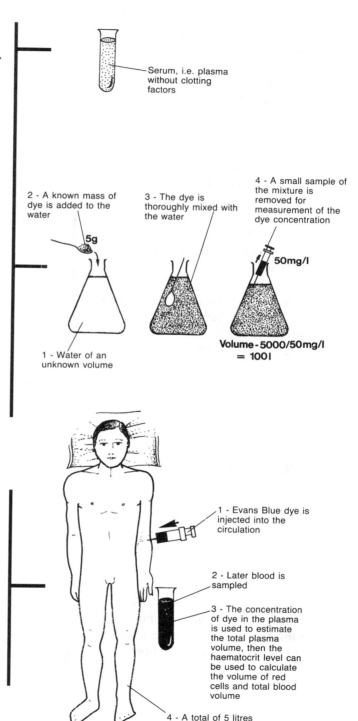

Serum, i.e. plasma without clotting factors

2 - A known mass of dye is added to the water

3 - The dye is thoroughly mixed with the water

4 - A small sample of the mixture is removed for measurement of the dye concentration

5g

50mg/l

1 - Water of an unknown volume

Volume - 5000/50mg/l = 100l

1 - Evans Blue dye is injected into the circulation

2 - Later blood is sampled

3 - The concentration of dye in the plasma is used to estimate the total plasma volume, then the haematocrit level can be used to calculate the volume of red cells and total blood volume

4 - A total of 5 litres of blood is present in a normal adult

A similar approach can be used to measure the size of other body fluid compartments. The **total body water** content is assessed by measuring the dilution of heavy water (D_2O) or tritiated water; in a normal 70 kg adult this is about 42 litres or 60% of body mass. The **extracellular fluid**, measured by using a marker such as inulin or sucrose which does not cross cell walls, totals about 15.5 litres or 22% of body mass. This extracellular fluid includes plasma, occupying 3.5 litres or 5% of body mass, and the **interstitial fluid** whose volume is obtained by subtracting plasma volume from extracellular fluid volume and amounts to 12 litres or 17% of body mass. The **intracellular fluid** volume is calculated by subtracting extracellular fluid from total body water, and is 26.5 litres or 38% of body mass.

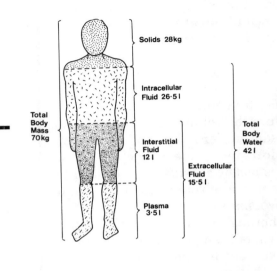

COMPOSITION OF PLASMA

The main constituent of plasma is water, in which the other contents are dissolved or suspended. The other constituents are known as **crystalloids** and **colloids**. The crystalloids are mainly ions, electrolytes or small, relatively simple organic molecules, while the colloids are much larger molecules such as proteins and complex mucopolysaccharides or lipids.

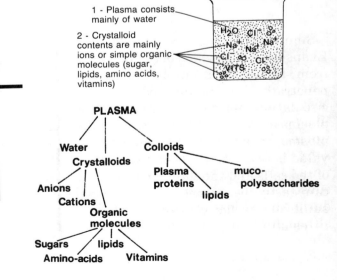

The approximate concentrations (in mmol/l) of the various electrolytes are shown in the table.

	Plasma	Interstitial	Cell
Na^+	142	145	10
K^+	4	4	160
Ca^{2+}	2	1	1
Mg^{2+}	1	1	13
Cl^-	103	114	3
HCO_3^-	27	31	10
HPO_4^{2-}	1	1	50
SO_4^{2-}	0.5	0.5	10
Organic anions	6	7	?
Proteins	2	<0.1	8

Note that although proteins only contribute 2 mmol/l, this actually represents a concentration of 60 g/l since the molecules are so large.

The most important ions in plasma are sodium and chloride, and in many instances a person's plasma can be replaced, substituted or augmented by a solution of 0.9% NaCl in water. This is 9 g/l or about 145 mmol/l. In terms of osmotically active particles this represents a solution of about 290 mosmol/l, since each molecule of crystalline NaCl dissociates in solution into one Na^+ ion and one Cl^- ion.

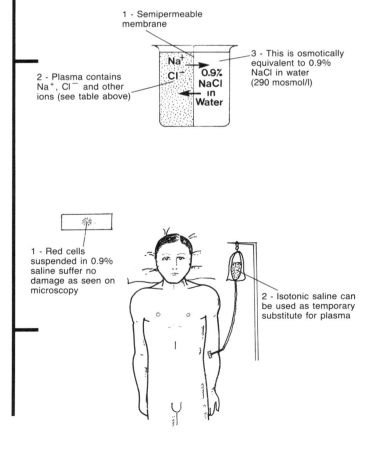

1 - Semipermeable membrane

2 - Plasma contains Na^+, Cl^- and other ions (see table above)

3 - This is osmotically equivalent to 0.9% NaCl in water (290 mosmol/l)

Na^+
Cl^-
0.9% NaCl in Water

1 - Red cells suspended in 0.9% saline suffer no damage as seen on microscopy

2 - Isotonic saline can be used as temporary substitute for plasma

Red blood cells removed from the body can be suspended without damage in a 0.9% saline solution (often called **normal** or more accurately **isotonic** saline); isotonic saline can also be infused into the body as a temporary substitute for plasma, for instance during blood loss or fluid restriction, although as water and sodium chloride can easily leave the circulation such substitution can only be temporary.

THE PLASMA PROTEINS

Each litre of plasma contains about 60−75 g of protein, or about 2 mmol/l; thus proteins are the most abundant **colloid** in the plasma. The various different proteins can be separated by the process of **electrophoresis**, in which a drop of plasma is placed on a strip of paper impregnated with a suitable solvent, and the ends of the paper are connected to the positive and negative terminals of a battery. As current flows through the paper, the proteins which are electrically charged move towards either the anode or the cathode, depending on their charge. The rate of movement depends on the size and also the shape of the molecule, as the paper offers some restriction to movement and the smallest or most compact molecules will move fastest. After a fixed interval the paper strip is removed from the apparatus and dried, then sprayed with a marker to stain the proteins. The density of the marker can be measured to get an estimate of the relative abundance of the various proteins.

The fastest moving, and also the most abundant protein is **albumin**, with a molecular weight of 69 000. It is a long, thin molecule, whereas the **globulins** are round, compact molecules. These are separated by electrophoresis into alpha, beta and gamma globulins. Between the beta and gamma globulins on the electrophoretic strip comes **fibrinogen**, a very long, thin molecule which is important in blood clotting. The alpha globulins have molecular weights from 200 000 to 300 000, while the beta and gamma globulins have molecular weights from 160 000 to one million. Fibrinogen has a molecular weight of 400 000.

1 - Proteins are the most abundant colloid in plasma

2 - Each litre of plasma contains about 60−75 g protein (2 mmol/l)

1 - Drop of plasma

2 - Strip of paper

3 - Battery

4 - The electrically charged proteins move towards the anode or cathode. Rate of movement depends on the size and shape of the molecule

5 - Spray

6 - The paper is removed from the battery and dried and sprayed with a marker to stain proteins

7 - The density of the marker staining the protein shows the abundance of proteins

1 - Concentration

2 - Fibrinogen, important in blood clotting, has a molecular weight of 400 000

3 - Albumin, the fastest moving and most abundant protein, has a molecular weight of 69 000

$\gamma \quad \beta \quad \alpha_2 \alpha_1$

4 - Globulins: alpha globulins weigh between 200 000 and 300 000, and beta and gamma globulins weigh between 160 000 and 1 million

1 - Albumin is a long, thin molecule

2 - Globulin is a round, compact molecule

3 - Fibrinogen is a very long, thin molecule

Functions of plasma proteins

Many proteins have very specific functions: **fibrinogen** and the other **clotting factors**, or the **gamma globulins** which are specific **antibodies** against infection, or some **carrier** molecules which bind and transport hormones like thyroxine or minerals like iron.

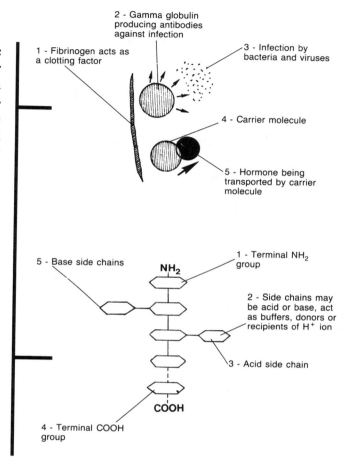

1 - Fibrinogen acts as a clotting factor

2 - Gamma globulin producing antibodies against infection

3 - Infection by bacteria and viruses

4 - Carrier molecule

5 - Hormone being transported by carrier molecule

All of them are capable of acting as **buffers**: since they are built up from amino acids they all have a terminal $-NH_2$ group at one end and a terminal $-COOH$ group at the other; many also have acidic or basic groups on their side chains. These groups can act as donors or recipients of hydrogen ions, depending on the pH of the solution. The mechanism of buffers will be more fully explained in the chapters on respiration and the kidney.

5 - Base side chains

1 - Terminal NH_2 group

2 - Side chains may be acid or base, act as buffers, donors or recipients of H^+ ion

3 - Acid side chain

4 - Terminal COOH group

All of the proteins, particularly albumin, can act as a pool of amino acids, and when certain tissues need more amino acids some of the plasma proteins become engulfed by cells of the **reticuloendothelial system** and broken down to their constituent amino acids, which are then returned to the circulation.

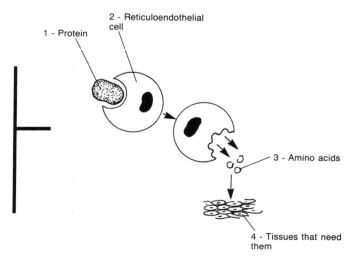

1 - Protein

2 - Reticuloendothelial cell

3 - Amino acids

4 - Tissues that need them

The **osmotic** function is one of the most vital roles of the plasma proteins, particularly albumin. While the true osmolarity of plasma against a genuine semipermeable membrane is about 290 mosmol/l, the walls of the blood capillaries are not true semipermeable membranes but are permeable to water and small molecules or ions. These substances pass easily out of and into blood vessels and have little effect on the control of fluid exchange across the capillary wall. Proteins do not cross the capillary wall, and if fluid leaves the capillary this renders the plasma more concentrated with proteins; this exerts an osmotic force tending to return fluid to the circulation. Although the concentration of plasma proteins is only a few milliosmoles per litre, the resulting osmotic force is sufficient to counteract the hydrostatic forces, pushing fluid out of the capillaries. This phenomenon is described in more detail in the chapter on the circulation.

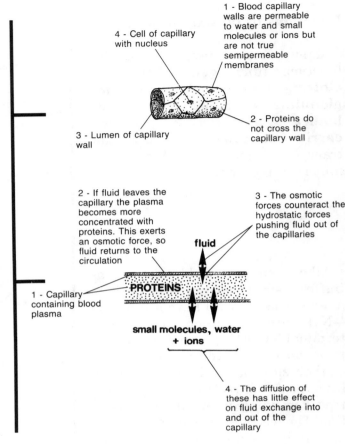

1 - Blood capillary walls are permeable to water and small molecules or ions but are not true semipermeable membranes

4 - Cell of capillary with nucleus

3 - Lumen of capillary wall

2 - Proteins do not cross the capillary wall

2 - If fluid leaves the capillary the plasma becomes more concentrated with proteins. This exerts an osmotic force, so fluid returns to the circulation

3 - The osmotic forces counteract the hydrostatic forces pushing fluid out of the capillaries

fluid

PROTEINS

1 - Capillary containing blood plasma

small molecules, water + ions

4 - The diffusion of these has little effect on fluid exchange into and out of the capillary

If the body becomes depleted of plasma proteins for some reason, such as malnutrition or disease, then the escape of fluid into the tissues is not prevented and swelling or **oedema** is the result.

The chief site of manufacture of plasma proteins is the liver, which makes about 4 g per hour or about 100 g per day. The other site of protein manufacture is the lymph nodes, which produce gamma globulins or antibodies at a rate depending upon the need for immune protection.

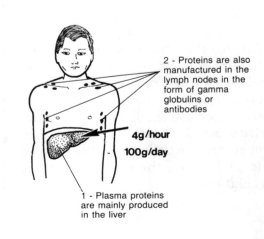

2 - Proteins are also manufactured in the lymph nodes in the form of gamma globulins or antibodies

4g/hour
100g/day

1 - Plasma proteins are mainly produced in the liver

THE FORMED ELEMENTS OF THE BLOOD

The formed elements are the red cells (erythrocytes), the white cells (leucocytes) and the platelets (thrombocytes). The leucocytes are further subdivided into numerous types depending on their histological appearance, staining reaction and function.

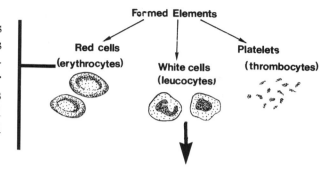

The red cells

The red cells or **erythrocytes** are the most abundant cells in the blood. They can be counted by taking a blood sample, diluting it by a known amount and then introducing a small volume into a special chamber on a microscope slide called a **haemocytometer**. This has a grid of fine squares etched on it, and the volume overlying each square is accurately known. The number of red cells occupying each of a large number of squares is counted, and after correcting for the dilution factors the number of cells in a given volume of blood is calculated.

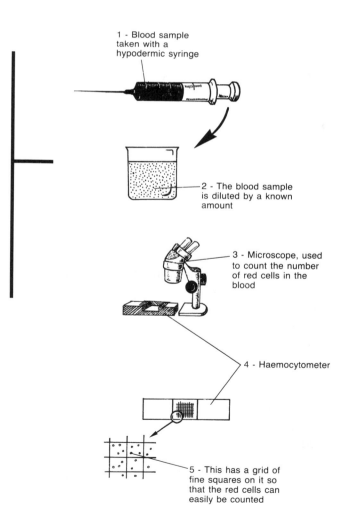

1 - Blood sample taken with a hypodermic syringe

2 - The blood sample is diluted by a known amount

3 - Microscope, used to count the number of red cells in the blood

4 - Haemocytometer

5 - This has a grid of fine squares on it so that the red cells can easily be counted

In modern hospital laboratories the red cells are counted automatically using a **Coulter counter**, which measures the optical transmission properties or the electrical conductivity of a suspension of cells as they pass the detector. Nevertheless, all medical and paramedical students should know how to use the manual method, in case they find themselves in remote conditions without access to expensive machines or in case the machine breaks down. The same applies to the measurement of haemoglobin and other blood indices.

The normal adult has, on average, five million red cells per cubic millimetre of blood, or 5×10^{12} per litre.

Mature red cells have no nucleus, but appear as biconcave discs with a maximum diameter of 7 μm; they are, however, sufficiently deformable to be able to pass through capillaries as narrow as 5 μm. Their main function is the transport of respiratory gases: oxygen from the lungs to the tissues and carbon dioxide from the tissues back to the lungs.

The transport function of the red cells is achieved by the protein **haemoglobin**, which is the chief constituent of the cells; it accounts for about one-third of the contents of the cells, the rest being mainly water and electrolytes.

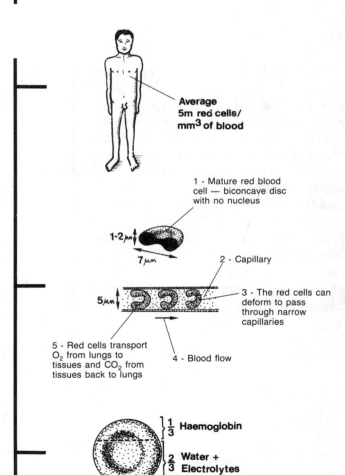

1 - Red blood cells move across the counter

2 - Electric current flows through gap

Average 5m red cells/ mm³ of blood

1 - Mature red blood cell — biconcave disc with no nucleus

1-2 μm

7 μm

2 - Capillary

5 μm

3 - The red cells can deform to pass through narrow capillaries

5 - Red cells transport O₂ from lungs to tissues and CO₂ from tissues back to lungs

4 - Blood flow

⅓ Haemoglobin

⅔ Water + Electrolytes

Haemoglobin is responsible for the red colour of the blood, and changes its colour according to the amount of oxygen present in the blood. If the blood is rich in oxygen it is coloured bright red, but if it is depleted of oxygen and has a high content of carbon dioxide it is a darker, almost purple colour. The structure of haemoglobin and its function in the carriage of the respiratory gases will be dealt with in the chapter on respiration.

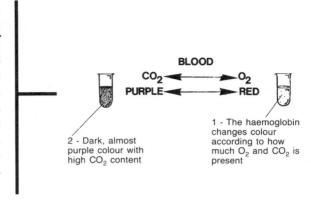

1 - The haemoglobin changes colour according to how much O_2 and CO_2 is present

2 - Dark, almost purple colour with high CO_2 content

Since haemoglobin is highly coloured, we can measure its concentration in blood by colorimetric methods. Unfortunately, it changes colour as it binds oxygen, so we need to convert it to a more stable form. One method, the **Sahli** method is to bubble carbon monoxide through the blood. This binds almost irreversibly with the haemoglobin, displacing oxygen and imparting a bright red cherry colour which is easily measured by comparing the sample to a standard with known concentration. (The original standard, representing 100% normal haemoglobin, was a sample of Dr Sahli's own blood!)

Another technique consists of adding acid to the blood, changing haemoglobin irreversibly to acid haematin, and comparing the resultant colour with a standard (Haldane's method).

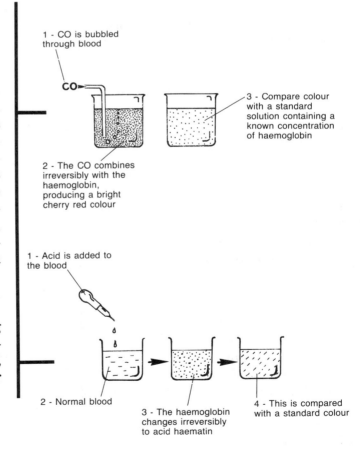

1 - CO is bubbled through blood

2 - The CO combines irreversibly with the haemoglobin, producing a bright cherry red colour

3 - Compare colour with a standard solution containing a known concentration of haemoglobin

1 - Acid is added to the blood

2 - Normal blood

3 - The haemoglobin changes irreversibly to acid haematin

4 - This is compared with a standard colour

The most satisfactory method, used in most hospital laboratories, is to rupture the cells with saponin (a detergent) to release the haemoglobin and then add ferricyanide to produce **cyanmethaemoglobin**, a stable molecule whose concentration is measured in a **colorimeter**. This detects how much light of a precise wavelength is absorbed by the sample, and is calibrated against known standards.

Knowing the haemoglobin concentration, red cell count and packed cell volume, we can calculate various secondary blood indices. These include the **mean corpuscular volume** (MCV), which is the haematocrit divided by the red cell count, and the **mean corpuscular haemoglobin concentration** (MCHC), which is the haemoglobin concentration divided by the haematocrit. These indices are valuable in the diagnosis of anaemia.

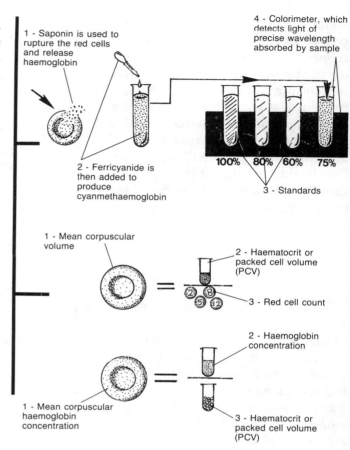

The white cells

The white cells or **leucocytes** are divided into **granulocytes**, which have granules in their cytoplasm and have multilobed nuclei which result in their being called **polymorphonuclear** cells, and **lymphocytes, monocytes** and **plasma cells**, which have no granules and have rather simpler nuclei.

The polymorphonuclear granulocytes or **polymorphs** are further subdivided according to their histochemical staining reaction into **neutrophils**, which do not bind either acidic or basic stains, **basophils**, which stain deep blue with basic stains and therefore have acidic material in their granules, and **eosinophils**, whose granules take up the acidic red dye eosin and therefore must contain basic or alkaline material.

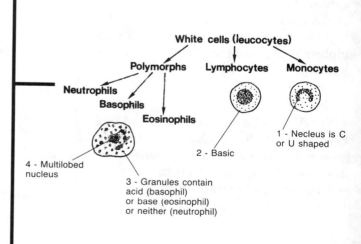

The granulocytes are slightly larger than the red cells, about 10 μm in diameter, and approximately spherical. The lymphocytes, which have a central densely staining nucleus and a bluish cytoplasm when stained with the usual histological stains, are slightly smaller, about 5−6 μm, and the monocytes look like rather large lymphocytes except that their nuclei are usually curved into a C or U shape; their diameter is about 10 μm.

The total number of white cells can be counted in a haemocytometer, in just the same way as red cells, but the white cells are much less abundant and so a much lower dilution factor must be used, and the cells must be stained with a dye which shows them up without displaying the red cells. The normal white cell count is 4000−10 000 per cubic millimetre (4−10 × 10^9 per litre), but can rise to much higher levels during infections or inflammations.

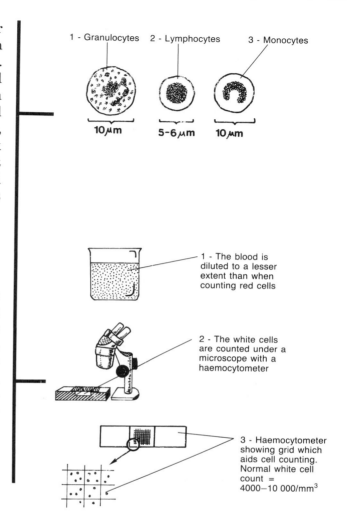

1 - Granulocytes   2 - Lymphocytes   3 - Monocytes

10 μm   5-6 μm   10 μm

1 - The blood is diluted to a lesser extent than when counting red cells

2 - The white cells are counted under a microscope with a haemocytometer

3 - Haemocytometer showing grid which aids cell counting. Normal white cell count = 4000−10 000/mm^3

It is important to know the relative abundance of the various sorts of leucocytes, as different types proliferate in different disease conditions. A drop of fresh capillary or venous blood is placed on a clean microscope slide, and the edge of another slide is used to smear the blood evenly in a thin layer along the surface of the slide.

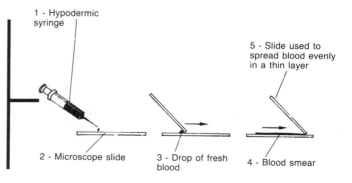

1 - Hypodermic syringe

5 - Slide used to spread blood evenly in a thin layer

2 - Microscope slide

3 - Drop of fresh blood

4 - Blood smear

After fixation and staining the blood smear is examined under the microscope using the high-power objective, and the distribution of cell types observed. It is usual to begin at one edge of the smear, and search across the slide, noting down the type of each cell encountered; when the opposite side of the smear is reached, the position of the slide is moved to scan a different area. This process is continued in a systematic way until 100 cells have been counted. The percentage of cells belonging to each type is calculated; such a description is known as the **differential white cell count** (DWCC). In modern laboratories the Coulter counter can perform the analysis automatically on a moving suspension of blood cells.

In a normal healthy person the most abundant white cell type is the neutrophil polymorph; the next most common is the lymphocyte; the other types are found rather infrequently.

Neutrophils	60–70%
Basophils	0–2%
Eosinophils	2–4%
Lymphocytes	20–30%
Monocytes	2–8%

1 - High-power objective of microscope

2 - After fixation and staining the blood smear is examined to note the distribution of cell types

3 - Search pattern

1 - White cells from blood suspension pass through the counter

2 - Electric current flows through gap

No. of Cells

100

1 - Differential white cell count (DWCC)

Neutrophils — Basophils — Eosinophils — Lymphocytes — Monocytes —

Functions of the leucocytes

Most of the leucocytes have a protective function; either they are scavengers, engulfing and destroying invading microorganisms and other debris, or they make or carry specific antibodies against foreign bodies or molecules. Many white cells are not really resident in the blood at all, but are merely found there while they make their way to some other tissue in the body where they are destined to exercise their protective function.

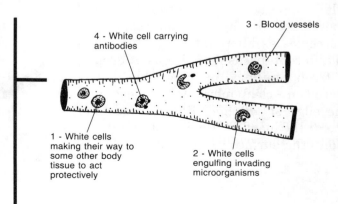

3 - Blood vessels

4 - White cell carrying antibodies

1 - White cells making their way to some other body tissue to act protectively

2 - White cells engulfing invading microorganisms

The **neutrophil** polymorphs are abundant, relatively non-specific protective cells which migrate in large numbers to a site of injury, invasion or infection, where they try to destroy the invaders by engulfing them.

They do this by **phagocytosis**, the thrusting out of finger-like projections or **pseudopodia** from the cytoplasm which surround the invader and draw it into the cell's substance, where it is attacked and dissolved by the enzymes which are contained in the cell's granules. Large numbers of neutrophils die in this process; their debris and that of their victims forms a yellow viscous liquid or **pus** at the site of infection, and neutrophils are often known as pus cells.

The **basophils** probably have no real function in the blood, but exert their true effects when they reach the peripheral tissues. When they are found in the tissues they are known as **mast cells** and are important as mediators of inflammation. Many substances and many antigen—antibody reactions cause the mast cells to release the contents of their granules into the interstitial fluid. The contents include several very potent chemicals such as histamine, substance P and heparin, which can profoundly alter local tissue blood flow, the permeability of capillaries or the coagulability of the blood.

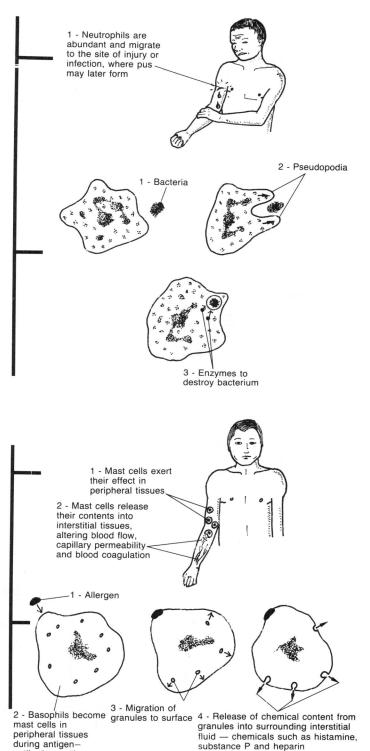

1 - Neutrophils are abundant and migrate to the site of injury or infection, where pus may later form

1 - Bacteria

2 - Pseudopodia

3 - Enzymes to destroy bacterium

1 - Mast cells exert their effect in peripheral tissues

2 - Mast cells release their contents into interstitial tissues, altering blood flow, capillary permeability and blood coagulation

1 - Allergen

2 - Basophils become mast cells in peripheral tissues during antigen—antibody reaction

3 - Migration of granules to surface

4 - Release of chemical content from granules into surrounding interstitial fluid — chemicals such as histamine, substance P and heparin

The function of **eosinophils** is still rather obscure. They are found in rather high numbers in the blood and tissues of individuals with allergic conditions like bronchial asthma, and in patients infested with worms or other parasites.

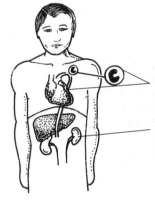

1 - Eosinophils are found in the blood and tissues in high numbers in cases of:

2 - Bronchial asthma

3 - Tapeworm infestation

The **monocytes**, like the basophils, are cells of passage through the blood, and exert their chief effects when they reach the tissues, where they become known as **histiocytes** or **macrophages** (literally 'large eaters').

1 - Monocytes in the blood vascular system

2 - In the tissues monocytes are known as histiocytes or macrophages and have greater phagocytic activity than neutrophils

Macrophages have a phagocytic function, engulfing and destroying bacteria and particles of dust or soot. The phagocytic capacity of macrophages is much greater than that of neutrophils; while a neutrophil can engulf and destroy about 5—10 bacteria, a macrophage can cope with up to 100. When they are confronted with particularly large or indigestible particles, groups of macrophages can become aggregated to form **giant cells** which surround and often destroy the invader. Macrophages contain several enzymes including **lipase**, which can destroy the fatty coats of many bacterial types, including the organisms responsible for tuberculosis and leprosy.

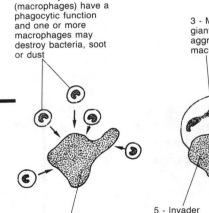

1 - Monocytes (macrophages) have a phagocytic function and one or more macrophages may destroy bacteria, soot or dust

3 - Multinucleated giant cell formed by aggregation of several macrophages

2 - Large invader

4 - Enzyme of macrophages can destroy fatty coat of bacteria

5 - Invader

The **lymphocytes** are concerned with the body's **immune** responses. When an organism or a foreign body invades the body, fragments are engulfed by the phagocytic cells and carried to the nearest lymph node, where special lymphocytes become transformed into **plasma cells** and manufacture large quantities of **antibodies** against the invader. These antibodies are released into the blood, and combine with the invading organisms or molecules (the **antigens**) and bring about their destruction, either by direct chemical attack, or by rendering them more susceptible to attack by phagocytic cells.

The first time that the body encounters a particular antigen, a moderate amount of antibody is manufactured, but a subsequent exposure to the same antigen in a previously **sensitized** individual causes a much greater response and the production of very large amounts of antibody.

Antibodies may be of two types: free in the plasma (soluble), or attached to cells. There are thus two types of lymphocytes: those which make soluble antibodies, and those which carry antibodies attached to their surfaces. For more details the student is referred to textbooks of microbiology or immunology.

The **platelets** are tiny fragments of cells whose function is to promote blood clotting; this function is described in detail later in this chapter.

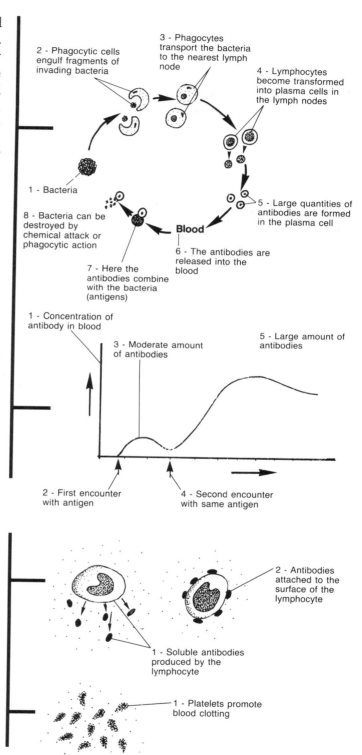

2 - Phagocytic cells engulf fragments of invading bacteria
3 - Phagocytes transport the bacteria to the nearest lymph node
4 - Lymphocytes become transformed into plasma cells in the lymph nodes
1 - Bacteria
8 - Bacteria can be destroyed by chemical attack or phagocytic action
5 - Large quantities of antibodies are formed in the plasma cell
Blood
6 - The antibodies are released into the blood
7 - Here the antibodies combine with the bacteria (antigens)

1 - Concentration of antibody in blood
3 - Moderate amount of antibodies
5 - Large amount of antibodies
2 - First encounter with antigen
4 - Second encounter with same antigen

2 - Antibodies attached to the surface of the lymphocyte
1 - Soluble antibodies produced by the lymphocyte
1 - Platelets promote blood clotting

THE FORMATION OF BLOOD CELLS

The process of **haemopoiesis** (the formation of blood cells) takes place at three main sites: bone marrow, the spleen and the lymph nodes. The lymphocytes are manufactured in the lymph nodes scattered throughout the body, monocytes originate in the spleen and bone marrow, and the rest of the formed elements of the blood are made in the bone marrow.

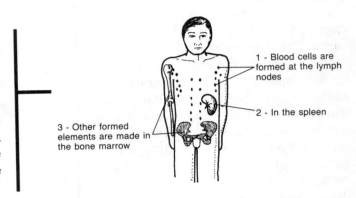

1 - Blood cells are formed at the lymph nodes

2 - In the spleen

3 - Other formed elements are made in the bone marrow

Bone marrow, found in the cavities at the centre of all bones, may be of two types: red or white. White marrow, found chiefly in the shafts of the long bones, consists largely of fibrous tissue and fat, and probably represents red marrow which has ceased to function. Red marrow, found in the flat bones such as the sternum and the pelvis in adults, but found also in the long bones of children, consists of a network of **trabeculae** — spikes of bone and fibrous tissue which support the lining of a series of blood-filled cavities or **sinusoids**. The cells lining the cavities are in a highly active state, constantly dividing and developing, to produce finally the mature cell types which will be released into the blood.

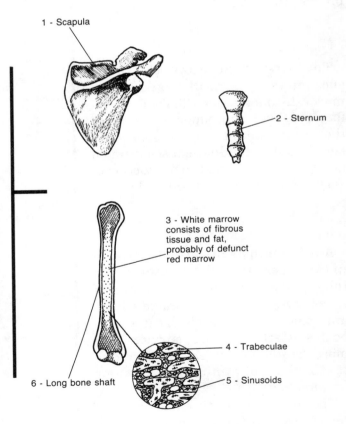

1 - Scapula

2 - Sternum

3 - White marrow consists of fibrous tissue and fat, probably of defunct red marrow

4 - Trabeculae

5 - Sinusoids

6 - Long bone shaft

In the marrow there are primitive stem cells called **haemocytoblasts** from which all other cell types are eventually derived. These can differentiate into **proerythroblasts** from which the red cells develop, **myeloblasts** from which the various granulocytes develop, **monoblasts** from which the monocytes develop, or **megakaryocytes** from which the platelets bud off as tiny fragments.

The proerythroblasts undergo several stages of development, through **normoblasts** of various types and **reticulocytes**, until mature erythrocytes are formed. It is during the normoblast stage that the nucleus is lost, and the reticulocyte is so called because only a faintly staining **reticulum** of nucleic acids remains in the cytoplasm.

During times of increased demand for red cells, for instance after blood loss, some immature reitculocytes may be released into the circulation as well as the red cells.

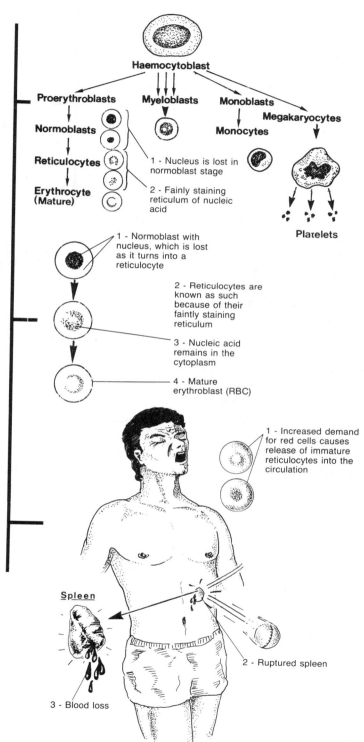

Haemocytoblast

Proerythroblasts   Myeloblasts   Monoblasts

Megakaryocytes

Normoblasts   Monocytes

Reticulocytes

1 - Nucleus is lost in normoblast stage

Erythrocyte (Mature)

2 - Fainly staining reticulum of nucleic acid

Platelets

1 - Normoblast with nucleus, which is lost as it turns into a reticulocyte

2 - Reticulocytes are known as such because of their faintly staining reticulum

3 - Nucleic acid remains in the cytoplasm

4 - Mature erythroblast (RBC)

1 - Increased demand for red cells causes release of immature reticulocytes into the circulation

Spleen

2 - Ruptured spleen

3 - Blood loss

The correct maturation of the various stages in the red cell series requires the presence of a number of key nutrients in the diet. Iron is necessary for the synthesis of the haem part of haemoglobin, and protein is required for the globin part, as well as for general synthetic pathways throughout the marrow. Vitamin B_{12} is needed for proper cell division and differentiation, and this substance is normally present in adequate quantities in a normal mixed diet. However, an **intrinsic factor** secreted from the stomach is needed for the absorption of the vitamin, and the individual who is deficient in intrinsic factor develops **pernicious anaemia**, with abnormal red cells called **megaloblasts** in his peripheral blood. The total number of red cells is reduced and hence the total oxygen-carrying capacity is reduced. Fortunately the condition is readily treatable with monthly injections of vitamin B_{12}. A similar megaloblastic anaemia can be caused by deficiency of folic acid in the diet; this is treated by dietary supplement.

The various groups of **granulocytes** are produced by differentiation of primitive cells into one of three lines (corresponding to neutrophils, basophils and eosinophils) and development through various stages known as **myelocytes** and **metamyelocytes**, with eventual appearance of the mature forms.

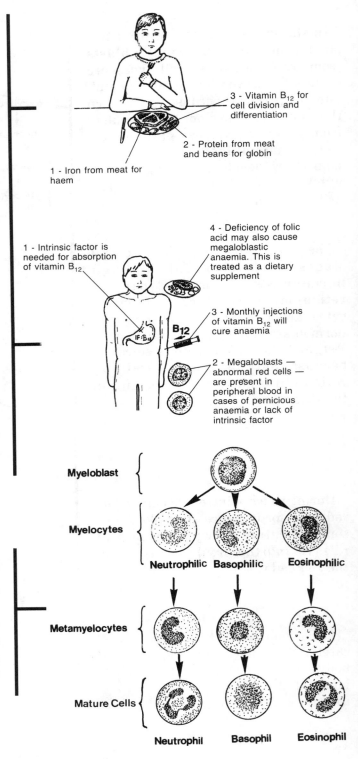

3 - Vitamin B_{12} for cell division and differentiation

2 - Protein from meat and beans for globin

1 - Iron from meat for haem

1 - Intrinsic factor is needed for absorption of vitamin B_{12}

4 - Deficiency of folic acid may also cause megaloblastic anaemia. This is treated as a dietary supplement

3 - Monthly injections of vitamin B_{12} will cure anaemia

2 - Megaloblasts — abnormal red cells — are present in peripheral blood in cases of pernicious anaemia or lack of intrinsic factor

B_{12}

Myeloblast

Myelocytes

Neutrophilic   Basophilic   Eosinophilic

Metamyelocytes

Mature Cells

Neutrophil   Basophil   Eosinophil

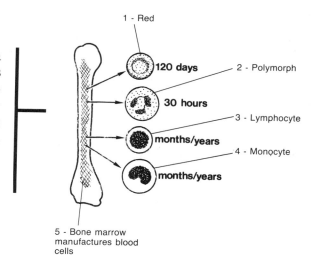

Red cells survive in the circulation for about 120 days; most polymorphs survive only about 30 hours; the lymphocytes and monocytes may survive for months or even years. It is necessary for the cells of the blood to be continuously replenished, and bone marrow is one of the most active and rapidly dividing tissues in the body.

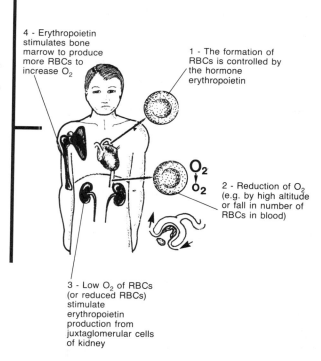

The formation of red cells is controlled by a hormone called **erythropoietin**. If the oxygen content of the blood is reduced, either by a fall in the number of red cells or by a decrease in the amount of available oxygen (such as would occur at high altitude) then this is detected by **juxtaglomerular** cells in the kidney, which release erythropoietin; this hormone stimulates the bone marrow to produce more red cells. A return to normal oxygen content will allow the kidney cells to stop producing erythropoietin until the next time the oxygen content falls.

The formation of leucocytes is also carefully controlled, and adjusted to the body's needs. However, the mechanisms of this control are not yet understood.

BLOOD GROUPS

Since the body has an efficient mechanism for recognizing and eliminating foreign proteins, it seems remarkable that it is possible to introduce any tissue or fluid from one individual into another. However, blood from certain individuals can be injected (**transfused**) into others, without any damage to the recipient. Blood from other individuals produces a catastrophic reaction in the recipient, in other words there are compatible and incompatible blood 'types' or 'groups'.

The reason why blood transfusion is possible at all is that there are only a few distinct groups of antigens present on the walls of red cells, and thus there is a relatively high chance of finding another individual with a compatible set of antigens and antibodies.

The most important set of blood group antigens belongs to the ABO system; this was the first system of blood groups to be discovered. A person in group A has A-type antigens on the cell walls of his erythrocytes; a person of group B has B-type antigens. A person of group A has pre-formed antibodies in his serum against B-type antigens; these antibodies are unusual in being present from birth — the person need never have been exposed to the B-type antigens. Similarly a person of group B has pre-formed anti-A antibodies in his serum. There are two further groups in this system: group AB in which both A-type and B-type antigens are present on the red cells (and obviously neither type of antibody is present in the serum), and group O which has neither type of antigen on the red cells but both types of antibody in the serum.

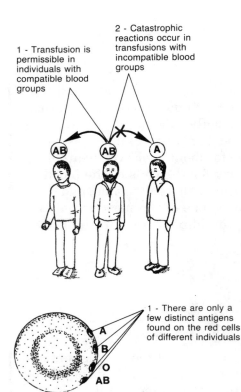

1 - Transfusion is permissible in individuals with compatible blood groups

2 - Catastrophic reactions occur in transfusions with incompatible blood groups

1 - There are only a few distinct antigens found on the red cells of different individuals

Group	Cells (antigen)	Serum (antibodies)
A	A	Anti-B
B	B	Anti-A
AB	A,B	—
O	—	Anti-A, Anti-B

1 - Antigens are present on the cell walls of RBCs

2 - These antibodies are present from birth and did not require exposure to any antigens

If an individual of group A is given blood of type B or even AB, then the antibodies in his serum attack the B-type antigens on the donor red cells and produce a **haemolytic** reaction, i.e. the red cells are broken down and destroyed. The contents are released into the plasma, and may cause illness.

The patient may begin to feel feverish, with a raised temperature and an acceleration of heart rate. The free haemoglobin in his blood may block up the fine capillaries throughout his body and may in particular block up the fine tubules in the kidney, causing irreversible and potentially fatal renal damage.

Similar events follow the giving of type A blood to a person in group B, or the giving of AB blood to someone in group O (or A or B). Fortunately it is possible to test for compatibility in the laboratory by mixing appropriate samples of known cells and serum with those of the potential donor and recipient; incompatibilities are revealed by the reaction of **agglutination**, or clumping together of the red cells. If donor and recipient are found to belong to the same blood group, it is still necessary to do a direct **cross-match** between the two samples of blood to ensure that haemolysis does not take place.

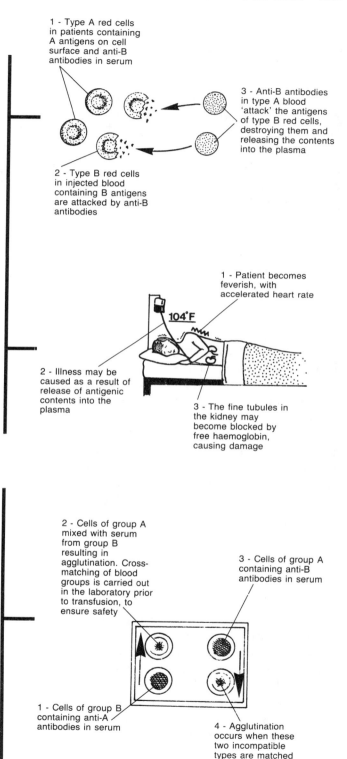

1 - Type A red cells in patients containing A antigens on cell surface and anti-B antibodies in serum

3 - Anti-B antibodies in type A blood 'attack' the antigens of type B red cells, destroying them and releasing the contents into the plasma

2 - Type B red cells in injected blood containing B antigens are attacked by anti-B antibodies

1 - Patient becomes feverish, with accelerated heart rate

104°F

2 - Illness may be caused as a result of release of antigenic contents into the plasma

3 - The fine tubules in the kidney may become blocked by free haemoglobin, causing damage

2 - Cells of group A mixed with serum from group B resulting in agglutination. Cross-matching of blood groups is carried out in the laboratory prior to transfusion, to ensure safety

3 - Cells of group A containing anti-B antibodies in serum

1 - Cells of group B containing anti-A antibodies in serum

4 - Agglutination occurs when these two incompatible types are matched

The blood groups are inherited in a fairly simple manner; a child receives a gene from each of its parents, and if both parents are homozygous for group A then the child will also be of group A. If one parent contributes an A gene and the other contributes a B gene then the child has blood group AB; if neither parent contributes a specific gene, the child will have group O. In European populations about 45% of people belong to group A, 43% to group O, 9% to group B and 3% to group AB. These proportions vary slightly among other racial groups.

Another clinically important blood group system is the **rhesus** system (so called because it was first discovered by injecting cells from rhesus monkeys into rabbits). A large proportion of people (85%) have the Rh antigen on their red cells, and are called Rh-positive. The remaining 15% are called Rh-negative and have no antigen, but also are not born with pre-formed antibodies against the Rh antigen.

Antibodies are only formed if the person becomes exposed to Rh-positive antigens; this is a fairly unlikely event except in the case of an Rh-negative mother who is carrying an Rh-positive fetus in her uterus. Fetal red cells may enter the mother's circulation during birth, pre- or post-partum haemorrhage, or abortion (miscarriage), and may sensitize the mother to produce antibodies against Rh-positive cells.

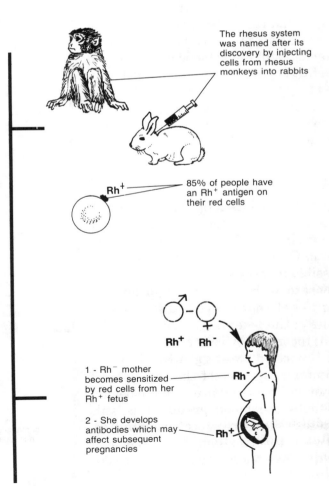

The rhesus system was named after its discovery by injecting cells from rhesus monkeys into rabbits

85% of people have an Rh+ antigen on their red cells

1 - Rh− mother becomes sensitized by red cells from her Rh+ fetus

2 - She develops antibodies which may affect subsequent pregnancies

This may not matter in the current pregnancy, but the fetus in a subsequent pregnancy may be attacked by the maternal antibodies, which may cross the placenta, enter the fetal circulation and cause lysis of the fetal red cells. The baby may die before birth, or may be born severely anaemic and very jaundiced (yellow) due to the breakdown of haemoglobin in the blood. An exchange transfusion, in which most of the baby's blood is replaced by fresh blood, may be required.

There are other blood group systems including the Kell and MN systems; these are of minor clinical importance, but may be useful in genetic tracing, for example to establish claims for paternity.

4 - Blood

1 - Maternal antibodies may enter the fetus via the placenta and cause lysis of the fetal red cells

2 - The baby may die or be born severely anaemic and jaundiced

3 - An exchange transfusion may be required

1 - Parents

2 - Child

3 - The normal ABO system may be insufficient in establishing paternal claims

4 - The MN system and the Kell system can be used to establish claims for paternity

HAEMOSTASIS

Haemostasis is the name given to the mechanisms which prevent blood loss when the body is injured, and prevent seepage of blood into the tissues from leaky blood vessels.

If there is damage to a blood vessel or to body tissues, a set of protective reactions is initiated; some of these reactions are non-specific, such as **vascular spasm** and the formation of **platelet plugs**; other reactions are highly specific and very complex, such as **blood clotting**.

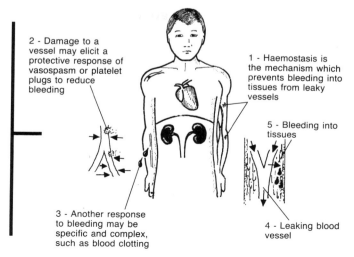

2 - Damage to a vessel may elicit a protective response of vasospasm or platelet plugs to reduce bleeding

1 - Haemostasis is the mechanism which prevents bleeding into tissues from leaky vessels

5 - Bleeding into tissues

3 - Another response to bleeding may be specific and complex, such as blood clotting

4 - Leaking blood vessel

Injury to a blood vessel causes spasm of the vessel wall; this reduces the flow of blood to the site of the injury, causing less blood to be lost and allowing the other protective mechanisms more time to be effective. The **bleeding time** is an indicator of the efficiency of the vascular reaction, and is measured by pricking a finger with a needle, and wiping the blood off at half-minute intervals until the bleeding stops.

The vascular spasm is caused partly by a direct stimulant effect on the smooth muscle of the vessel wall; by nervous reflexes, possibly involving the pain pathways; by the release of vasoconstrictor substances from damaged cells in the vessel wall and surrounding tissues; and by the release of a potent vasoconstrictor (serotonin) from the blood platelets. The greater the amount of tissue damage, the greater the degree of vascular spasm. This is one reason why a crushing or tearing injury may actually bleed less than a clean cut with a knife or scalpel.

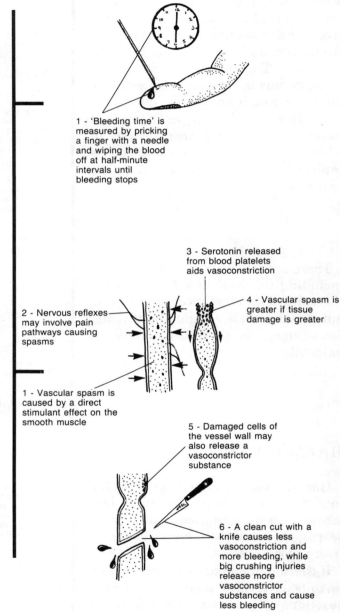

1 - 'Bleeding time' is measured by pricking a finger with a needle and wiping the blood off at half-minute intervals until bleeding stops

3 - Serotonin released from blood platelets aids vasoconstriction

4 - Vascular spasm is greater if tissue damage is greater

2 - Nervous reflexes may involve pain pathways causing spasms

1 - Vascular spasm is caused by a direct stimulant effect on the smooth muscle

5 - Damaged cells of the vessel wall may also release a vasoconstrictor substance

6 - A clean cut with a knife causes less vasoconstriction and more bleeding, while big crushing injuries release more vasoconstrictor substances and cause less bleeding

Injury to the endothelium of blood vessels causes the formation of a platelet plug, which makes a temporary seal for the defect, rather like sandbags are used to produce temporary seals in breached river banks or sea walls. The vascular endothelium is not normally a water-wettable surface, but any defect in the wall allows platelets to make contact with underlying wettable structures like collagen. The platelets liberate chemicals which attract other platelets to migrate to the site of injury, and become sticky; they stick both to the wall of the vessel and to one another. Eventually they congeal, their cell walls break down, and they form a cohesive mass which plugs the gap in the vessel.

The altered platelets also release chemicals which initiate the definitive clotting mechanism, eventually producing a more permanent seal. Clotting consists of the deposition of strands of the protein **fibrin** around the platelet plug, trapping yet more platelets, as well as red and white blood cells. After some hours the fibrin meshwork becomes tighter, binding all of the constituents of the clot together and forming a really effective seal which permanently repairs the defect in the vessel wall.

Later the clot is attacked and broken down by enzymes known as **fibrinolysins**, and is invaded by capillaries and fibroblasts; the vesssel wall is remodelled and its former profile is eventually restored.

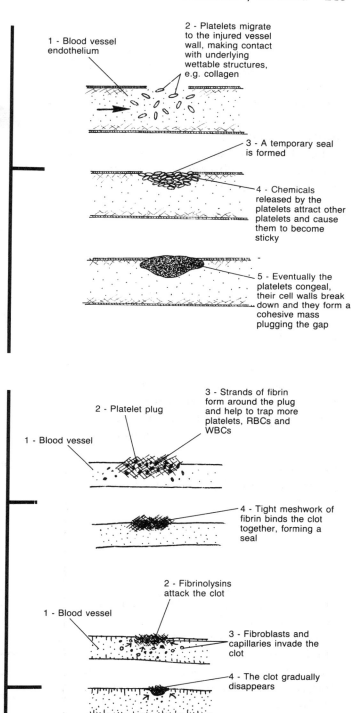

1 - Blood vessel endothelium

2 - Platelets migrate to the injured vessel wall, making contact with underlying wettable structures, e.g. collagen

3 - A temporary seal is formed

4 - Chemicals released by the platelets attract other platelets and cause them to become sticky

5 - Eventually the platelets congeal, their cell walls break down and they form a cohesive mass plugging the gap

1 - Blood vessel

2 - Platelet plug

3 - Strands of fibrin form around the plug and help to trap more platelets, RBCs and WBCs

4 - Tight meshwork of fibrin binds the clot together, forming a seal

1 - Blood vessel

2 - Fibrinolysins attack the clot

3 - Fibroblasts and capillaries invade the clot

4 - The clot gradually disappears

5 - The vessel wall returns to its former profile

The **clotting time** is measured by taking a sample of blood into a glass tube (a water-wettable surface), placing the tube into a water-bath at 37 °C, and inverting the tube every 15 seconds until the blood no longer flows in the tube. The time is, naturally, determined by the efficacy of the whole clotting process.

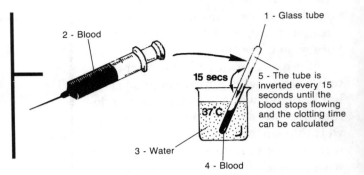

2 - Blood

1 - Glass tube

15 secs

37 C

5 - The tube is inverted every 15 seconds until the blood stops flowing and the clotting time can be calculated

3 - Water

4 - Blood

Clotting

The fundamental reaction of blood clotting is the conversion of the soluble plasma protein **fibrinogen** to the insoluble protein **fibrin**. This reaction is catalyzed by the enzyme **thrombin**, which is not normally present in plasma, but is formed from the inactive precursor **prothrombin**, another plasma protein.

FIBRINOGEN ⟶ FIBRIN
[soluble]   [insoluble]

THROMBIN
[active enzyme]

PROTHROMBIN
[inactive precursor]

The action of thrombin is to remove the terminal part of the fibrinogen molecule, rather like removing the cap of a pen. This exposes an active site on the fibrinogen molecule, allowing large numbers of molecules to become joined together, forming long protein strands of insoluble fibrin. This process is known as **polymerization**.

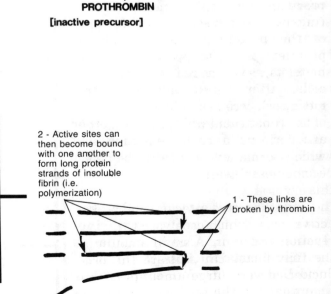

2 - Active sites can then become bound with one another to form long protein strands of insoluble fibrin (i.e. polymerization)

1 - These links are broken by thrombin

The conversion of prothrombin to thrombin may be initiated by one of two mechanisms, an 'extrinsic' pathway and an 'intrinsic' pathway. In the extrinsic pathway, damage inflicted on tissues surrounding blood vessels causes release of various proteins and lipids which are together known as 'tissue thromboplastin', and which can initiate clotting very rapidly, within 15 seconds.

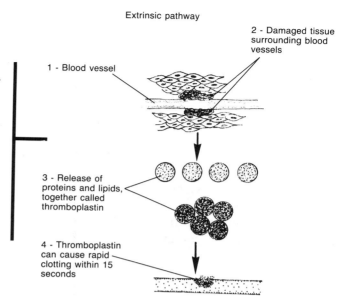

Extrinsic pathway

1 - Blood vessel

2 - Damaged tissue surrounding blood vessels

3 - Release of proteins and lipids, together called thromboplastin

4 - Thromboplastin can cause rapid clotting within 15 seconds

In the intrinsic pathway, blood comes into contact with a water-wettable surface such as collagen (or the glass of a test-tube, but not plastic, silicone or paraffin); this contact starts a **'cascade'** or chain reaction — a sequence of enzymic conversions which leads eventually to the formation of thrombin. This pathway is rather slower than the extrinsic pathway, taking 2−3 minutes to produce clotting.

The term 'cascade' refers to a sequence of chemical reactions in which one inactive precursor (or factor) becomes changed to an active enzyme; this enzyme catalysts the conversion of the next inactive precursor into its active form, which catalyses the next reaction and so on. A small amount of the first factor can initiate the production of very large amounts of the final factor in the sequence. Many of these reactions require the presence of calcium ions as a cofactor.

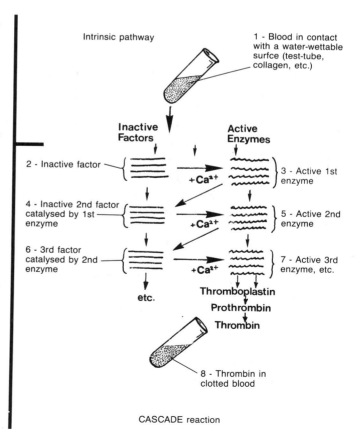

Intrinsic pathway

1 - Blood in contact with a water-wettable surfce (test-tube, collagen, etc.)

Inactive Factors

Active Enzymes

2 - Inactive factor

$+Ca^{2+}$

3 - Active 1st enzyme

4 - Inactive 2nd factor catalysed by 1st enzyme

$+Ca^{2+}$

5 - Active 2nd enzyme

6 - 3rd factor catalysed by 2nd enzyme

$+Ca^{2+}$

7 - Active 3rd enzyme, etc.

etc.

Thromboplastin

Prothrombin

Thrombin

8 - Thrombin in clotted blood

CASCADE reaction

THE CLOTTING FACTORS

Factor	Alternative name
I	Fibrinogen
II	Prothrombin
III	Thromboplastin
IV	Calcium
V	Pro-accelerin
VI	(does not exist)
VII	Pro-convertin
VIII	Anti-haemophilic globulin
IX	Christmas factor
X	Stuart-Power factor
XI	Plasma thromboplastin antecedent
XII	Hageman factor
XIII	Fibrin-stabilizing factor

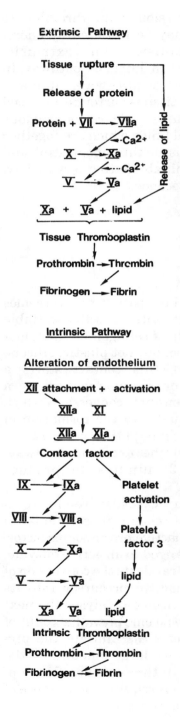

The actual details of blood clotting are quite complicated; a very large number of clotting factors have been discovered (see table), and they have been given numbers which are in the approximate order of their discovery. Some of the factors such as calcium, fibrinogen and thrombin are usually referred to by name rather than number, and some of the numbered factors have alternative names. Thus factor VIII is also known as anti-haemophilic globulin (AHG) and factor IX is known as Christmas factor, named after the patient in whom its lack was first discovered.

Most of the clotting factors are plasma proteins, manufactured in the liver, and often requiring the presence of cofactors for their formation. For instance, vitamin K is required for the synthesis of prothrombin by the liver.

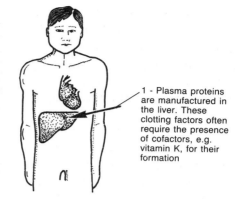

1 - Plasma proteins are manufactured in the liver. These clotting factors often require the presence of cofactors, e.g. vitamin K, for their formation

Why does not blood clot all the time?

If there is a small area of localized damage to a blood vessel, there may be a high local concentration of clotting factors, but the blood flowing past tends to wash them away and dilutes them in the general circulation, making them ineffective.

There needs to be quite a large injury before local concentration of clotting factors becomes high enough to cause clotting.

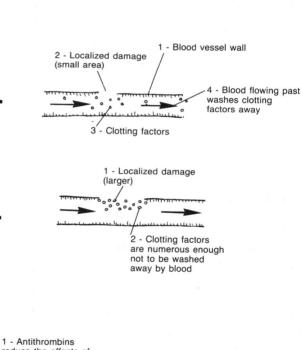

2 - Localized damage (small area)
1 - Blood vessel wall
4 - Blood flowing past washes clotting factors away
3 - Clotting factors

1 - Localized damage (larger)
2 - Clotting factors are numerous enough not to be washed away by blood

As the clotting factors are produced, a series of **antithrombins** are produced at the same time; these tend to reduce but not abolish the effects of the clotting factors. They are rather like the brakes of a car, preventing it from running out of control.

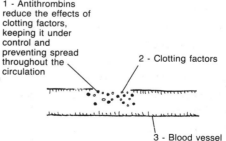

1 - Antithrombins reduce the effects of clotting factors, keeping it under control and preventing spread throughout the circulation
2 - Clotting factors
3 - Blood vessel

Some of the activated clotting factors also catalyse the conversion of **plasminogen** (another plasma protein) to **plasmin**, a proteolytic enzyme which breaks down fibrin. Thus fibrin may become broken down almost as rapidly as it is formed.

Normally in the body any tendency to clot spontaneously is prevented by these processes; however, when there is injury the stimulus to clotting becomes much greater, the protective mechanisms are overcome, and the blood clots. The anti-clotting mechanisms still serve to control the rate of clotting, and prevent it from spreading throughout the circulation.

1 - A plasma protein

2 - Clotting factors act as a catalyst

3 - A proteolytic enzyme which breaks down fibrin

Plasminogen ⟶ **Plasmin**

6 - Fibrin

4 - Broken-down fibrin

5 - Plasmin, an enzyme which breaks down fibrin

1 - Blood must be prevented from clotting following removal from the body since it is needed for transfusion or various laboratory tests

Anticoagulation

It is often necessary to prevent blood from clotting following its removal from the body, if it is to be used for transfusion or if various laboratory tests are to be performed. There are also clinical conditions in which it is necessary to prevent blood from clotting within the body.

One useful *in vitro* method is to remove or absorb the calcium ions, by the addition of citrate (for transfusion), oxalate or chelating agents like EDTA (ethylenediaminetetraacetic acid). This technique is obviously not suitable *in vivo*, as calcium has many other important roles and its removal from the blood of a living individual would be lethal.

2 - Certain clinical conditions (e.g. thrombosis) may also require that the blood is prevented from clotting within the body

3 - Blood clot

1 - Citrate, oxalate or EDTA is added to the blood to remove or absorb the calcium ions and prevent blood clotting (suitable for *in vivo* purposes only)

2 - Blood

Another technique is to add to the blood a molecule which has a high electric charge, which combines with molecules of fibrin and other clotting factors and causes them to repel each other, preventing their aggregation into long chains and thus preventing clotting. This is the mode of action of **heparin**, a naturally occurring anticoagulant found in the liver and the mast cells.

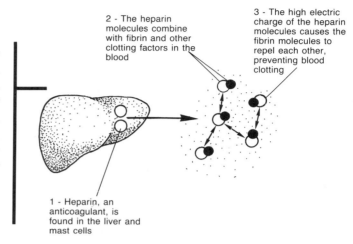

2 - The heparin molecules combine with fibrin and other clotting factors in the blood

3 - The high electric charge of the heparin molecules causes the fibrin molecules to repel each other, preventing blood clotting

1 - Heparin, an anticoagulant, is found in the liver and mast cells

A third approach is to give a drug which interferes with the sythesis of clotting factors in the liver. This approach only works for long-term anti-coagulation, and would be quite ineffective in preventing clotting *in vitro*. For example, **warfarin** is a vitamin K antagonist which prevents the formation of prothrombin, and is widely used for anticoagulant therapy in patients following coronary or cerebral artery thrombosis or pulmonary embolism. In all patients undergoing anticoagulant therapy it is essential to keep a careful check on the clotting time or the rate of prothrombin production.

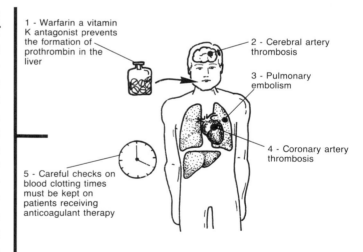

1 - Warfarin a vitamin K antagonist prevents the formation of prothrombin in the liver

2 - Cerebral artery thrombosis

3 - Pulmonary embolism

4 - Coronary artery thrombosis

5 - Careful checks on blood clotting times must be kept on patients receiving anticoagulant therapy

The Circulation

The circulatory system, comprising the heart and the peripheral blood vessels, is concerned with distributing the blood around tbe body to all of the tissues according to their needs, and with passing blood returned from the tissues through the lungs in order to replenish it with fresh gases.

The heart is the pump driving the system; it has muscular contractile walls and a series of valves which ensure that blood flows in only one direction.

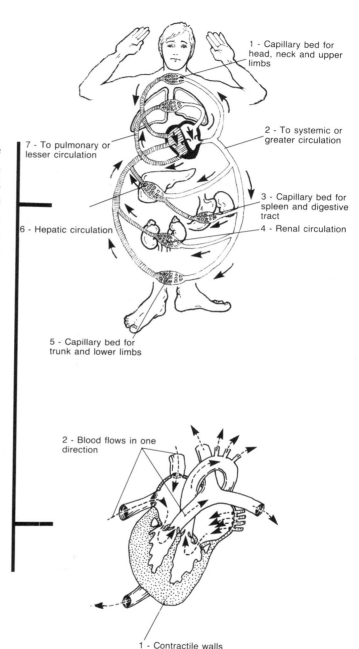

1 - Capillary bed for head, neck and upper limbs

2 - To systemic or greater circulation

3 - Capillary bed for spleen and digestive tract

4 - Renal circulation

7 - To pulmonary or lesser circulation

6 - Hepatic circulation

5 - Capillary bed for trunk and lower limbs

2 - Blood flows in one direction

1 - Contractile walls

The blood is pumped into the major arteries, whence it is distributed through smaller and smaller branching arteries, then through arterioles into the capillaries; here the major exchange of nutrients, gases and waste products occurs between blood and tissues. The blood from capillaries is collected into venules which join together to form small veins, and these drain into bigger and bigger veins which eventually empty into the heart through the superior and inferior venae cavae. By the time the blood reaches the veins, much of the energy imparted by the heart has dissipated, so many veins have valves to ensure that the blood keeps flowing in the right direction.

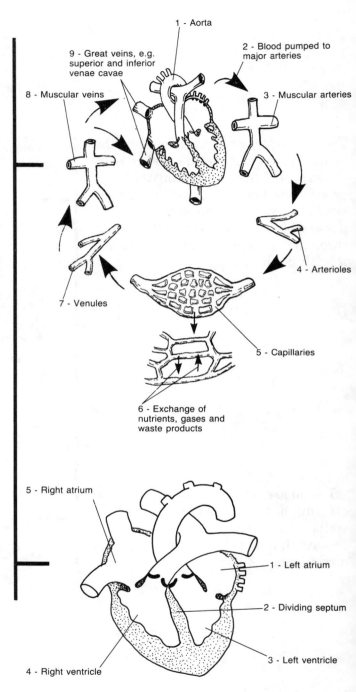

1 - Aorta
2 - Blood pumped to major arteries
3 - Muscular arteries
4 - Arterioles
5 - Capillaries
6 - Exchange of nutrients, gases and waste products
7 - Venules
8 - Muscular veins
9 - Great veins, e.g. superior and inferior venae cavae

5 - Right atrium
1 - Left atrium
2 - Dividing septum
3 - Left ventricle
4 - Right ventricle

The heart has four chambers, arranged as a pair on the right and a pair on the left side of a muscular dividing **septum**.

The two chambers on the right, the atrium and the ventricle, are concerned with collecting the used systemic blood returning in the great veins and pumping it out into the pulmonary artery and through the lungs.

The atrium and ventricle on the left side collect the replenished blood returning from the lungs through the pulmonary veins and pump it out through the aorta (the major artery) to supply the whole of the body.

There are valves between each atrium and its ventricle, and between each ventricle and its corresponding major artery.

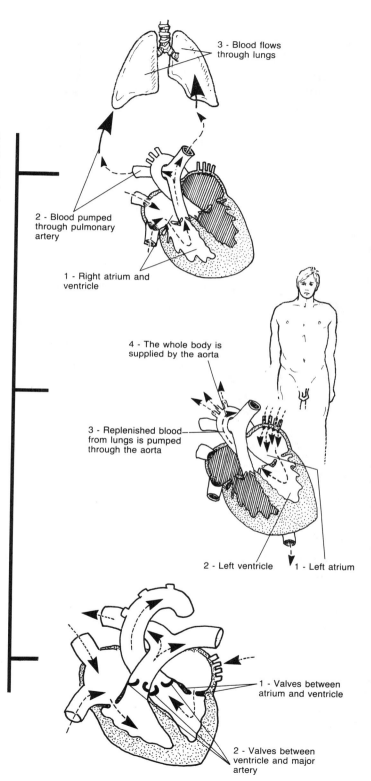

3 - Blood flows through lungs

2 - Blood pumped through pulmonary artery

1 - Right atrium and ventricle

4 - The whole body is supplied by the aorta

3 - Replenished blood from lungs is pumped through the aorta

2 - Left ventricle

1 - Left atrium

1 - Valves between atrium and ventricle

2 - Valves between ventricle and major artery

The right atrioventricular valve is called the **tricuspid** valve because it has three leaflets, and the atrioventricular valve on the left is known as the **mitral** valve because it looks like a bishop's hat. The right ventricular outlet valve is the **pulmonary** valve, and the left one is the **aortic** valve.

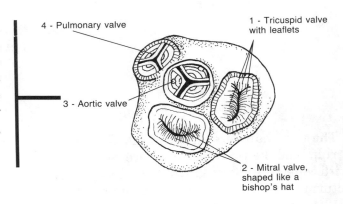

4 - Pulmonary valve

1 - Tricuspid valve with leaflets

3 - Aortic valve

2 - Mitral valve, shaped like a bishop's hat

INITIATION OF THE HEART BEAT

The heart is composed of specialized striated muscle which contracts and relaxes in a rhythmic fashion.

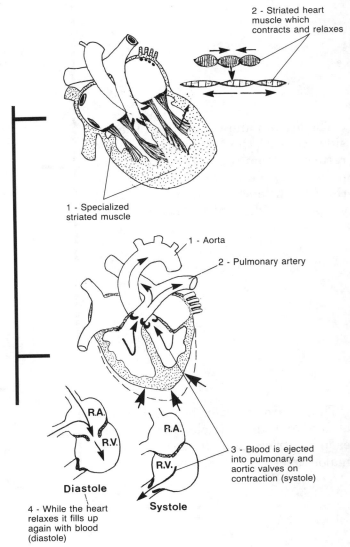

2 - Striated heart muscle which contracts and relaxes

1 - Specialized striated muscle

While it contracts (systole) it squeezes blood out through the pulmonary and aortic valves; while it relaxes (diastole) it fills up again with blood returning it to the veins.

1 - Aorta

2 - Pulmonary artery

R.A.

R.V.

Diastole

R.A.

R.V.

Systole

3 - Blood is ejected into pulmonary and aortic valves on contraction (systole)

4 - While the heart relaxes it fills up again with blood (diastole)

The rhythmic contraction and relaxation is brought about by the initiation and spread of electrical impulses throughout the heart muscle. The electrical events occur independently of any intervention from the nervous system; they are intrinsic properties of the heart muscle itself.

There is a negative potential difference between the inside of each cell and the bathing fluid (the membrane potential); the membrane is **polarized**.

When any cell of the heart muscle (myocardium) is electrically excited above a certain **threshold** level it discharges an electrical impulse or **action potential**; the membrane is **depolarized**, and the inside of the cells becomes positive with respect to the outside.

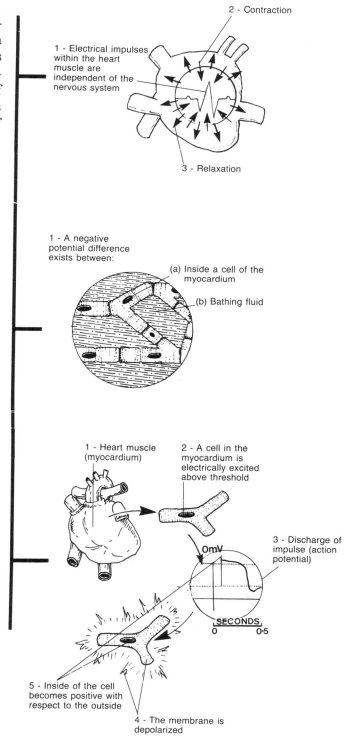

1 - Electrical impulses within the heart muscle are independent of the nervous system

2 - Contraction

3 - Relaxation

1 - A negative potential difference exists between:

(a) Inside a cell of the myocardium

(b) Bathing fluid

1 - Heart muscle (myocardium)

2 - A cell in the myocardium is electrically excited above threshold

3 - Discharge of impulse (action potential)

0mV

SECONDS
0   0·5

5 - Inside of the cell becomes positive with respect to the outside

4 - The membrane is depolarized

An impulse in one cell can spread to adjacent cells through the **intercalated discs** or low-resistance contacts between cell membranes. The mechanisms of the action potential are described much more fully in the chapters on the nervous and muscular systems.

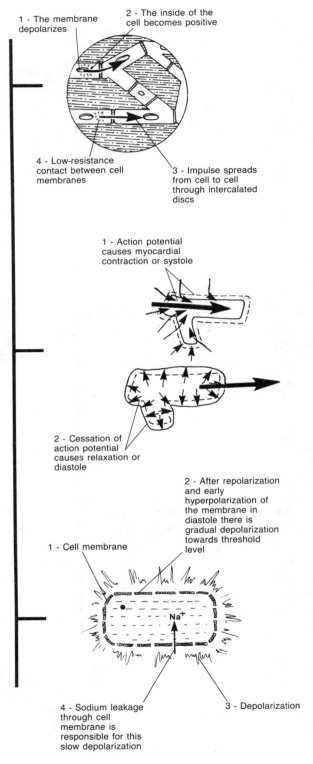

1 - The membrane depolarizes

2 - The inside of the cell becomes positive

4 - Low-resistance contact between cell membranes

3 - Impulse spreads from cell to cell through intercalated discs

1 - Action potential causes myocardial contraction or systole

The action potential in each myocardial cell causes contraction or systole; the cessation of the action potential allows relaxation or diastole.

2 - Cessation of action potential causes relaxation or diastole

2 - After repolarization and early hyperpolarization of the membrane in diastole there is gradual depolarization towards threshold level

1 - Cell membrane

The membrane potential of the myocardial cell is not stationary during diastole: after repolarization and an initial hyperpolarization there is a gradual depolarizatiion towards the threshold level, caused by a slow inward leak of sodium ions as the membrane's permeability for these ions increases.

Na$^+$

4 - Sodium leakage through cell membrane is responsible for this slow depolarization

3 - Depolarization

Different parts of the heart, and different groups of myocardial cells, vary in the rate at which the membrane becomes depolarized during diastole. The ventricular cells depolarize rather slowly, the atrial cells a little faster.

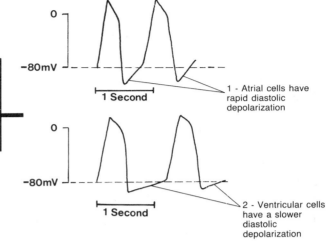

-80mV

1 Second

1 - Atrial cells have rapid diastolic depolarization

0

-80mV

1 Second

2 - Ventricular cells have a slower diastolic depolarization

SPREAD OF THE CARDIAC IMPULSE

The region of the heart which has the highest rate of spontaneous diastolic depolarization, and which therefore acts as the **pacemaker**, is the **sino-atrial node** (so called because it represents all that is left of the **sinus venosus**, a primitive pre-atrial chamber of the fetal heart). This node is situated in the wall of the right atrium near the site of entry of the superior and inferior venae cavae.

Since the rate of spontaneous depolarization is highest here, the cells reach threshold for depolarization earlier than their neighbours, and the action potentials which result trigger off action potentials in the other cells.

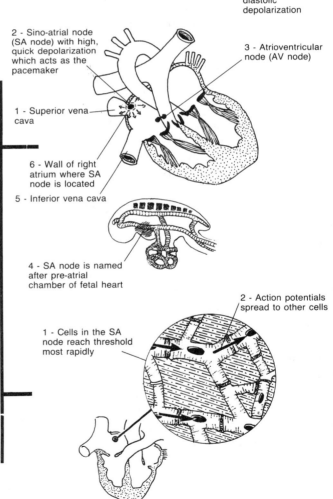

2 - Sino-atrial node (SA node) with high, quick depolarization which acts as the pacemaker

3 - Atrioventricular node (AV node)

1 - Superior vena cava

6 - Wall of right atrium where SA node is located

5 - Interior vena cava

4 - SA node is named after pre-atrial chamber of fetal heart

2 - Action potentials spread to other cells

1 - Cells in the SA node reach threshold most rapidly

Electrical impulses originating in the sino-atrial node are conducted from cell to cell through the atrial muscle via the intercalated discs which connect the cells; the arrival of the impulse at any given atrial cell causes that cell to contract. There is no direct pathway for spread of the impulse from atrial to ventricular muscle, as the upper chambers are separated from the lower by a fibrous ring which forms a supporting framework for the atrioventricular valves. There is a single site where it is possible for impulses to cross from atria to ventricles: this is known as the **atrioventricular node** and is found in the inter-atrial septum near the junction with the ventricles, in the wall of the right atrium.

The electrical impulse is delayed for a short time in the atrioventricular node, as the conduction velocity of this group of specialized muscle cells is rather slower than that of the bulk of the myocardium. The impulse then passes to a group of rapidly conducting fibres called the **bundle of His**, which lies in the interventricular septum, running down towards the apex of the heart and then splitting into bundles of **Purkinje fibres**, which spread up the epicardial surfaces of both ventricles. The purpose of the His–Purkinje system is to carry the impulse rapidly to all regions of the ventricle; the impulse spreads from the Purkinje fibres to the underlying ventricular myocardium at a slower rate, but because the conducting system has distributed the impulse so rapidly the electrical activation of the whole ventricular muscle mass occurs almost simultaneously. The arrival of the electrical impulse at any given ventricular cell triggers the onset of contraction.

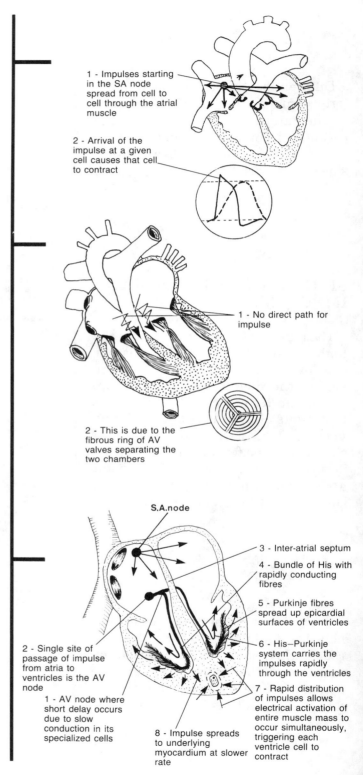

1 - Impulses starting in the SA node spread from cell to cell through the atrial muscle

2 - Arrival of the impulse at a given cell causes that cell to contract

1 - No direct path for impulse

2 - This is due to the fibrous ring of AV valves separating the two chambers

S.A. node

3 - Inter-atrial septum

4 - Bundle of His with rapidly conducting fibres

5 - Purkinje fibres spread up epicardial surfaces of ventricles

6 - His–Purkinje system carries the impulses rapidly through the ventricles

7 - Rapid distribution of impulses allows electrical activation of entire muscle mass to occur simultaneously, triggering each ventricle cell to contract

2 - Single site of passage of impulse from atria to ventricles is the AV node

1 - AV node where short delay occurs due to slow conduction in its specialized cells

8 - Impulse spreads to underlying myocardium at slower rate

If there were no rapid conduction system, the impulse would have to pass from one ordinary cell to the next throughout the myocardium, with the result that the apex of the ventricle would be activated to contract a long time after the base: the ventricle would not contract in a coordinated manner.

CONTROL OF THE HEART RATE

The action of the cardiac pacemaker, and hence the heart rate, can be influenced by certain nerves and hormones. The vagus (parasympathetic) nerve, arising from the brain stem, sends fibres to the region of the sino-atrial and atrioventricular nodes. Impulses in the vagus nerve cause the release of acetylcholine from the nerve endings, and this transmitter reduces the rate of diastolic depolarization in the sino-atrial node, lengthening the interval between cardiac impulses and slowing the heart rate.

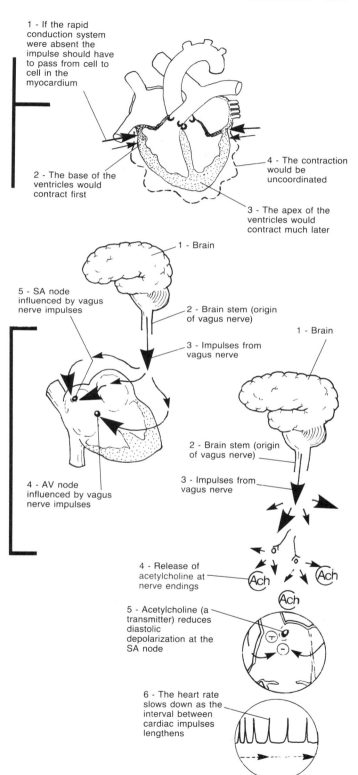

1 - If the rapid conduction system were absent the impulse should have to pass from cell to cell in the myocardium

2 - The base of the ventricles would contract first

3 - The apex of the ventricles would contract much later

4 - The contraction would be uncoordinated

1 - Brain

2 - Brain stem (origin of vagus nerve)

3 - Impulses from vagus nerve

5 - SA node influenced by vagus nerve impulses

4 - AV node influenced by vagus nerve impulses

1 - Brain

2 - Brain stem (origin of vagus nerve)

3 - Impulses from vagus nerve

4 - Release of acetylcholine at nerve endings

5 - Acetylcholine (a transmitter) reduces diastolic depolarization at the SA node

6 - The heart rate slows down as the interval between cardiac impulses lengthens

Sympathetic nerves reaching the heart supply all parts of the myocardium, but particularly the nodal areas; impulses in these nerves release noradrenaline, which accelerates the rate of diastolic depolarization, shortens the interval between cardiac impulses and speeds the heart rate.

Adrenaline released from the adrenal gland during excitement or fear has an effect similar to noradrenaline.

It is very important to emphasize that the heart is not dependent upon its nerves for the *initiation* of the heart beat; the completely denervated heart (or even a disembodied, isolated heart in a test-tube) will beat quite spontaneously, as rhythmicity is an intrinsic property of the myocardium.

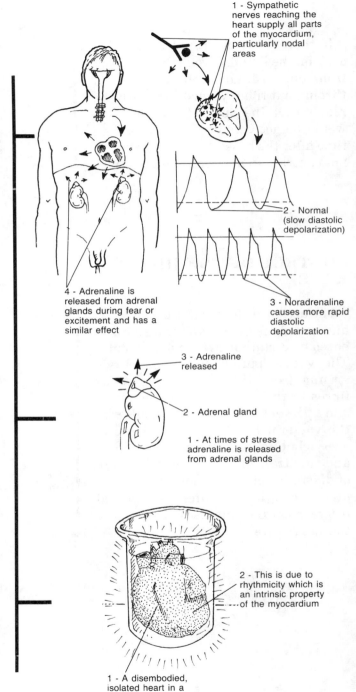

1 - Sympathetic nerves reaching the heart supply all parts of the myocardium, particularly nodal areas

2 - Normal (slow diastolic depolarization)

3 - Noradrenaline causes more rapid diastolic depolarization

4 - Adrenaline is released from adrenal glands during fear or excitement and has a similar effect

3 - Adrenaline released

2 - Adrenal gland

1 - At times of stress adrenaline is released from adrenal glands

2 - This is due to rhythmicity which is an intrinsic property of the myocardium

1 - A disembodied, isolated heart in a test-tube will still beat quite spontaneously

However, the nerves are very important in regulating, modifying and controlling the function of the heart, allowing its rate to be adjusted in accordance with the body's needs.

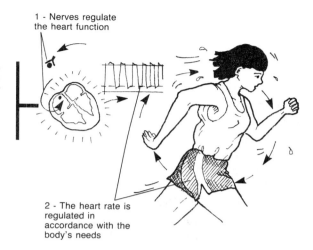

1 - Nerves regulate the heart function

2 - The heart rate is regulated in accordance with the body's needs

THE ELECTROCARDIOGRAM

The passage of the electrical impulse through the heart produces a disturbance in the body's electrical field which can be detected with electrodes on the body's surface.

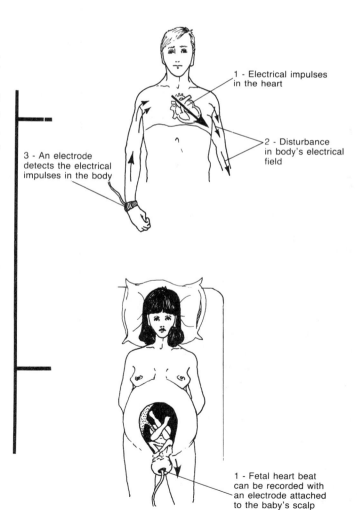

1 - Electrical impulses in the heart

2 - Disturbance in body's electrical field

3 - An electrode detects the electrical impulses in the body

In principle the electrocardiogram can be recorded from anywhere on the surface (for instance the fetal heart beat can be recorded with an electrode attached to the scalp as the baby's head passes through the birth canal), but there are particular sites where the waveform is recorded with greatest advantage.

1 - Fetal heart beat can be recorded with an electrode attached to the baby's scalp

By convention, electrodes are placed on the wrists and ankles; lead I is taken between the two wrists, lead II is between right arm and left leg, and lead III is taken between the left arm and leg. There are numerous other leads, which simply examine the cardiac waveform from different points of view and thereby allow us to build up a three-dimensional picture of the way in which current spreads within the heart.

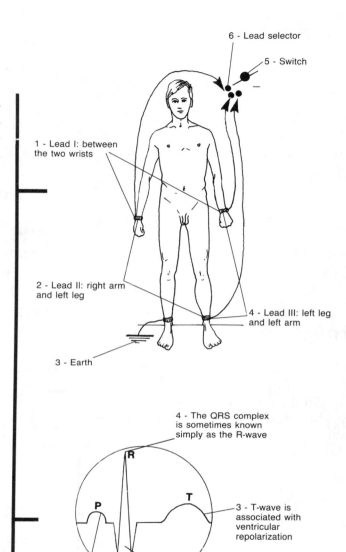

6 - Lead selector

5 - Switch

1 - Lead I: between the two wrists

2 - Lead II: right arm and left leg

4 - Lead III: left leg and left arm

3 - Earth

No matter which lead is used to record the electrocardiogram (ECG, or in the USA, EKG) there are particular components which can always be recognized. The first wave is a small deflection known as the P-wave; this is followed by a highly complicated QRS complex which usually has a downward, then an upward and then another downward deflection, but may have more or fewer changes in direction — often one speaks merely of the R-wave; then there is a T-wave, and after a long pause comes the P-wave of the next cardiac cycle.

The P-wave is associated with atrial depolarization, the QRS complex with ventricular depolarization and the T-wave with ventricular repolarization. There is no visible ECG wave associated with atrial repolarization, first because this event produces only a tiny disturbance in the electric field, and second because it occurs during the QRS complex and is therefore masked by the much larger electrical event.

4 - The QRS complex is sometimes known simply as the R-wave

3 - T-wave is associated with ventricular repolarization

2 - The complicated QRS wave is associated with ventricular depolarization

1 - The P-wave is associated with atrial depolarization

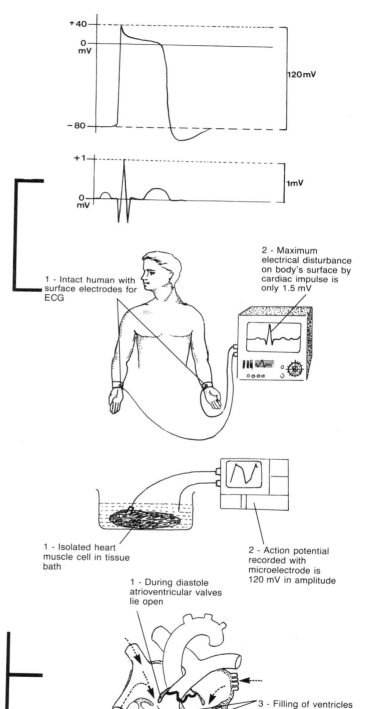

While the action potential recorded across the cardiac cell membrane with a microelectrode may be up to 120 mV in amplitude, the maximum electrical disturbance recorded at the body's surface due to the cardiac impulse is only about 1.5 mV.

1 - Intact human with surface electrodes for ECG

2 - Maximum electrical disturbance on body's surface by cardiac impulse is only 1.5 mV

1 - Isolated heart muscle cell in tissue bath

2 - Action potential recorded with microelectrode is 120 mV in amplitude

EVENTS IN THE CARDIAC CYCLE

During diastole the pressure in the relaxed ventricles is low, and the atrioventricular valves lie open. Blood flows from the veins into the right atrium and ventricle largely under the impetus given to it by the previous contraction, and most of the filling of the ventricle occurs passively.

1 - During diastole atrioventricular valves lie open

2 - Blood flows into right atrium and ventricle largely from impetus of previous contraction

3 - Filling of ventricles generally occurs passively

Following the onset of atrial depolarization, the atria contract and eject a certain amount of blood into the ventricles; there is also a small amount of reflux of blood into the great veins.

1 - Atria contract at onset of atrial depolarization

4 - Small reflux of blood into the great veins

2 - Some blood is ejected into the ventricle

3 - Ventricles relaxed

120 mm Hg

0

◄TIME►
SECONDS

0

1

Aortic pressure

Ventricular pressure

Atrial pressure

As the ventricles begin to contract, their pressure rises and soon exceeds the pressure in the atria; this closes the atrioventricular valves and for a period both the inlet and outlet valves of the ventricles are closed, so that pressure rises rapidly without any change in ventricular volume. This is known as the **isovolumic** or isometric phase of contraction.

2 - For a time inlet and outlet valves are closed

1 - Ventricles begin to contract

3 - Interventricular pressures rise but not ventricular volume. This is known as the isovolumic phase

Eventually the ventricular pressure exceeds that in the aorta or pulmonary artery, and the aortic and pulmonary valves open. This allows blood to flow out of ventricles — the **ejection** phase of systole. The blood ejected into the large arteries distends their elastic walls, and a proportion of the ejected volume is stored in the arteries during systole.

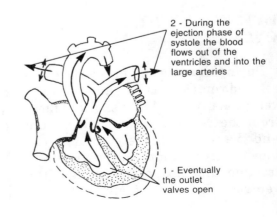

2 - During the ejection phase of systole the blood flows out of the ventricles and into the large arteries

1 - Eventually the outlet valves open

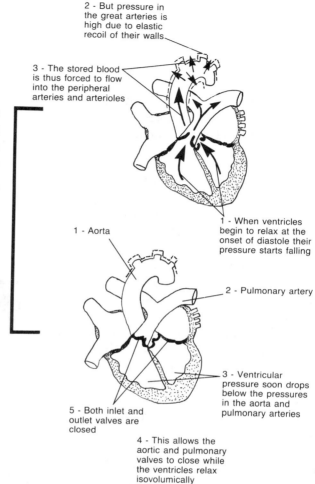

2 - But pressure in the great arteries is high due to elastic recoil of their walls

3 - The stored blood is thus forced to flow into the peripheral arteries and arterioles

1 - When ventricles begin to relax at the onset of diastole their pressure starts falling

1 - Aorta

2 - Pulmonary artery

3 - Ventricular pressure soon drops below the pressures in the aorta and pulmonary arteries

5 - Both inlet and outlet valves are closed

4 - This allows the aortic and pulmonary valves to close while the ventricles relax isovolumically

As the ventricles begin to relax at the onset of diastole their pressure starts to fall, but the pressure in the great arteries is kept high by the elastic recoil of their walls, forcing the stored blood to flow into the more peripheral arteries and arterioles. Ventricular pressure soon drops below the pressures in the aorta and pulmonary arteries. This allows the aortic and pulmonary valves to close, and for a while the ventricles relax isovolumically, with both outlet and inlet valves closed.

Eventually the pressure falls below atrial pressure and the atrioventricular valves open, to allow ventricular filling to begin again.

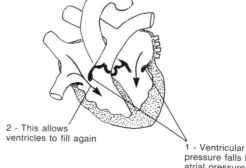

2 - This allows ventricles to fill again

1 - Ventricular pressure falls below atrial pressure and atrioventricular valves open

When a valve closes, turbulence is induced in the flowing bloodstream and vibration occurs in the cardiac muscle.

These events produce sounds which can be heard through a stethoscope placed on the chest wall. The heart sounds are *not* caused by the leaflets of the valves slapping together: a moment's thought about the flimsy nature of the valves should make it obvious that they are structurally incapable of making a slapping noise. The sound is simply due to interruption of the smooth flow of blood. The first heart sound occurs at the time of closure of the atrioventricular valves, and has a low-pitched quality often described as 'lub'. The second heart sound occurs at the time of closure of the aortic and pulmonary valves, and has a higher-pitched quality referred to as 'dub' or 'dup'. The two heart sounds are often described together as 'lub—dub'.

FACTORS INFLUENCING CARDIAC OUTPUT

Cardiac output is defined as the volume of blood flowing out of either the left or the right side of the heart per minute. It is calculated by multiplying the **stroke volume** or volume ejected during each heartbeat by the heart rate. The heart rate is determined by the action of the nerves controlling the pacemaker.

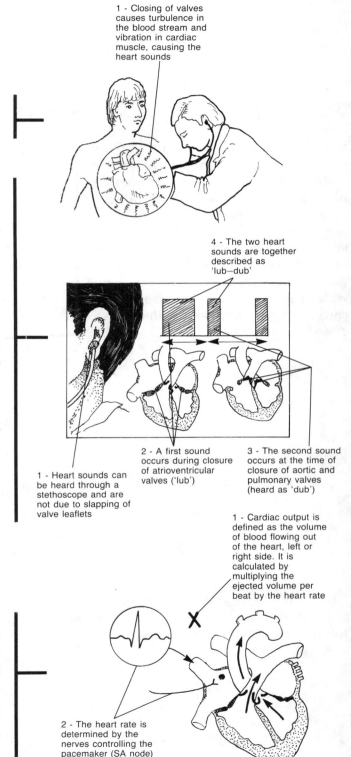

1 - Closing of valves causes turbulence in the blood stream and vibration in cardiac muscle, causing the heart sounds

4 - The two heart sounds are together described as 'lub—dub'

1 - Heart sounds can be heard through a stethoscope and are not due to slapping of valve leaflets

2 - A first sound occurs during closure of atrioventricular valves ('lub')

3 - The second sound occurs at the time of closure of aortic and pulmonary valves (heard as 'dub')

1 - Cardiac output is defined as the volume of blood flowing out of the heart, left or right side. It is calculated by multiplying the ejected volume per beat by the heart rate

2 - The heart rate is determined by the nerves controlling the pacemaker (SA node)

The stroke volume is determined by the **venous return** and the **contractility** of the myocardium.

Venous return determines stroke volume, as the heart can only pump out the blood that comes into it; if venous return decreases then stroke volume must inevitably fall. If venous return increases then stroke volume rises; this occurs because of the mechanical property of muscle, which contracts more forcefully if the cells are stretched, as a greater opportunity is afforded for cross-bridge formation between the sliding filaments. These properties are summed up in Starling's famous 'law of the heart': the more the ventricles are stretched the more forcefully they contract.

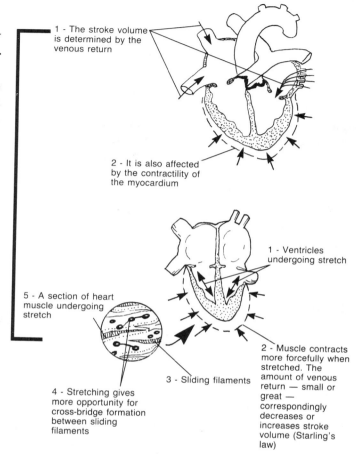

1 - The stroke volume is determined by the venous return

2 - It is also affected by the contractility of the myocardium

1 - Ventricles undergoing stretch

5 - A section of heart muscle undergoing stretch

3 - Sliding filaments

2 - Muscle contracts more forcefully when stretched. The amount of venous return — small or great — correspondingly decreases or increases stroke volume (Starling's law)

4 - Stretching gives more opportunity for cross-bridge formation between sliding filaments

If only a small volume of blood returns to the heart during a particular diastolic period, the ventricular muscle is stretched only slightly, and the force of contraction is small; the volume ejected is correspondingly small. If a large volume of blood is returned during diastole then the muscle is stretched by a great deal, and contracts forcefully, ejecting a large volume. In both cases, the volume of blood remaining in the ventricles at the end of systole is about the same.

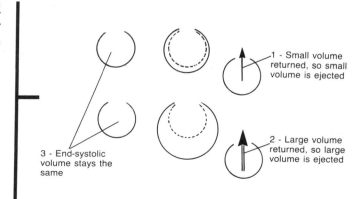

1 - Small volume returned, so small volume is ejected

2 - Large volume returned, so large volume is ejected

3 - End-systolic volume stays the same

If the ventricles become over-filled, so that the muscle fibres are over-stretched, then the force of contraction is reduced. This is partly due to the effect on the myofilaments, which are pulled out to such a length that the opportunity for cross-bridge formation is reduced. It is also due to the physical effect on the curvature of the heart: by the law of Laplace, the pressure in a hollow sphere or cylinder is inversely proportional to the radius, so as the radius increases the ability to develop pressure declines. An over-filled heart which is unable to eject all of the blood entering it is said to be in **cardiac failure**.

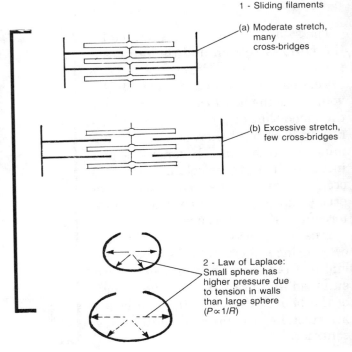

1 - Sliding filaments
(a) Moderate stretch, many cross-bridges
(b) Excessive stretch, few cross-bridges
2 - Law of Laplace: Small sphere has higher pressure due to tension in walls than large sphere ($P \propto 1/R$)

The contractile properties of the myocardium can be influenced by nerves and hormones. In the presence of noradrenaline (from sympathetic nerves) or adrenaline (from the adrenal gland) the muscle contracts more forcefully for a given amount of stretch; in other words, if the ventricle is filled by a certain amount, it contracts more strongly than the unstimulated heart. It ejects a bigger proportion of the total volume contained in the heart; the end-systolic volume is smaller and the stroke volume is increased. Thus noradrenaline and adrenaline have a twofold effect on the cardiac output; they both speed up the heart and increase the stroke volume.

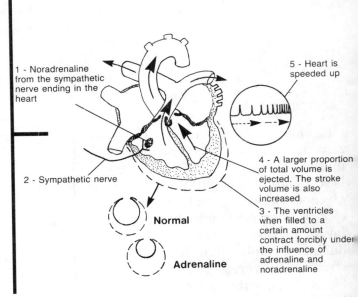

1 - Noradrenaline from the sympathetic nerve ending in the heart
2 - Sympathetic nerve
5 - Heart is speeded up
4 - A larger proportion of total volume is ejected. The stroke volume is also increased
3 - The ventricles when filled to a certain amount contract forcibly under the influence of adrenaline and noradrenaline
Normal
Adrenaline

MEASUREMENT OF CARDIAC OUTPUT

Cardiac output can be measured directly by fitting the aorta or pulmonary artery with a flow-meter, or by collecting the blood leaving the heart.

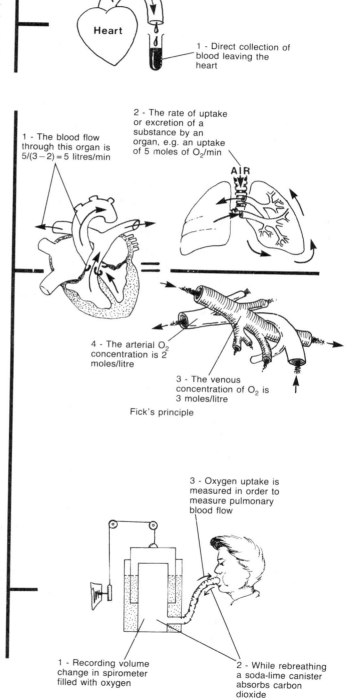

1 - Direct collection of blood leaving the heart

These techniques are not particularly convenient for applying to the intact patient or experimental subject, and more indirect means usually have to be used. One class of methods makes use of the **Fick principle**: the blood flow through an organ can be calculated from the rate of uptake or excretion of a substance by the organ, divided by the arteriovenous concentration difference. For example, if the blood flowing through the lungs takes up 5 moles of oxygen per minute, with an arterial oxygen concentration of 2 moles per litre and a venous concentration of 3 moles per litre, then the blood flow is $5/(3-2)$ or 5 litres per minute.

1 - The blood flow through this organ is $5/(3-2) = 5$ litres/min

2 - The rate of uptake or excretion of a substance by an organ, e.g. an uptake of 5 moles of O_2/min

AIR

4 - The arterial O_2 concentration is 2 moles/litre

3 - The venous concentration of O_2 is 3 moles/litre

Fick's principle

In order to measure pulmonary blood flow (which equals the output from the right side of the heart) by this technique, it is necessary to measure oxygen uptake (by recording the volume change in a spirometer filled with oxygen while rebreathing through a soda-lime canister to absorb carbon dioxide).

3 - Oxygen uptake is measured in order to measure pulmonary blood flow

1 - Recording volume change in spirometer filled with oxygen

2 - While rebreathing a soda-lime canister absorbs carbon dioxide

It is also necessary to measure the concentrations of oxygen in mixed venous and arterial blood. Arterial blood can be sampled from any peripheral artery, but mixed venous blood can only be obtained from the right atrium, ventricle or pulmonary artery. This requires the passage of a catheter up a peripheral vein and into the heart; it is thus obvious that measurement of cardiac output is not a trivial procedure.

Another group of techniques for estimating cardiac output makes use of **indicator dilution**. A known mass of dye or other indicator is injected into the bloodstream close to the heart, and the concentration of dye in the artrial blood is recorded as a function of time.

The area under the curve of dye concentration can be related to the **blood flow**, provided allowance is made for recirculation of the dye; it is often more convenient and accurate to plot the dye concentration on a logarithmic scale.

This type of technique requires fewer invasive procedures than the Fick principle, but still needs continuous monitoring of arterial concentrations, which can be inconvenient.

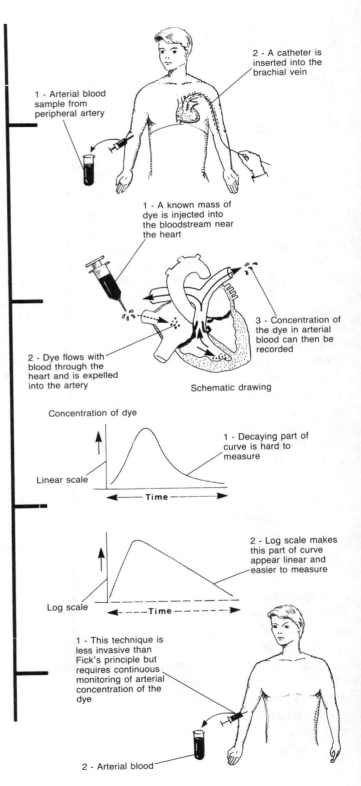

1 - Arterial blood sample from peripheral artery

2 - A catheter is inserted into the brachial vein

1 - A known mass of dye is injected into the bloodstream near the heart

2 - Dye flows with blood through the heart and is expelled into the artery

3 - Concentration of the dye in arterial blood can then be recorded

Schematic drawing

Concentration of dye

Linear scale

Time

1 - Decaying part of curve is hard to measure

Log scale

Time

2 - Log scale makes this part of curve appear linear and easier to measure

1 - This technique is less invasive than Fick's principle but requires continuous monitoring of arterial concentration of the dye

2 - Arterial blood

THE PERIPHERAL CIRCULATION

Once it leaves the heart, the blood flows to the rest of the body through a series of tubes; we should now consider the factors which regulate the flow of fluid through a tube.

The first of these is the pressure difference between the two ends of the tube, for if the pressure is the same at both ends then fluid cannot flow. The second is the resistance to fluid flow. Some of this resistance is due to the properties of the fluid, and some is due to the properties of the tube. A long tube has more resistance than a short one; a narrow tube has more resistance than a wide one.

The resistance of a tube is directly proportional to the length, but is inversely proportional to the **fourth power** of the radius, i.e.

$$\text{Resistance} = k \cdot \frac{\text{length}}{\text{radius}^4}$$

where k is a constant.

In other words, if the radius of a vessel is doubled, the resistance is reduced to one-sixteenth of its value. The circulation is very sensitive to small changes in the calibre of blood vessels, particularly the arterioles or 'resistance' vessels.

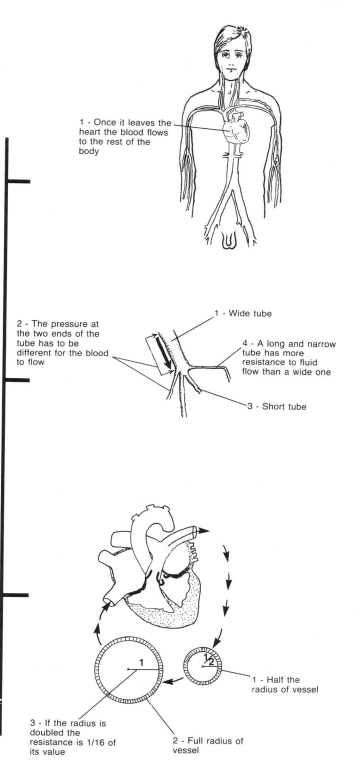

1 - Once it leaves the heart the blood flows to the rest of the body

2 - The pressure at the two ends of the tube has to be different for the blood to flow

1 - Wide tube

4 - A long and narrow tube has more resistance to fluid flow than a wide one

3 - Short tube

1 - Half the radius of vessel

3 - If the radius is doubled the resistance is 1/16 of its value

2 - Full radius of vessel

Resistance to flow in a tube also depends on whether or not the flow is turbulent. At low flow rates in smooth-walled tubes the 'layers' of fluid slip easily past each other, with concentric layers of fluid flowing in a parallel way. If flow becomes rapid, intermittent or disturbed, or there is a narrowing or obstruction or irregularity in the vessel wall, the turbulent flow occurs and causes a huge increase in the resistance to flow down that tube.

The properties of the **fluid** which determine resistance include the **viscosity**, or its thickness and stickiness. Blood is basically a watery solution whose viscosity is not much greater than that of water, but the presence of plasma proteins produces a slight increase in viscosity, and the presence of the formed elements produces a large increase. If the red cells form rouleaux then the viscosity increases even more. Patients with too many red cells (suffering from **polycythaemia**) have abnormally viscous blood and may in consequence develop hypertension; so too may patients who produce abnormally large amounts of gamma-globulin.

Simple, ideal solutions exhibit the same viscosity no matter what the size of the tube or the rate of flow. Blood has some properties which depart significantly from the ideal; for example the viscosity is less in small blood vessels than in large ones.

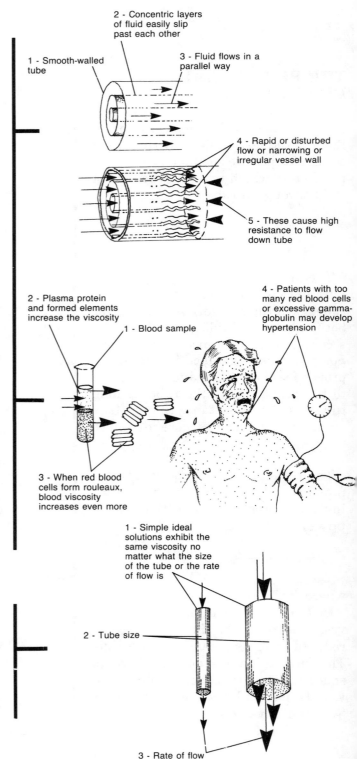

2 - Concentric layers of fluid easily slip past each other

1 - Smooth-walled tube

3 - Fluid flows in a parallel way

4 - Rapid or disturbed flow or narrowing or irregular vessel wall

5 - These cause high resistance to flow down tube

2 - Plasma protein and formed elements increase the viscosity

1 - Blood sample

4 - Patients with too many red blood cells or excessive gamma-globulin may develop hypertension

3 - When red blood cells form rouleaux, blood viscosity increases even more

1 - Simple ideal solutions exhibit the same viscosity no matter what the size of the tube or the rate of flow is

2 - Tube size

3 - Rate of flow

The reason for this is that blood cells are particles of finite size; no cell can approach closer to the side of the tube than its own radius, so there is a region at the edge of the vessel where the blood is relatively depleted of cells and therefore less viscous.

This effect is much more important in small vessels than in large ones, and the side branches of smaller vessels will actually receive blood with fewer cells, as a consequence of this 'plasma skimming'.

The pressure in a blood vessel is the consequence of the fluid inside pressing outwards on the walls; pressure is force per unit area and is measured in pascals (Pa) or kilopascals (kPa). Some measurements, such as blood pressure, are still expressed in millimetres of mercury (mmHg), i.e. the height of a column of mercury which can be supported by the pressure under investigation, but most pressures should be expressed in the SI unit, which is the pascal. One pascal is the pressure produced by a force of one newton per square metre.

A newton is the force required to accelerate a mass of 1 kg by 1 metre per second per second (1 kg.m.s^{-2}).

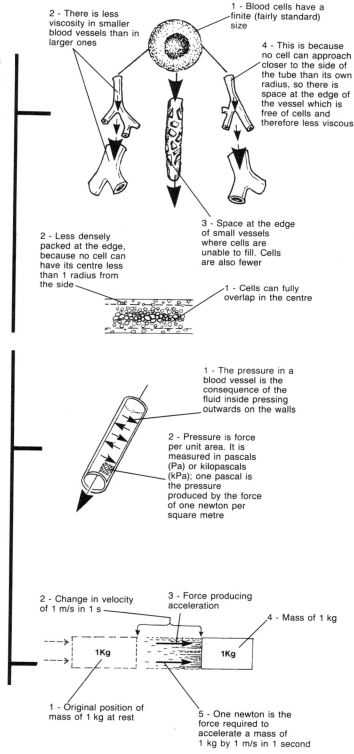

1 - Blood cells have a finite (fairly standard) size

2 - There is less viscosity in smaller blood vessels than in larger ones

4 - This is because no cell can approach closer to the side of the tube than its own radius, so there is space at the edge of the vessel which is free of cells and therefore less viscous

2 - Less densely packed at the edge, because no cell can have its centre less than 1 radius from the side

3 - Space at the edge of small vessels where cells are unable to fill. Cells are also fewer

1 - Cells can fully overlap in the centre

1 - The pressure in a blood vessel is the consequence of the fluid inside pressing outwards on the walls

2 - Pressure is force per unit area. It is measured in pascals (Pa) or kilopascals (kPa); one pascal is the pressure produced by the force of one newton per square metre

2 - Change in velocity of 1 m/s in 1 s

3 - Force producing acceleration

4 - Mass of 1 kg

1Kg

1Kg

1 - Original position of mass of 1 kg at rest

5 - One newton is the force required to accelerate a mass of 1 kg by 1 m/s in 1 second

The pressure in arteries is developed during systole by the force of the ventricular contraction, and during diastole is maintained by the elastic recoil of the arterial wall.

It can be measured by inserting a tube into an artery and connecting it to a manometer (either a mercury-filled tube or an electronic transducer), and this technique is widely used in experimental physiology and in high-dependency or intensive care monitoring. However, it is inconvenient for routine clinical measurement, and an indirect method for measurement of arterial pressure is widely used.

An airtight bag or cuff is wrapped around a limb — typically the upper arm — and inflated via a bulb until the pressure in the bag is high enough to occlude the blood vessels in the arm. The pressure in the bag is registered with a mercury or aneroid manometer. If the pressure in the bag is gradually released, it eventually falls below the pressure in the artery, and some blood can flow through the artery for part of the cardiac cycle.

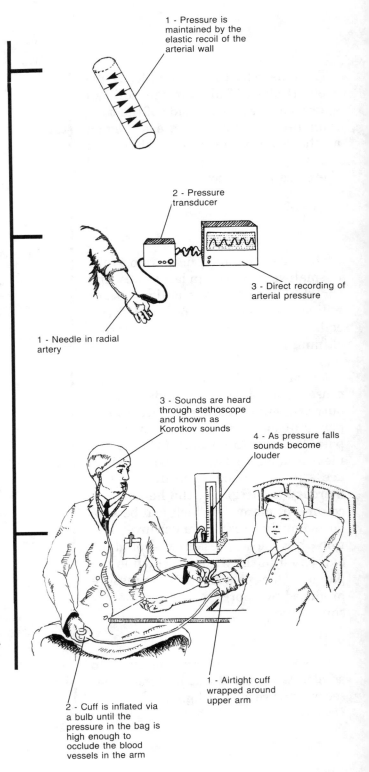

1 - Pressure is maintained by the elastic recoil of the arterial wall

2 - Pressure transducer

3 - Direct recording of arterial pressure

1 - Needle in radial artery

3 - Sounds are heard through stethoscope and known as Korotkov sounds

4 - As pressure falls sounds become louder

1 - Airtight cuff wrapped around upper arm

2 - Cuff is inflated via a bulb until the pressure in the bag is high enough to occlude the blood vessels in the arm

As the blood flows only intermittently, it causes turbulence and this is detected as a tapping sound with a stethoscope placed over the artery just distal to the cuff. As the pressure in the bag is released still further, blood is able to flow for more and more of the cycle, and the sounds become louder. When the pressure falls below diastolic pressure, flow can occur for the whole of the cycle and at this stage the sounds heard through the stethoscope become muffled; they do not entirely disappear until pressure is released to a much lower value, as the blood flow is still rather irregular and turbulent so long as pressure is applied to the arm. The sounds heard through the stethoscope are called the **Korotkov** sounds.

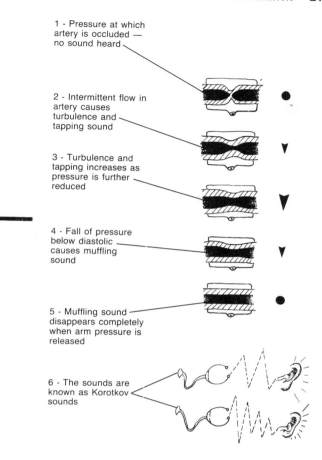

1 - Pressure at which artery is occluded — no sound heard

2 - Intermittent flow in artery causes turbulence and tapping sound

3 - Turbulence and tapping increases as pressure is further reduced

4 - Fall of pressure below diastolic causes muffling sound

5 - Muffling sound disappears completely when arm pressure is released

6 - The sounds are known as Korotkov sounds

The systolic pressure is taken as the pressure (during release of the cuff) when tapping sounds are first heard; the diastolic pressure is that pressure at which the sounds become muffled (though in the United States the diastolic is regarded as the pressure at which the Korotkov sounds disappear entirely).

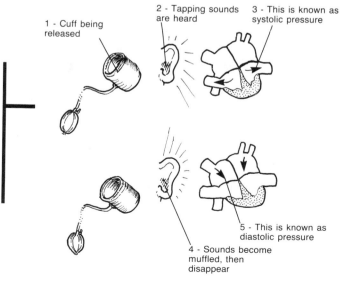

1 - Cuff being released

2 - Tapping sounds are heard

3 - This is known as systolic pressure

4 - Sounds become muffled, then disappear

5 - This is known as diastolic pressure

1 - The pressure at which the sounds appear is the systolic blood pressure

2 - The point at which the sounds become muffled is called Korotkov phase 4

3 - The point at which the sounds disappear completely is called Korotkov phase 5

The blood pressure is conventionally recorded as the systolic over the diastolic, eg 120/80 mmHg. The figures do not represent a fraction or a process of division, but are simply a convenient notation for writing down the systolic and diastolic pressures.

Systolic pressure

mmHg

120

80

Diastolic pressure

0

mmHg
120
80
0

Pulse pressure

The difference between systolic and diastolic pressures is called **pulse pressure**; the mean pressure is calculated by adding one-third of the pulse pressure to the diastolic value, and represents the effective pressure which is applied, on average, to the vascular beds.

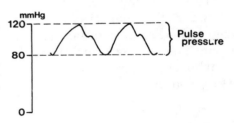

Systolic

Pulse pressure

Diastolic

0

1/3 pulse pressure

Mean pressure = diastolic + 1/3 pulse pressure

The **perfusion pressure** for a given vascular bed, such as the vessels of a particular organ, is the mean arterial pressure less the venous pressure.

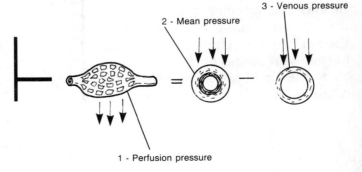

3 - Venous pressure

2 - Mean pressure

1 - Perfusion pressure

The arterial and venous pressures are influenced by hydrostatic pressure. The arteries in the foot are subjected to the normal arterial pressure plus the pressure due to the column of blood between the heart and the foot; the veins are similarly subject to the pressure in the central veins plus the hydrostatic pressure due to a similar column of blood.

The perfusion pressure should usually be exactly the same as for an organ at heart level, as the hydrostatic pressure is applied equally to the arteries and veins.

If there is a change in the hydrostatic pressure, as when a seated person stands up, the veins which are more distensible than arteries become widened by the extra pressure, so that some blood pools in the veins and the venous return to the heart is transiently reduced. Eventually the extra capacity of the veins becomes filled up and the venous return reverts to normal, but in the meantime the circulatory reflexes have to act in order to maintain the blood pressure constant (see below).

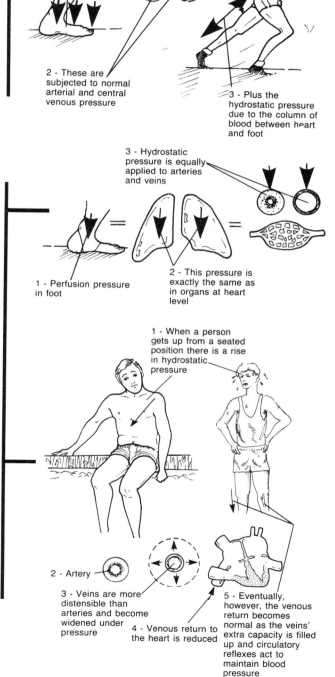

1 - Pressure on arteries and veins in feet

2 - These are subjected to normal arterial and central venous pressure

3 - Plus the hydrostatic pressure due to the column of blood between heart and foot

3 - Hydrostatic pressure is equally applied to arteries and veins

1 - Perfusion pressure in foot

2 - This pressure is exactly the same as in organs at heart level

1 - When a person gets up from a seated position there is a rise in hydrostatic pressure

2 - Artery

3 - Veins are more distensible than arteries and become widened under pressure

4 - Venous return to the heart is reduced

5 - Eventually, however, the venous return becomes normal as the veins' extra capacity is filled up and circulatory reflexes act to maintain blood pressure

The blood vessels above the heart are subjected to a lower hydrostatic pressure, and in fact may be at a negative pressure. In these circumstances the veins with their rather flaccid walls collapse: this can easily be observed by raising one's own arm from an initially low position with distended veins to a position above the heart, when the walls collapse.

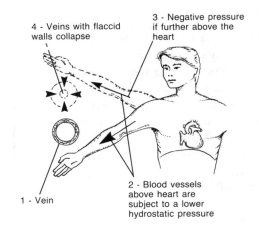

4 - Veins with flaccid walls collapse

3 - Negative pressure if further above the heart

2 - Blood vessels above heart are subject to a lower hydrostatic pressure

1 - Vein

This means that the pressure in the veins is hardly ever truly negative, but is simply reduced to zero. Meanwhile the arteries are subjected to the mean arterial pressure less the pressure due to the height of the fluid column above the heart, and the net effect is that the perfusion pressure in vascular beds above the heart is reduced; arterial pressure is lowered but venous pressure cannot fall below zero. This is why the use of hand tools such as screwdrivers or ceiling paint brushes above the head is so much harder than their use in the normal position over a work-bench.

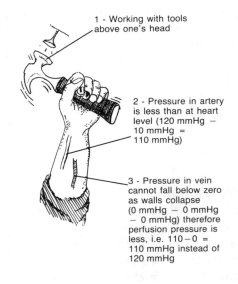

1 - Working with tools above one's head

2 - Pressure in artery is less than at heart level (120 mmHg − 10 mmHg = 110 mmHg)

3 - Pressure in vein cannot fall below zero as walls collapse (0 mmHg − 0 mmHg − 0 mmHg) therefore perfusion pressure is less, i.e. 110−0 = 110 mmHg instead of 120 mmHg

The arterial blood pressure is produced by the blood ejected from the heart trying to flow through the resistance offered by the peripheral vessels. In other words:

$$\frac{\text{blood}}{\text{pressure}} = \frac{\text{cardiac}}{\text{output}} \times \frac{\text{peripheral}}{\text{resistance}}$$

The factors influencing cardiac output have already been considered; we shall now examine the control of the peripheral resistance.

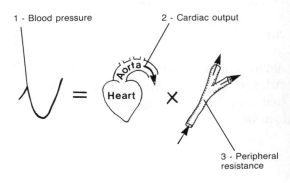

1 - Blood pressure   2 - Cardiac output

3 - Peripheral resistance

CONTROL OF THE ARTERIOLES

The arterioles, placed at the entrance to the microcirculatory bed, control the blood flow through the capillaries and hence through the main exchange area of the body. Since the total cross-sectional area of the arterioles is much smaller than the cross-section of the arteries, capillaries or veins, the arterioles contribute a very large part of the total resistance to blood flow in the circulation, and changes in their diameter can cause profound changes in the total vascular resistance.

The calibre of the arterioles is controlled by the smooth muscle in their wall, which is subject to a number of influences including **nerves**, circulating **hormones** and local **metabolites**.

The most important influence is the sympathetic (part of the autonomic) nervous system. Postganglionic non-myelinated axons arising from the paravertebral or splanchnic ganglia run along the walls of the arteries, or occasionally in mixed or splanchnic nerves, until they reach the target arterioles. The nerve endings typically release noradrenaline to produce constriction, but some of them release acetylcholine, which dilates the vessels.

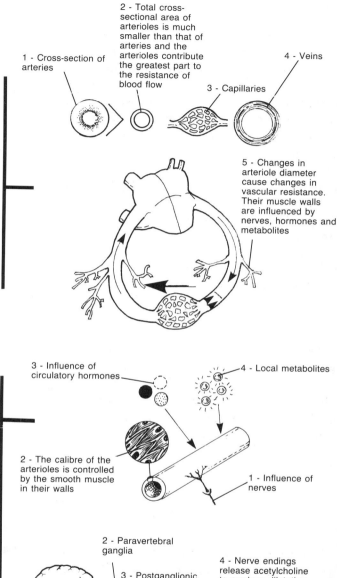

1 - Cross-section of arteries

2 - Total cross-sectional area of arterioles is much smaller than that of arteries and the arterioles contribute the greatest part to the resistance of blood flow

3 - Capillaries

4 - Veins

5 - Changes in arteriole diameter cause changes in vascular resistance. Their muscle walls are influenced by nerves, hormones and metabolites

3 - Influence of circulatory hormones

4 - Local metabolites

2 - The calibre of the arterioles is controlled by the smooth muscle in their walls

1 - Influence of nerves

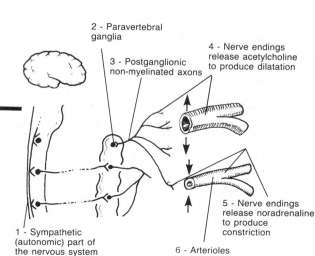

2 - Paravertebral ganglia

3 - Postganglionic non-myelinated axons

4 - Nerve endings release acetylcholine to produce dilatation

1 - Sympathetic (autonomic) part of the nervous system

5 - Nerve endings release noradrenaline to produce constriction

6 - Arterioles

The blood vessels of the skin are controlled almost exclusively by vasoconstrictor fibres, so that dilatation is produced simply by the release of nervous constrictor activity. Some dilatation of skin blood vessels is brought about as a by-product of the sweating mechanism. When cholinergic sympathetic fibres activate the sweat glands, the glandular activity causes the release of proteolytic enzymes which act on tissue proteins to produce **bradykinin**, a powerful vasodilator which relaxes the cutaneous blood vessels. This mechanism is similar to that which produces the vasodilatation in the salivary gland.

The blood vessels supplying **muscles** are partly controlled by noradrenic vasoconstrictor fibres, and partly by cholinergic dilator fibres. The vessels of the viscera are largely controlled by noradrenergic constrictors.

A number of **hormones** act on blood vessels. These include **adrenaline**, liberated from the adrenal gland during fear, exercise or excitement. As well as speeding the heart the hormone constricts blood vessels in the skin and viscera while dilating the vessels in the muscles; the differences between the actions of adrenaline and noradrenaline are explained in the chapter on the autonomic nervous system.

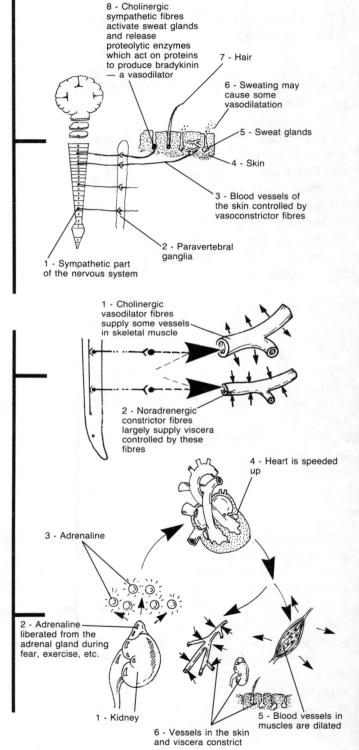

8 - Cholinergic sympathetic fibres activate sweat glands and release proteolytic enzymes which act on proteins to produce bradykinin — a vasodilator

7 - Hair

6 - Sweating may cause some vasodilatation

5 - Sweat glands

4 - Skin

3 - Blood vessels of the skin controlled by vasoconstrictor fibres

2 - Paravertebral ganglia

1 - Sympathetic part of the nervous system

1 - Cholinergic vasodilator fibres supply some vessels in skeletal muscle

2 - Noradrenergic constrictor fibres largely supply viscera controlled by these fibres

4 - Heart is speeded up

3 - Adrenaline

2 - Adrenaline liberated from the adrenal gland during fear, exercise, etc.

1 - Kidney

6 - Vessels in the skin and viscera constrict

5 - Blood vessels in muscles are dilated

The **antidiuretic hormone** released from the posterior part of the pituitary gland has its primary effect on the kidney, but it is also a potent vasoconstrictor; hence its alternative name, **vasopressin**. Another potent constrictor of arterioles is **angiotensin**, formed in the blood as a result of renin release from the kidney.

A number of local influences act on blood vessels, altering the circulation in accordance with local needs. As a muscle contracts and does work, its requirement for blood supply increases; there is a local depletion of tissue oxygen and an accumulation of carbon dioxide, and both of these factors increase the blood flow by producing a direct dilator effect on blood vessels. There is an accumulation of lactic acid in contracting muscle and other active tissues, and the resulting decrease in pH also causes vasodilatation by a direct effect on the arterioles.

The effects of a local oxygen lack (hypoxia), an excess of carbon dioxide (hypercapnia) or a fall in pH can be seen even in isolated blood vessels removed from the person or animal.

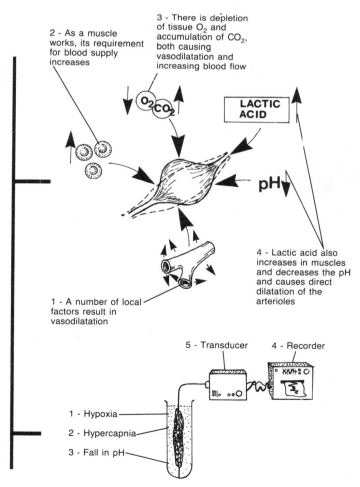

1 - Posterior part of pituitary gland

2 - Release of antidiuretic hormone of posterior pituitary gland

5 - Renin released from kidney results in the formation of angiotensin, another potent vasoconstrictor

Renin

3 - This has a primary effect on the kidney

4 - But it is also a potent vasoconstrictor, hence its alternative name, vasopressin

2 - As a muscle works, its requirement for blood supply increases

3 - There is depletion of tissue O_2 and accumulation of CO_2, both causing vasodilatation and increasing blood flow

O_2 CO_2 LACTIC ACID   pH

4 - Lactic acid also increases in muscles and decreases the pH and causes direct dilatation of the arterioles

1 - A number of local factors result in vasodilatation

5 - Transducer   4 - Recorder

1 - Hypoxia
2 - Hypercapnia
3 - Fall in pH

These influences all cause relaxation of arterial smooth muscle (except for the pulmonary artery which responds in the opposite manner to hypoxia). A fall in temperature causes constriction and warming produces dilatation; these phenomena will be familiar to anyone who has put a hand into cold or hot water.

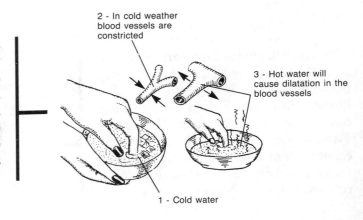

2 - In cold weather blood vessels are constricted

3 - Hot water will cause dilatation in the blood vessels

1 - Cold water

THE MICROCIRCULATION

The arterioles lead into the extensively branching network of capillaries. The capillaries have no muscle in their walls, so their blood flow is determined entirely by the state of opening or closure of the arterioles. The pattern can be extremely variable; the direction of flow in some of the capillaries can actually be reversed, depending on whether the appropriate arterioles are closed or open. The blood flows rather slowly through capillaries; the diameter is about 5 μm, and the erythrocytes, being 7 μm across, become deformed as they pass through.

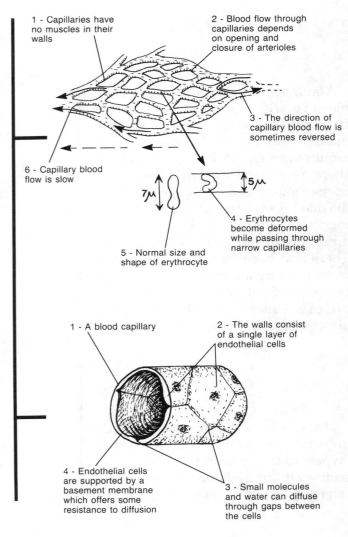

1 - Capillaries have no muscles in their walls

2 - Blood flow through capillaries depends on opening and closure of arterioles

3 - The direction of capillary blood flow is sometimes reversed

6 - Capillary blood flow is slow

4 - Erythrocytes become deformed while passing through narrow capillaries

5 - Normal size and shape of erythrocyte

7μ

5μ

The capillaries consist of a single layer of endothelial cells supported on a basement membrane and surrounded by some strands of connective tissue. The endothelial cells have gaps between them through which small molecules and water can diffuse; the real barrier to diffusion is the basement membrane layer surrounding the capillary.

1 - A blood capillary

2 - The walls consist of a single layer of endothelial cells

4 - Endothelial cells are supported by a basement membrane which offers some resistance to diffusion

3 - Small molecules and water can diffuse through gaps between the cells

Fluid is forced out of the capillary by the hydrostatic pressure transmitted from the arteries; at the venous end of the capillary the pressure is lower, but the net pressure gradient is still outwards. As fluid flows out of the capillary, it leaves behind the plasma proteins, so that the blood becomes relatively concentrated. This sets up an osmotic gradient, tending to attract fluid back into the capillary. The balance between outward hydrostatic pressure and inward osmotic pressure determines whether the net movement of fluid is out of or into the capillary.

Some of the fluid leaving the capillary remains in the interstitial space, and some protein escapes from the capillary. This excess fluid and protein enter the **lymphatic** capillaries, which are blind-ending vessels lying in the interstitium.

The lymphatic vessels have valves, and smooth muscle in their walls. They are capable of pumping fluid away from the tissues, through the lymph nodes (where the lymph is filtered) and via larger and larger lymphatic vessels into the **thoracic duct**, which empties into the subclavian vein.

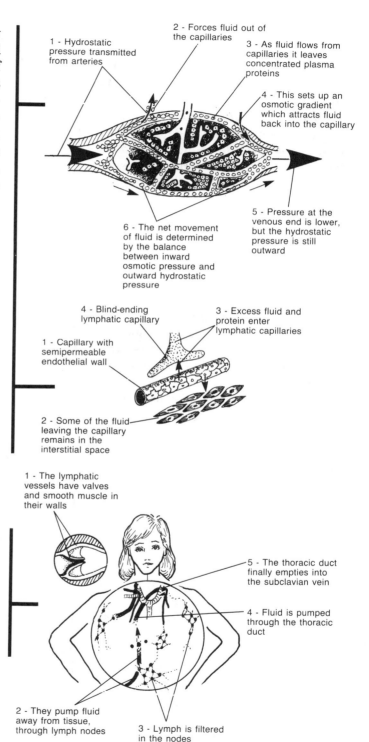

1 - Hydrostatic pressure transmitted from arteries

2 - Forces fluid out of the capillaries

3 - As fluid flows from capillaries it leaves concentrated plasma proteins

4 - This sets up an osmotic gradient which attracts fluid back into the capillary

5 - Pressure at the venous end is lower, but the hydrostatic pressure is still outward

6 - The net movement of fluid is determined by the balance between inward osmotic pressure and outward hydrostatic pressure

4 - Blind-ending lymphatic capillary

3 - Excess fluid and protein enter lymphatic capillaries

1 - Capillary with semipermeable endothelial wall

2 - Some of the fluid leaving the capillary remains in the interstitial space

1 - The lymphatic vessels have valves and smooth muscle in their walls

5 - The thoracic duct finally empties into the subclavian vein

4 - Fluid is pumped through the thoracic duct

2 - They pump fluid away from tissue, through lymph nodes

3 - Lymph is filtered in the nodes

If excessive fluid accumulates in the tissues, the condition is called **oedema**. This can arise if capillary pressure is abnormally high, due to arterial hypertension or venous blockage; if osmotic pressure is low due to plasma protein deficiency; or if the lymphatic vessels are blocked by tumours, infections or parasites.

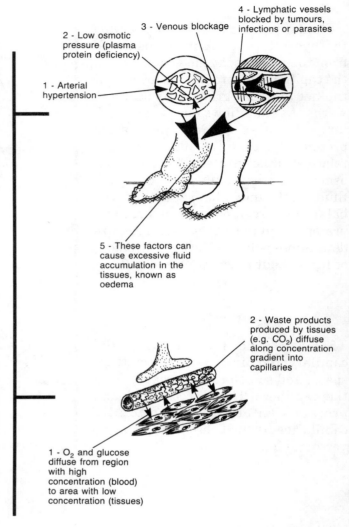

2 - Low osmotic pressure (plasma protein deficiency)

3 - Venous blockage

4 - Lymphatic vessels blocked by tumours, infections or parasites

1 - Arterial hypertension

5 - These factors can cause excessive fluid accumulation in the tissues, known as oedema

Substances are exchanged across the capillary wall in response to the concentration gradients. As the tissues use up oxygen, the concentration is lower than in the capillary blood, so oxygen diffuses out of the blood and into the tissues. The tissues produce carbon dioxide, which diffuses into the capillary blood. The concentration of nutrients such as glucose is higher in the blood than in the tissues, so they diffuse out, while the waste products of metabolism which accumulate in the tissues diffuse into the capillaries.

2 - Waste products produced by tissues (e.g. CO_2) diffuse along concentration gradient into capillaries

1 - O_2 and glucose diffuse from region with high concentration (blood) to area with low concentration (tissues)

The rate of supply of substances to the tissues depends not only on the concentration gradient but also on the rate of blood flow. Even if there is only a small concentration difference, there can be a high rate of diffusion if blood flow is high, as the supply of the substance in the blood is rapidly replenished. If blood flow is low, there needs to be a large gradient for much diffusion to occur.

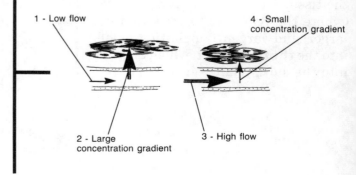

1 - Low flow

4 - Small concentration gradient

2 - Large concentration gradient

3 - High flow

THE VENULES AND VEINS

The blood leaving the capillaries is collected into venules and veins, which constitute the low-pressure side of the circulation. The walls of these vessels have smooth muscle controlled by sympathetic nerves, but changes in vascular tone at this level have little effect on circulatory resistance. The main effect of constriction or dilatation of veins is on the **capacity** of the circulation; there is a considerable volume of fluid stored in the relaxed veins, and if they are made to constrict a large amount of this blood can be rapidly returned to the heart, producing an effect rather like a rapid blood transfusion. There is a temporary increase in venous return, resulting in a rise in cardiac output.

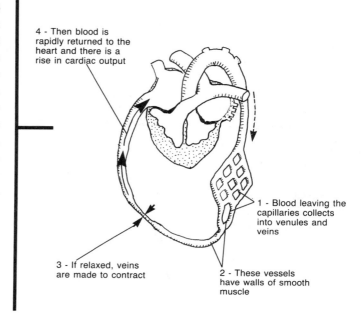

4 - Then blood is rapidly returned to the heart and there is a rise in cardiac output

1 - Blood leaving the capillaries collects into venules and veins

3 - If relaxed, veins are made to contract

2 - These vessels have walls of smooth muscle

Since pressures are low in the venous system, these vessels are provided with valves which prevent retrograde flow of blood. The forward impetus which remains after blood has passed through the small blood vessels is augmented by a number of other influences: the contraction of muscles squeezes veins; the movement of viscera in the abdomen has a small propulsive effect; the rhythmic pressure changes in the thorax during respiration have a major effect in persuading blood in the great veins to return to the heart.

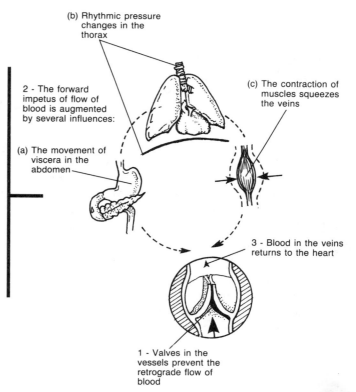

(b) Rhythmic pressure changes in the thorax

2 - The forward impetus of flow of blood is augmented by several influences:

(c) The contraction of muscles squeezes the veins

(a) The movement of viscera in the abdomen

3 - Blood in the veins returns to the heart

1 - Valves in the vessels prevent the retrograde flow of blood

CARDIOVASCULAR REFLEXES

One of the most important autonomic reflexes is concerned with regulation of the blood pressure. The carotid artery, which carries blood to the head, and particularly to the brain, has an area of dilatation near to its bifurcation into internal and external branches. This **carotid sinus** is richly endowed with stretch receptors in its wall, which are sensitive to distension of the artery; they are pressure receptors or **baroreceptors**. If pressure in the arteries rises, the carotid sinus becomes distended and impulses are discharged at a greater rate in the sensory **carotid sinus nerve**, which joins the hypoglossal nerve (cranial nerve XII).

The carotid sinus nerve enters the medulla oblogata of the brain stem, and the fibres go to the **cardiac** and **vasomotor** centres in the medulla. As the impulse discharge rate increases, the cardiac (vagal) centre is stimulated and more impulses travel down the vagus nerve, slowing the heart. At the same time the vasomotor centre is inhibited, so that fewer impulses travel out along the sympathetic nerves throughout the body, and the peripheral arterioles relax. The result of these two actions is that cardiac output falls and peripheral resistance is reduced, so the blood pressure comes down towards its normal value.

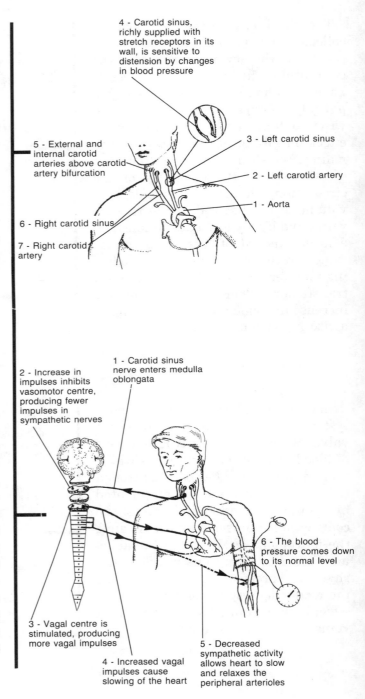

4 - Carotid sinus, richly supplied with stretch receptors in its wall, is sensitive to distension by changes in blood pressure

5 - External and internal carotid arteries above carotid artery bifurcation

3 - Left carotid sinus

2 - Left carotid artery

1 - Aorta

6 - Right carotid sinus

7 - Right carotid artery

2 - Increase in impulses inhibits vasomotor centre, producing fewer impulses in sympathetic nerves

1 - Carotid sinus nerve enters medulla oblongata

6 - The blood pressure comes down to its normal level

3 - Vagal centre is stimulated, producing more vagal impulses

4 - Increased vagal impulses cause slowing of the heart

5 - Decreased sympathetic activity allows heart to slow and relaxes the peripheral arterioles

If pressure in the carotid sinus falls, the baroreceptors are stimulated less and the carotid sinus nerve discharges less frequently. The inhibition of the vasomoter centre ceases while the vagus nerve discharges less often; the heart rate and cardiac output consequently rise while the peripheral vessels constrict, raising the blood pressure.

This baroreceptor reflex is a prime example of a homeostatic mechanism, with a negative feedback loop. The baroreceptors are the detectors, the control centres are in the medulla, the effectors are the heart and peripheral blood vessels, and the controlled variable is the arterial blood pressure.

The carotid sinus baroreceptors are very favourably situated in the main arterial trunk supplying the brain, as this is the organ which above all requires to have a steady, ideal blood pressure. There are also some baroreceptors in the arch of the aorta; they function in essentially the same way as the receptors of the carotid sinus.

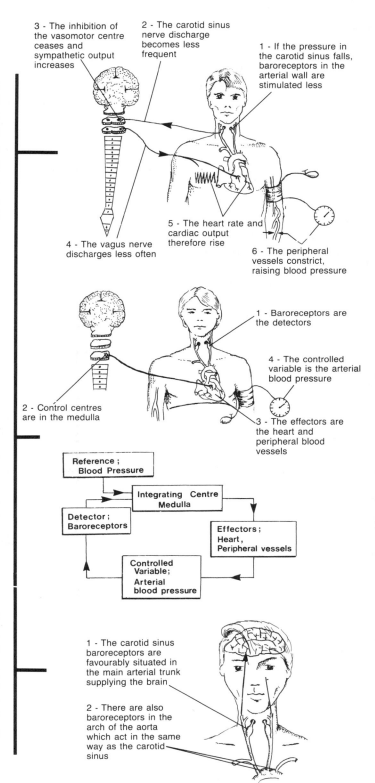

3 - The inhibition of the vasomotor centre ceases and sympathetic output increases

2 - The carotid sinus nerve discharge becomes less frequent

1 - If the pressure in the carotid sinus falls, baroreceptors in the arterial wall are stimulated less

5 - The heart rate and cardiac output therefore rise

4 - The vagus nerve discharges less often

6 - The peripheral vessels constrict, raising blood pressure

1 - Baroreceptors are the detectors

4 - The controlled variable is the arterial blood pressure

2 - Control centres are in the medulla

3 - The effectors are the heart and peripheral blood vessels

Reference ; Blood Pressure

Integrating Centre Medulla

Detector ; Baroreceptors

Effectors ; Heart, Peripheral vessels

Controlled Variable ; Arterial blood pressure

1 - The carotid sinus baroreceptors are favourably situated in the main arterial trunk supplying the brain

2 - There are also baroreceptors in the arch of the aorta which act in the same way as the carotid sinus

The baroreceptor reflex is important in the moment-by-moment maintenance of the arterial blood pressure. It helps the body to cope with the pressure changes associated with alterations in posture; if one stands up suddenly after sitting or lying down, the pooling of blood in the lower veins produces a transient reduction of venous return and a consequent lowering of cardiac output and hence blood pressure, and this is detected by the baroreceptors, which cause tachycardia and peripheral vasoconstriction.

A reduction of venous return because of acute haemorrhage or because of flying in an aircraft during a tight turning manoeuvre produces similar reflex changes.

Lying down causes the reverse postural effects and hence the reverse operation of the baroreceptor reflex.

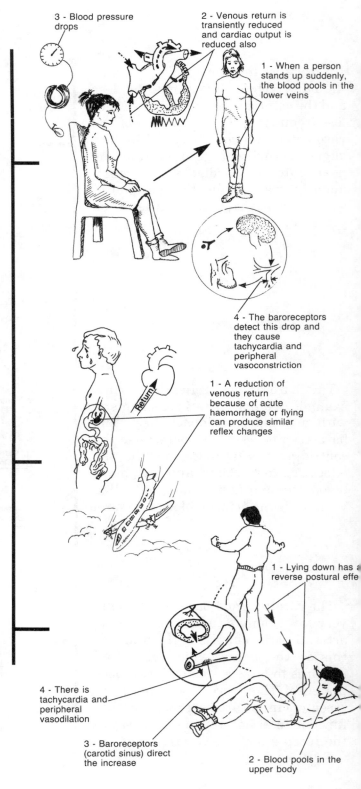

3 - Blood pressure drops

2 - Venous return is transiently reduced and cardiac output is reduced also

1 - When a person stands up suddenly, the blood pools in the lower veins

4 - The baroreceptors detect this drop and they cause tachycardia and peripheral vasoconstriction

1 - A reduction of venous return because of acute haemorrhage or flying can produce similar reflex changes

1 - Lying down has a reverse postural effe

4 - There is tachycardia and peripheral vasodilation

3 - Baroreceptors (carotid sinus) direct the increase

2 - Blood pools in the upper body

Close to the carotid sinus is a small, highly vascular organ known as the **carotid body**; there is an **aortic body** near the arch of the aorta with similar structure and function. These organs are **chemoreceptors**, responding to the level of oxygen dissolved in the blood. If the blood carries less oxygen than normal, the chemoreceptors discharge very rapidly, influencing the cardiac and vasomotor centres to cause cardiac acceleration and peripheral vasoconstriction. The consequent rise in blood pressure represents an attempt to compensate by increased blood flow for the reduced level of oxygen in the blood. However, the main role of the carotid and aortic body chemoreceptors is in the regulation of pulmonary ventilation, and they are described more fully in the chapter on the respiratory system.

There are several other areas in the circulation which contribute to reflexes. In the low-pressure, venous side of the circulation there are stretch receptors which have been called 'volume' receptors because distension of veins or of the right atrium itself is associated with changes in the total plasma volume. Stimulation of these receptors by distension of the great **veins** causes peripheral arterioles to dilate and the heart rate to slow. There are reflexes mediated by receptors in the lungs and in the peripheral veins; the function of many of these reflexes is still obscure.

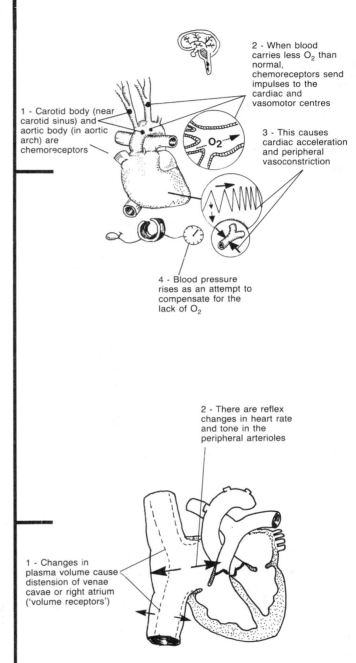

1 - Carotid body (near carotid sinus) and aortic body (in aortic arch) are chemoreceptors

2 - When blood carries less O_2 than normal, chemoreceptors send impulses to the cardiac and vasomotor centres

3 - This causes cardiac acceleration and peripheral vasoconstriction

4 - Blood pressure rises as an attempt to compensate for the lack of O_2

2 - There are reflex changes in heart rate and tone in the peripheral arterioles

1 - Changes in plasma volume cause distension of venae cavae or right atrium ('volume receptors')

HUMORAL INFLUENCES ON THE CIRCULATION

The nervous system is of paramount importance in the short-term regulation of the circulation, but the longer-term regulation is accomplished largely by the modification of vascular fluid volume and by a number of hormonal mechanisms.

If the volume of the blood increases, venous filling pressure and hence venous return are larger and cardiac output is increased. As a consequence the filtration rate in the kidney is larger and excretion of water increases; this results in a fall in blood volume, venous return and cardiac output. Distension of the right atrium also causes the secretion of **atrial natriuretic hormone**, which stimulates the kidney to excrete sodium and water; this results in the loss of fluid from the circulation.

If blood volume falls, the reverse mechanisms act to retain fluid and keep as much as possible in the circulation.

If the perfusion pressure to the kidneys falls, this is detected by a series of cells in the renal vessels known as the **juxtaglomerular apparatus**, and they secrete a hormone known as **renin** (not to be confused with rennin, the enzyme in the stomach which curdles milk). Renin acts on protein precursor substances in the blood to produce **angiotensin**, a very powerful **vasoconstrictor** substance which raises blood pressure. The net result is to restore perfusion pressure in that kidney.

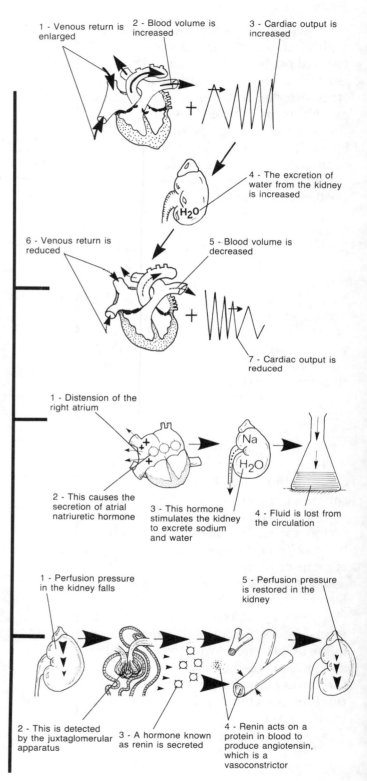

1 - Venous return is enlarged
2 - Blood volume is increased
3 - Cardiac output is increased
4 - The excretion of water from the kidney is increased
6 - Venous return is reduced
5 - Blood volume is decreased
7 - Cardiac output is reduced

1 - Distension of the right atrium
2 - This causes the secretion of atrial natriuretic hormone
3 - This hormone stimulates the kidney to excrete sodium and water
4 - Fluid is lost from the circulation

1 - Perfusion pressure in the kidney falls
2 - This is detected by the juxtaglomerular apparatus
3 - A hormone known as renin is secreted
4 - Renin acts on a protein in blood to produce angiotensin, which is a vasoconstrictor
5 - Perfusion pressure is restored in the kidney

Unfortunately, if the decreased perfusion pressure was caused by a narrowing of one renal artery, the consequence is that the rest of the circulation is subjected to a greatly increased blood pressure, which can cause cardiac strain, cerebral **haemorrhage** and damage to the normal kidney.

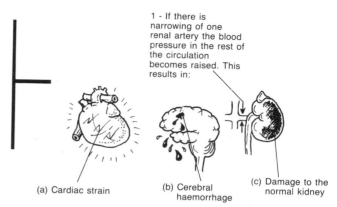

1 - If there is narrowing of one renal artery the blood pressure in the rest of the circulation becomes raised. This results in:

(a) Cardiac strain

(b) Cerebral haemorrhage

(c) Damage to the normal kidney

Many of the endocrine hormones cause indirect effects on the circulation. Thyroxine, by stimulating tissue metabolism, increases peripheral blood flow and hence cardiac output.

1 - Thyroxine stimulates tissue metabolism

3 - Cardiac output increases

2 - Peripheral blood flow is increased

Antidiuretic hormone and oxytocin from the posterior pituitary gland have an incidental vasoconstrictor effect although this is not their main physiological action.

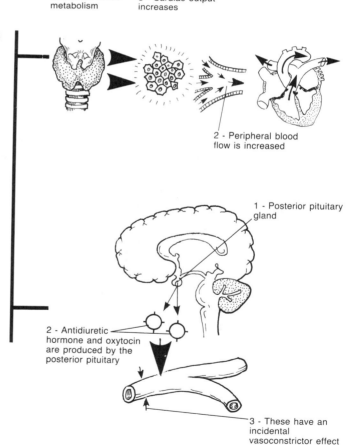

1 - Posterior pituitary gland

2 - Antidiuretic hormone and oxytocin are produced by the posterior pituitary

3 - These have an incidental vasoconstrictor effect

The hormones of pregnancy (oestrogen and progesterone) cause an increase in metabolism and cardiac output, but also relax veins, make them more distensible and predispose to the formation of haemorrhoids and varicose veins.

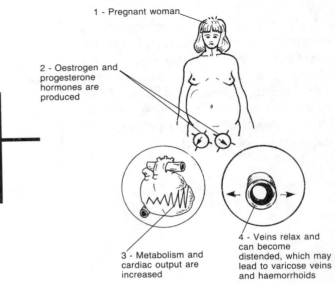

1 - Pregnant woman

2 - Oestrogen and progesterone hormones are produced

3 - Metabolism and cardiac output are increased

4 - Veins relax and can become distended, which may lead to varicose veins and haemorrhoids

CIRCULATION TO SPECIAL REGIONS

The coronary circulation

The heart muscle has its own arterial blood supply, through the coronary arteries which originate at the beginning of the aorta just at the base of the leaflets of the aortic valve. There are two arteries: one of these largely supplies the left ventricular muscle, and the other supplies the right side of the heart including the all-important sino-atrial and atrioventricular nodes.

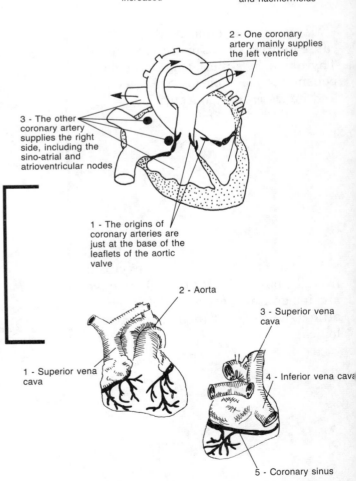

2 - One coronary artery mainly supplies the left ventricle

3 - The other coronary artery supplies the right side, including the sino-atrial and atrioventricular nodes

1 - The origins of coronary arteries are just at the base of the leaflets of the aortic valve

1 - Superior vena cava

2 - Aorta

3 - Superior vena cava

4 - Inferior vena cava

5 - Coronary sinus

In many other arteries, a large proportion of the flow of blood occurs during ventricular systole. However, during systole the coronary blood vessels are squeezed by the ventricular muscle, reducing blood flow, and a major part of coronary flow has to occur during diastole. This is one reason why the heart becomes less efficient at very high heart rates; the duration of diastole is reduced, and the opportunity for blood flow is decreased, so the oxygen supply to the heart is compromised.

The arterioles in the coronary circulation respond to many of the influences regulating the circulation elsewhere, but these influences seem to be less strong in the heart, so that generalized vasoconstricting processes tend to spare the coronary circulation. This is of course a reflection of the high priority which has to be given to the coronary circulation.

The blood coming out of the coronary capillaries is collected in venules and veins; eventually these join to form the **coronary sinus**, a large vein which empties directly into the right atrium. There are also some small veins in the myocardium, the **Thebesian veins**, which drain directly into the ventricular cavities.

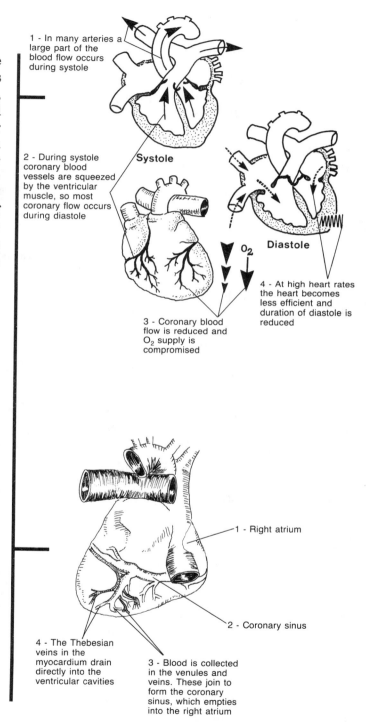

1 - In many arteries a large part of the blood flow occurs during systole

2 - During systole coronary blood vessels are squeezed by the ventricular muscle, so most coronary flow occurs during diastole

Systole

Diastole

O_2

4 - At high heart rates the heart becomes less efficient and duration of diastole is reduced

3 - Coronary blood flow is reduced and O_2 supply is compromised

1 - Right atrium

2 - Coronary sinus

4 - The Thebesian veins in the myocardium drain directly into the ventricular cavities

3 - Blood is collected in the venules and veins. These join to form the coronary sinus, which empties into the right atrium

The cerebral circulation

The blood vessels of the brain arise from a complicated network of arteries, the **circle of Willis** (see the chapters on the nervous system). Each area of brain is supplied with its own blood vessels, with little interconnection.

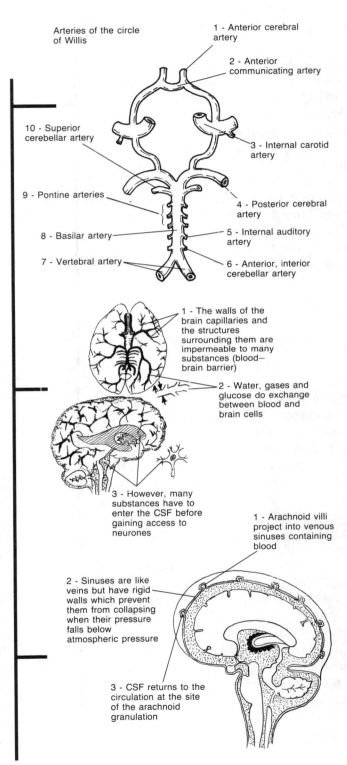

Arteries of the circle of Willis

1 - Anterior cerebral artery

2 - Anterior communicating artery

10 - Superior cerebellar artery

3 - Internal carotid artery

9 - Pontine arteries

4 - Posterior cerebral artery

8 - Basilar artery

5 - Internal auditory artery

7 - Vertebral artery

6 - Anterior, interior cerebellar artery

The walls of the brain capillaries and the structures surrounding them are rather impermeable to many substances (the blood—brain barrier) so the exchange of materials across the capillary wall is rather limited. Water, gases and glucose do exchange directly between blood and the brain cells, but many substances have to enter the cerebrospinal fluid (CSF) before they can gain access to the neurones.

The veins draining the brain and other cranial structures join the cerebral sinuses — large tubular spaces between layers of the dura mater and periosteum in the lining of the skull cavity. These sinuses are lined with endothelium like blood vessels elsewhere, but unlike other veins they have relatively rigid walls and are thus kept from collapsing when the pressure within them falls below atmospheric pressure. The sinuses have arachnoid granulations in their walls, and these are the sites where CSF returns to the circulation. The sinuses empty into the jugular veins, which eventually join the superior vena cava.

1 - The walls of the brain capillaries and the structures surrounding them are impermeable to many substances (blood—brain barrier)

2 - Water, gases and glucose do exchange between blood and brain cells

3 - However, many substances have to enter the CSF before gaining access to neurones

1 - Arachnoid villi project into venous sinuses containing blood

2 - Sinuses are like veins but have rigid walls which prevent them from collapsing when their pressure falls below atmospheric pressure

3 - CSF returns to the circulation at the site of the arachnoid granulation

The cerebral blood vessels are not greatly influenced by sympathetic nerves or circulating vasoactive substances; one might argue that cerebral blood flow is controlled by regulating the whole of the rest of the circulation, so that the blood pressure (and hence the cerebral perfusion pressure) is kept constant. The blood vessels in the brain are, however, very susceptible to the influences of hypoxia and hypercapnia, which cause considerable vasodilatation and hence can produce cerebral oedema.

Patients who have severe head injury are often intubated with an endotracheal tube and artificially hyperventilated to prevent this vasodilatation and its consequent severe cerebral oedema.

Part of the cerebral circulation is unusual in having a portal system. The veins leaving the median eminence of the hypothalamus pass down the pituitary stalk and enter the anterior lobe of the pituitary gland, where they break up again in capillaries. These portal vessels carry **releasing factors** from the hypothalamus to control the function of the hormone-producing cells of the pituitary gland (see the chapter on the endocrine system).

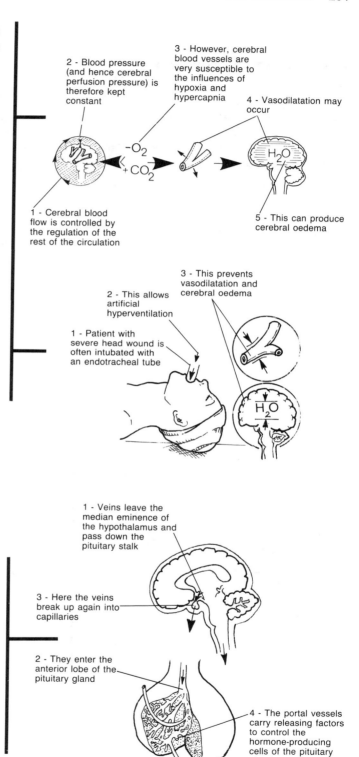

2 - Blood pressure (and hence cerebral perfusion pressure) is therefore kept constant

3 - However, cerebral blood vessels are very susceptible to the influences of hypoxia and hypercapnia

4 - Vasodilatation may occur

$-O_2$
$+CO_2$

H_2O

1 - Cerebral blood flow is controlled by the regulation of the rest of the circulation

5 - This can produce cerebral oedema

3 - This prevents vasodilatation and cerebral oedema

2 - This allows artificial hyperventilation

1 - Patient with severe head wound is often intubated with an endotracheal tube

H_2O

1 - Veins leave the median eminence of the hypothalamus and pass down the pituitary stalk

3 - Here the veins break up again into capillaries

2 - They enter the anterior lobe of the pituitary gland

4 - The portal vessels carry releasing factors to control the hormone-producing cells of the pituitary gland

Pulmonary and bronchial circulation

All of the output from the right ventricle flows through the lungs; there is thus not much scope for regulation by the lung vessels of the total flow through them. In fact the pulmonary vessels are not very densely innervated, though noradrenaline and adrenaline can produce pulmonary vasoconstriction.

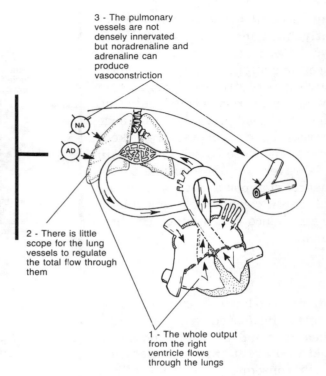

3 - The pulmonary vessels are not densely innervated but noradrenaline and adrenaline can produce vasoconstriction

2 - There is little scope for the lung vessels to regulate the total flow through them

1 - The whole output from the right ventricle flows through the lungs

There is, however, scope for **regional** modification of pulmonary flow. If an area of lung were under-ventilated, it would make sense for blood flow to that area to be restricted to allow the blood to flow through better ventilated, more useful areas of the lung. This does occur, and pulmonary arterial smooth muscle differs from all other vascular muscles in that hypoxia constricts, and a normal to high oxygen concentration dilates the vessels.

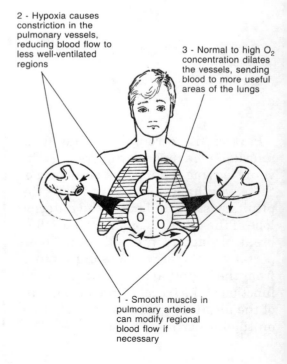

2 - Hypoxia causes constriction in the pulmonary vessels, reducing blood flow to less well-ventilated regions

3 - Normal to high O_2 concentration dilates the vessels, sending blood to more useful areas of the lungs

1 - Smooth muscle in pulmonary arteries can modify regional blood flow if necessary

The blood in the pulmonary arteries is deoxygenated and therefore useless in nourishing and sustaining the cells of the bronchial tree and the lung parenchyma. Although some oxygen can diffuse from the lumen into the cells of the smaller airways, even this is usually inadequate and so the airways are supplied by their own blood vessels, the **bronchial arteries**, which bring fresh arterial blood to the lung tissue.

Circulation to the gut and liver

The arteries supplying the gastro-intestinal tract (the coeliac and the superior and inferior mesenteric arteries) break up into smaller and smaller branches, the **arcuate arteries**, which run in quite a dramatic manner in the mesentery. Individual segments of gut are supplied from small terminal branches arising from the tops of the arches and splitting into tiny arterioles and capillaries in the gut wall.

The blood supply to the alimentary system is unusual in that the blood leaving the capillaries collects into veins which enter the liver as the **hepatic portal vein**. The blood is then distributed through **sinusoids** or blood-filled spaces throughout the liver so that the nutrients absorbed from the gut are brought into immediate and intimate contact with the liver cells for chemical processing. The sinusoids then drain into the hepatic veins, which join the inferior vena cava.

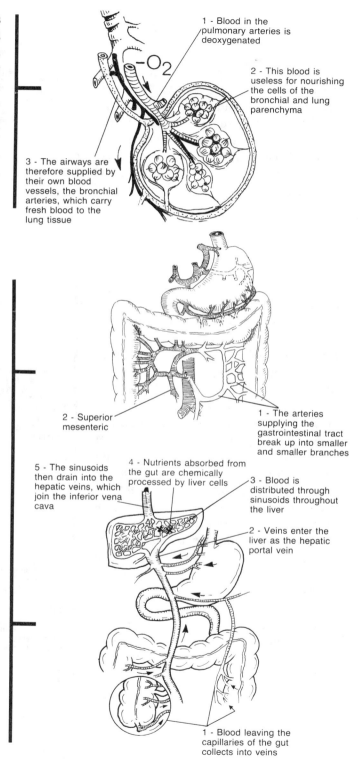

1 - Blood in the pulmonary arteries is deoxygenated

2 - This blood is useless for nourishing the cells of the bronchial and lung parenchyma

3 - The airways are therefore supplied by their own blood vessels, the bronchial arteries, which carry fresh blood to the lung tissue

1 - The arteries supplying the gastrointestinal tract break up into smaller and smaller branches

2 - Superior mesenteric

5 - The sinusoids then drain into the hepatic veins, which join the inferior vena cava

4 - Nutrients absorbed from the gut are chemically processed by liver cells

3 - Blood is distributed through sinusoids throughout the liver

2 - Veins enter the liver as the hepatic portal vein

1 - Blood leaving the capillaries of the gut collects into veins

The blood in the portal vein, having already passed through a capillary bed, is deoxygenated and inadequate for the metabolic needs of the rather active liver cells. There is therefore a separate arterial blood supply via the **hepatic artery**, which brings oxygenated blood directly to the cells of the liver.

The arterioles of the gut are responsive to the same influences as blood vessels elsewhere; sympathetic noradrenergic nerves constrict them, and the release of vasoconstrictor tone dilates them. There is a variety of other substances released around the gut, many of which are vasoactive. Some of them are hormones such as gastrin, whose primary task is the regulation of gastrointestinal secretion but which may incidentally produce vasoconstriction or dilatation; others such as vasoactive intestinal peptide (VIP) may be released from autonomic nerves as a true neurotransmitter to some other organ, and have an incidental vasodilator action. Almost all hormones and neurotransmitters can be shown to have some action on blood vessels, but many of these actions occur only at high concentrations and are not necessarily part of the body's normal mechanism.

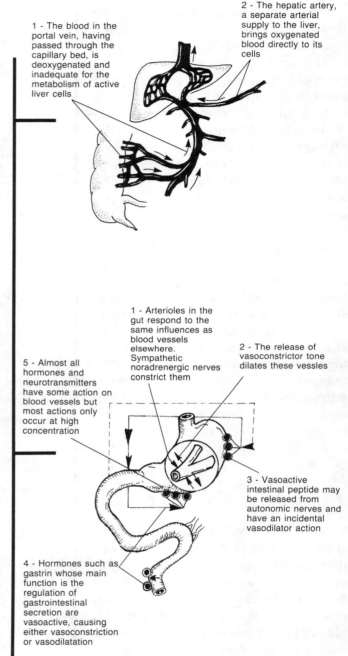

1 - The blood in the portal vein, having passed through the capillary bed, is deoxygenated and inadequate for the metabolism of active liver cells

2 - The hepatic artery, a separate arterial supply to the liver, brings oxygenated blood directly to its cells

1 - Arterioles in the gut respond to the same influences as blood vessels elsewhere. Sympathetic noradrenergic nerves constrict them

2 - The release of vasoconstrictor tone dilates these vessels

3 - Vasoactive intestinal peptide may be released from autonomic nerves and have an incidental vasodilator action

4 - Hormones such as gastrin whose main function is the regulation of gastrointestinal secretion are vasoactive, causing either vasoconstriction or vasodilatation

5 - Almost all hormones and neurotransmitters have some action on blood vessels but most actions only occur at high concentration

The visceral vessels, like the vessels of the skin, are constricted by circulating adrenaline, so that during the body's 'fight or flight' response the skin and viscera are vasoconstricted while the muscle blood vessels dilate. The blood is thus enabled to flow to those regions where it is most needed during the emergency.

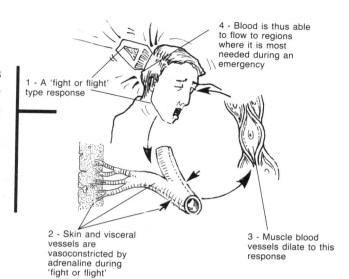

1 - A 'fight or flight' type response

4 - Blood is thus able to flow to regions where it is most needed during an emergency

2 - Skin and visceral vessels are vasoconstricted by adrenaline during 'fight or flight'

3 - Muscle blood vessels dilate to this response

Circulation to the kidney

This topic will be covered more fully in the chapter on the kidney. The blood flow through the kidney is far in excess of the organ's metabolic needs, and represents up to one quarter of the resting cardiac output. This is because the kidney's main function is to filter, purify and otherwise process the blood flowing through it, requiring only a modest amount of nutrition itself.

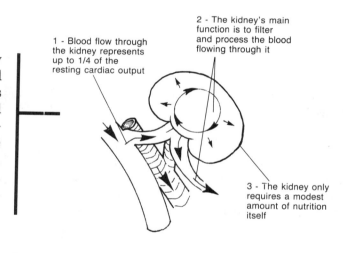

1 - Blood flow through the kidney represents up to 1/4 of the resting cardiac output

2 - The kidney's main function is to filter and process the blood flowing through it

3 - The kidney only requires a modest amount of nutrition itself

The renal arteries split into interlobar arteries which run between the major lobes. These branch into arciform or arcuate arteries which course at right angles to the interlobar arteries, running between the renal cortex and the medulla. They give off the interlobular arteries which run radially outward in the cortex and give off the afferent arterioles. After supplying the nephron (see the chapter on the kidney) the vessels collect through interlobular, arcuate and interlobar veins to form the main renal vein.

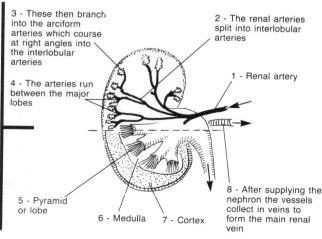

3 - These then branch into the arciform arteries which course at right angles into the interlobular arteries

4 - The arteries run between the major lobes

2 - The renal arteries split into interlobular arteries

1 - Renal artery

5 - Pyramid or lobe

6 - Medulla   7 - Cortex

8 - After supplying the nephron the vessels collect in veins to form the main renal vein

The circulations of fish and amphibia, but not of mammals or humans, include a renal portal system, where the veins draining the tail or lower limbs empty into the kidney so that the waste products of hind-limb metabolism can be eliminated immediately. There is, of course, still the normal renal arterial system, which is probably the most important component of the renal blood flow in these primitive creatures.

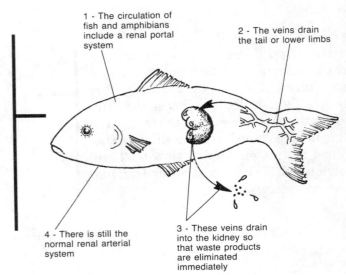

1 - The circulation of fish and amphibians include a renal portal system

2 - The veins drain the tail or lower limbs

4 - There is still the normal renal arterial system

3 - These veins drain into the kidney so that waste products are eliminated immediately

Circulatory adjustments to exercise

During muscular exercise, the body's requirements for oxygen and glucose, and the production of carbon dioxide and other waste products, can increase by up to twenty times. The cardiac output must increase by at least five or six times.

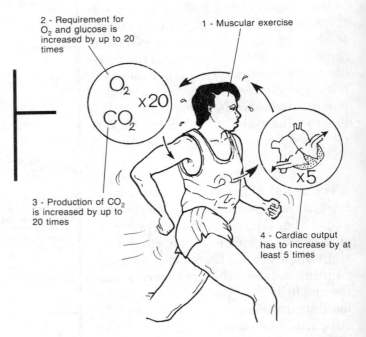

2 - Requirement for O_2 and glucose is increased by up to 20 times

1 - Muscular exercise

3 - Production of CO_2 is increased by up to 20 times

4 - Cardiac output has to increase by at least 5 times

Several mechanisms contribute to this adjustment. The anticipation of exertion can cause the adrenal gland to secrete large amounts of adrenaline; this speeds the heart and increases its contractile force, and adjusts the peripheral vessels by dilating muscle vessels while constricting skin and visceral vessels.

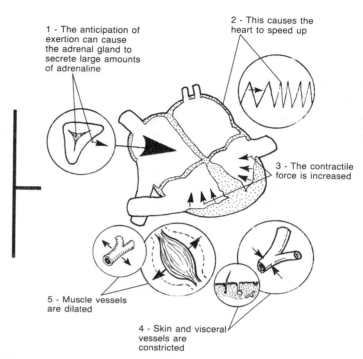

1 - The anticipation of exertion can cause the adrenal gland to secrete large amounts of adrenaline

2 - This causes the heart to speed up

3 - The contractile force is increased

5 - Muscle vessels are dilated

4 - Skin and visceral vessels are constricted

The adrenal gland's functions are augmented by the actions of the sympathetic nerves on the heart and blood vessels. Once the muscles start to contract they consume oxygen and generate carbon dioxide, lactic acid and heat, causing locally mediated vasodilatation; if the peripheral resistance falls as a consequence, then baroreceptor reflexes try to maintain pressure by further stimulating the heart. The contraction of muscles squeezes veins in their vicinity, increasing venous return to the heart and helping to maintain cardiac output.

The onset of exercise also stimulates pulmonary ventilation, as there would be little point in increasing cardiac output without increasing oxygen supply.

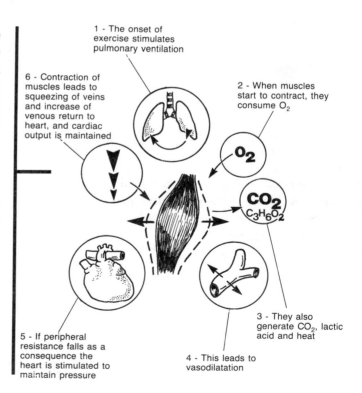

1 - The onset of exercise stimulates pulmonary ventilation

2 - When muscles start to contract, they consume O_2

6 - Contraction of muscles leads to squeezing of veins and increase of venous return to heart, and cardiac output is maintained

3 - They also generate CO_2, lactic acid and heat

4 - This leads to vasodilatation

5 - If peripheral resistance falls as a consequence the heart is stimulated to maintain pressure

Circulatory adjustments to heat and cold

When the body experiences cold, the thermoregulatory system causes the skin blood vessels to constrict; the resulting increase in peripheral resistance is compensated for by vasodilatation in the splanchnic and other vascular beds. If there is shivering, the increased metabolic rate requires a higher blood flow in the muscles, and there is an increase in cardiac output and in muscle blood flow.

In the heat, the vasodilatation in the skin causes a fall in peripheral resistance, and in order to compensate there is an increase in cardiac output brought about by a reflex tachycardia and a vasoconstriction in the muscular and splanchnic regions.

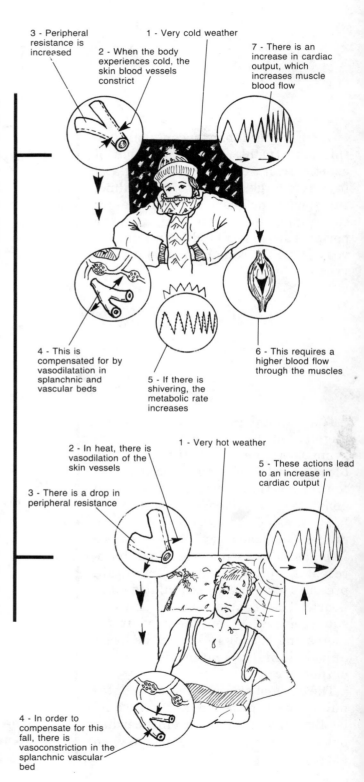

3 - Peripheral resistance is increased

1 - Very cold weather

2 - When the body experiences cold, the skin blood vessels constrict

7 - There is an increase in cardiac output, which increases muscle blood flow

4 - This is compensated for by vasodilatation in splanchnic and vascular beds

5 - If there is shivering, the metabolic rate increases

6 - This requires a higher blood flow through the muscles

2 - In heat, there is vasodilation of the skin vessels

1 - Very hot weather

5 - These actions lead to an increase in cardiac output

3 - There is a drop in peripheral resistance

4 - In order to compensate for this fall, there is vasoconstriction in the splanchnic vascular bed

Circulatory adjustments to injury and stress

If the body suffers injury and blood loss, the venous return to the heart decreases and cardiac output falls. This situation is known as **shock**, and produces a characteristic clinical picture. In response to the falling blood pressure there is reflex tachycardia, producing the typical 'rapid thready pulse'. There is skin vasoconstriction and the peripheries feel cold and may appear pale or blue. Many of these effects are the result of a massive outpouring of adrenaline from the adrenal gland together with activation of the sympathetic nervous system.

If the compensatory mechanisms are insuffient to maintain blood pressure, the perfusion of the heart by the coronary arteries becomes insufficient for the requirements of the myocardium; this leads to a decline in the force of cardiac contraction and hence in cardiac output, which produces a further decrease in blood pressure and myocardial perfusion, and further cardiac impairment. It is evident that replacement of lost fluid and restoration of the cardiac output must be a high priority in the treatment of injury and shock.

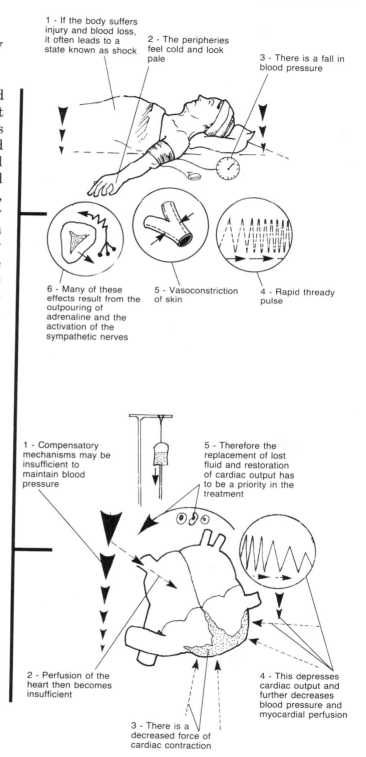

1 - If the body suffers injury and blood loss, it often leads to a state known as shock

2 - The peripheries feel cold and look pale

3 - There is a fall in blood pressure

6 - Many of these effects result from the outpouring of adrenaline and the activation of the sympathetic nerves

5 - Vasoconstriction of skin

4 - Rapid thready pulse

1 - Compensatory mechanisms may be insuffient to maintain blood pressure

5 - Therefore the replacement of lost fluid and restoration of cardiac output has to be a priority in the treatment

2 - Perfusion of the heart then becomes insufficient

3 - There is a decreased force of cardiac contraction

4 - This depresses cardiac output and further decreases blood pressure and myocardial perfusion

Respiration

The function of the respiratory system is to bring atmospheric air close to the blood, allowing oxygen to be taken up into the blood and carbon dioxide to be given up and removed from the body. The circulatory system transports the aerated blood to the tissues where the oxygen is used in **tissue respiration**, the metabolic reactions liberating energy for the vital functions of the various cells.

The most important organs are the lungs, where the exchange or gases takes place. The lungs consist of huge numbers of tiny air sacs, or **alveoli**, connected to the outside air through an extensive system of conducting tubes or airways.

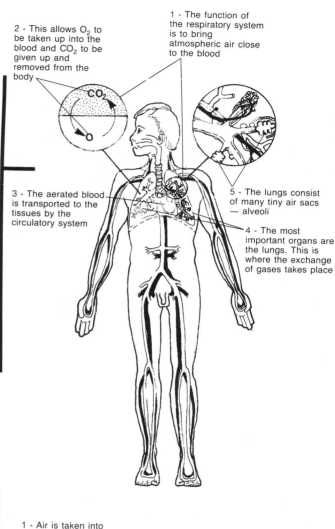

1 - The function of the respiratory system is to bring atmospheric air close to the blood

2 - This allows O_2 to be taken up into the blood and CO_2 to be given up and removed from the body

3 - The aerated blood is transported to the tissues by the circulatory system

5 - The lungs consist of many tiny air sacs — alveoli

4 - The most important organs are the lungs. This is where the exchange of gases takes place

Air is taken into the body through the mouth and nose. These join at the back to form the pharynx, which soon branches into two tubes: the oesophagus, leading to the digestive system, and the larynx, leading to the respiratory system. The two tubes are partly separated by the flap-like **epiglottis**, which deflects food into the oesophagus. The larynx is a cartilaginous 'voice-box' containing the vocal cords or glottis, a pair of muscular flaps which can come together to protect the airway from inhaled food; they can also be made to vibrate and generate the sounds of speech and song.

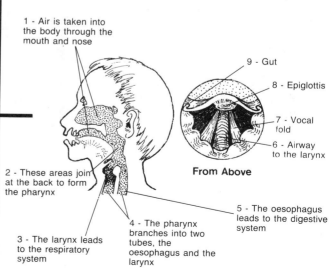

1 - Air is taken into the body through the mouth and nose

2 - These areas join at the back to form the pharynx

3 - The larynx leads to the respiratory system

4 - The pharynx branches into two tubes, the oesophagus and the larynx

5 - The oesophagus leads to the digestive system

9 - Gut

8 - Epiglottis

7 - Vocal fold

6 - Airway to the larynx

From Above

The larynx leads into the trachea, a long tube with cartilaginous and muscular walls. The cartilages are incomplete rings, 'C' shaped with the opening posteriorly; the gap in the 'C' is bridged by smooth muscle which can adjust the tension in the walls and hence the calibre of the airways. The trachea bifurcates at the **carina** into the right and left main **bronchi**, supplying the two lungs. Within the lungs each main bronchus divides into successively smaller and smaller bronchi until the airways are so small that they become **bronchioles**.

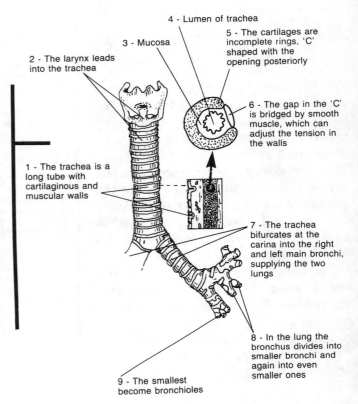

The bronchi, like the trachea, consist of cartilaginous plates connected by bands of smooth muscle. In the larger bronchi the cartilages retain their 'C' shape, but in the smaller bronchi they are simply irregular flat plates embedded in the circular smooth muscle of the bronchial wall.

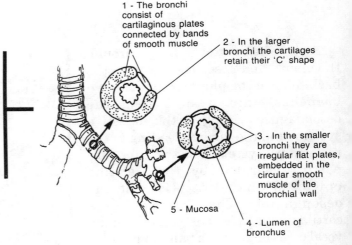

The whole of the tracheobronchial tree is lined with pseudostratified ciliated columnar epithelium liberally supplied with mucus-secreting goblet cells. The microscopic cilia of the epithelial cells waft particles trapped in the mucus out towards the mouth.

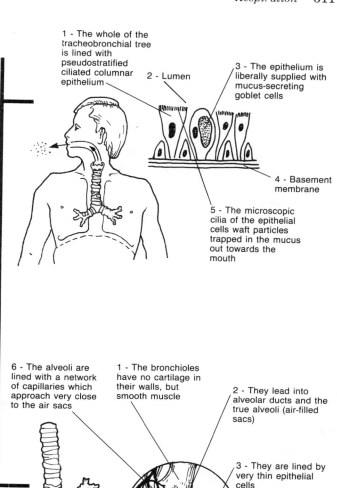

1 - The whole of the tracheobronchial tree is lined with pseudostratified ciliated columnar epithelium

2 - Lumen

3 - The epithelium is liberally supplied with mucus-secreting goblet cells

4 - Basement membrane

5 - The microscopic cilia of the epithelial cells waft particles trapped in the mucus out towards the mouth

The bronchioles have no cartilage in their walls, but are well endowed with smooth muscle. They lead into the alveolar ducts and the true alveoli, which are air-filled sacs (lined by very thin epithelial cells) where the respiratory gas exchange takes place. The surface area of the alveoli of the two lungs is enormous, being about 70 m^2 or the size of a tennis court. The alveoli are lined with an extensive network of capillaries, which approach very close to the air sacs and allow the easy diffusion of gases.

6 - The alveoli are lined with a network of capillaries which approach very close to the air sacs

1 - The bronchioles have no cartilage in their walls, but smooth muscle

2 - They lead into alveolar ducts and the true alveoli (air-filled sacs)

3 - They are lined by very thin epithelial cells

4 - Respiratory gas exchange takes place here

5 - The surface area of the alveoli of the two lungs is approximately 70 m^2

The blood from the right ventricle is brought to the lungs by the right and left branches of the pulmonary artery. The arteries enter each lung at the **hilum** (or stalk) close to the main bronchus.

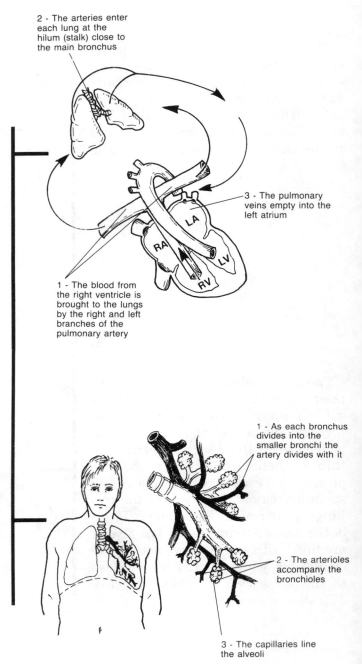

2 - The arteries enter each lung at the hilum (stalk) close to the main bronchus

3 - The pulmonary veins empty into the left atrium

1 - The blood from the right ventricle is brought to the lungs by the right and left branches of the pulmonary artery

As each bronchus divides into lobar and then segmental bronchi, so the artery divides to accompany it. Eventually the arterioles accompany the bronchioles, and the capillaries line the alveoli. The pulmonary venules collect into larger and larger veins until the two pulmonary veins from each lung empty into the left atrium.

1 - As each bronchus divides into the smaller bronchi the artery divides with it

2 - The arterioles accompany the bronchioles

3 - The capillaries line the alveoli

THE AIR IN THE LUNGS: THE LUNG VOLUMES

The process of breathing occurs constantly throughout life, and most of the time it proceeds without the individual having to think about it. Air is rhythmically drawn into the lungs and then expelled; the air drawn in and out is known as the **tidal** air, and the volume breathed in and out in each breath is called the tidal volume.

The lungs are not completely filled during each inspiration, and not all of the air is expelled from the lungs during each expiration. Instead a small proportion of the air in the lung is exchanged during each respiratory cycle.

The lung volumes can be studied by allowing the subject to breathe in and out of a **spirometer**, a large cylindrical reservoir filled with air or oxygen. The open end of the cylinder is immersed in water, and as the subject breathes in and out the bell goes down and up in the water, and can be made to record on a piece of moving paper. The tidal volume during normal shallow breathing may easily be demonstrated and measured: there are small regular fluctuations on the spirometer trace. If the subject breathes in very deeply the spirometer moves a long way, and if he breathes out forcefully the spirometer moves a large distance in the opposite direction.

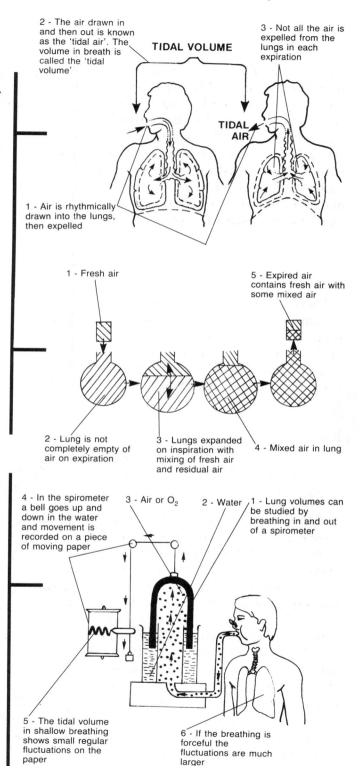

TIDAL VOLUME

TIDAL AIR

2 - The air drawn in and then out is known as the 'tidal air'. The volume in breath is called the 'tidal volume'

3 - Not all the air is expelled from the lungs in each expiration

1 - Air is rhythmically drawn into the lungs, then expelled

1 - Fresh air

5 - Expired air contains fresh air with some mixed air

2 - Lung is not completely empty of air on expiration

3 - Lungs expanded on inspiration with mixing of fresh air and residual air

4 - Mixed air in lung

4 - In the spirometer a bell goes up and down in the water and movement is recorded on a piece of moving paper

3 - Air or O₂

2 - Water

1 - Lung volumes can be studied by breathing in and out of a spirometer

5 - The tidal volume in shallow breathing shows small regular fluctuations on the paper

6 - If the breathing is forceful the fluctuations are much larger

If a maximal breath is taken in, and then the air is forcibly expelled until no more can be breathed out, the total volume is known as the **vital capacity**. Even at the end of a maximal expiration there is some air left in the lungs; this is the **residual volume**. The amount of air left in the lungs at the end of a normal tidal expiration is the **functional residual capacity**.

There is also an inspiratory reserve volume, an expiratory reserve volume, and a total lung capacity. Note that each **volume** is a single simple component, while the **capacities** are each made up of two or more volumes.

For example:

$$\begin{matrix} \text{functional} \\ \text{residual} \\ \text{capacity} \end{matrix} = \begin{matrix} \text{residual} \\ \text{volume} \end{matrix} + \begin{matrix} \text{expiratory} \\ \text{reserve} \\ \text{volume} \end{matrix}$$

If the subject attempts to expel his vital capacity as rapidly and forcefully as possible, he can usually breathe out about 75–80% of the vital capacity in the first second. This is known as the **forced expiratory volume in one second** or the FEV_1 (usually expressed as a percentage). This simple test is used clinically to distinguish between diseases where there is obstruction to airflow (where FEV_1 is reduced but vital capacity is normal) and diseases where there is restriction of lung expansion, where vital capacity is reduced but FEV_1 is a normal percentage.

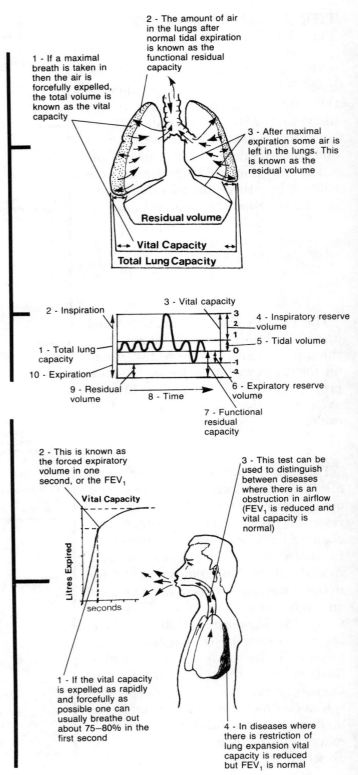

1 - If a maximal breath is taken in then the air is forcefully expelled, the total volume is known as the vital capacity

2 - The amount of air in the lungs after normal tidal expiration is known as the functional residual capacity

3 - After maximal expiration some air is left in the lungs. This is known as the residual volume

Residual volume

Vital Capacity

Total Lung Capacity

2 - Inspiration
1 - Total lung capacity
10 - Expiration
9 - Residual volume
8 - Time
3 - Vital capacity
4 - Inspiratory reserve volume
5 - Tidal volume
6 - Expiratory reserve volume
7 - Functional residual capacity

2 - This is known as the forced expiratory volume in one second, or the FEV_1

3 - This test can be used to distinguish between diseases where there is an obstruction in airflow (FEV_1 is reduced and vital capacity is normal)

Vital Capacity

Litres Expired

seconds

1 - If the vital capacity is expelled as rapidly and forcefully as possible one can usually breathe out about 75–80% in the first second

4 - In diseases where there is restriction of lung expansion vital capacity is reduced but FEV_1 is normal

THE MUSCLES OF RESPIRATION

The lungs lie in the chest, a bony cage of ribs which are moved by various muscles. At the bottom of the chest, separating it from the abdomen, is the dome-shaped **diaphragm**.

Contraction of this muscle, which is attached to the ribs at its margins, causes the dome to move down and enlarges the chest cavity along the axis of the body. Between the ribs are the external and internal **intercostal** muscles, whose contraction moves the ribs upwards and outwards, increasing the diameter of the chest. Both of these sets of muscles enlarge the chest cavity, reducing the pressure within it. This allows the pressure of the atmosphere to drive air into the lungs (inspiration).

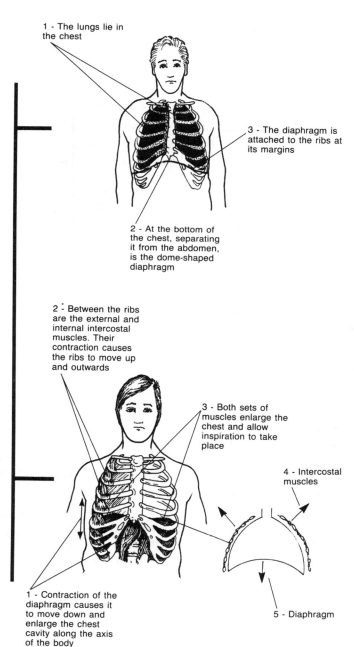

1 - The lungs lie in the chest

3 - The diaphragm is attached to the ribs at its margins

2 - At the bottom of the chest, separating it from the abdomen, is the dome-shaped diaphragm

2 - Between the ribs are the external and internal intercostal muscles. Their contraction causes the ribs to move up and outwards

3 - Both sets of muscles enlarge the chest and allow inspiration to take place

4 - Intercostal muscles

5 - Diaphragm

1 - Contraction of the diaphragm causes it to move down and enlarge the chest cavity along the axis of the body

The act of inspiration stretches tissues in the lungs and the chest wall, but when the active contraction of the inspiratory muscles ceases, the elastic recoil of these structures forces air out of the lungs. Expiration is normally a passive process, requiring no expenditure of muscular effort.

If forceful expiration is required, for instance when large amounts of air are needed for exercise, or when airflow is limited in diseases of the airways like asthma, then certain **accessory expiratory muscles** are called into play. The most important are the muscles of the abdominal wall, which contract and force the abdominal contents against the diaphragm, making it move up into the chest to compress the lungs.

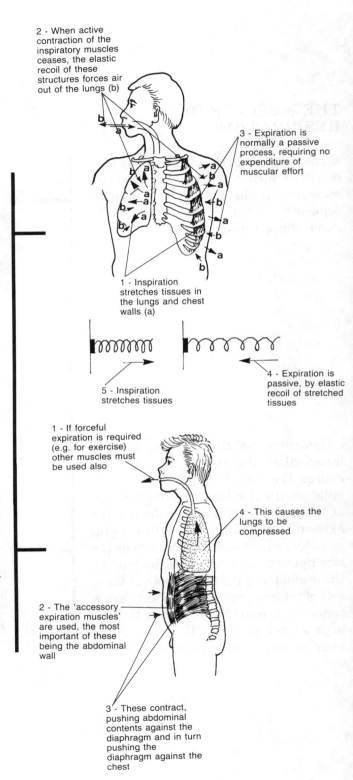

2 - When active contraction of the inspiratory muscles ceases, the elastic recoil of these structures forces air out of the lungs (b)

3 - Expiration is normally a passive process, requiring no expenditure of muscular effort

1 - Inspiration stretches tissues in the lungs and chest walls (a)

5 - Inspiration stretches tissues

4 - Expiration is passive, by elastic recoil of stretched tissues

1 - If forceful expiration is required (e.g. for exercise) other muscles must be used also

4 - This causes the lungs to be compressed

2 - The 'accessory expiration muscles' are used, the most important of these being the abdominal wall

3 - These contract, pushing abdominal contents against the diaphragm and in turn pushing the diaphragm against the chest

Either the diaphragm or the intercostal muscles alone are sufficient for normal quiet breathing. The diaphragm is controlled by the **phrenic nerve**, which originates in the neck (cervical spinal segments 3, 4 and 5) and runs down the centre of the chest.

If a patient suffers a spinal injury resulting in paralysis, the injury is often below the level of the phrenic nerve, so that contraction of the diaphragm is still possible although the intercostal muscles may be paralysed. Conversely, if the phrenic nerve becomes accidentally cut or otherwise injured, the intercostal muscles controlled by their segmental nerves are still able to maintain respiration.

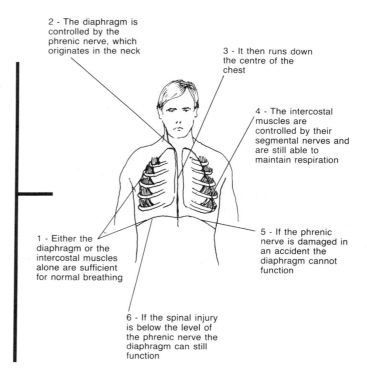

2 - The diaphragm is controlled by the phrenic nerve, which originates in the neck

3 - It then runs down the centre of the chest

4 - The intercostal muscles are controlled by their segmental nerves and are still able to maintain respiration

1 - Either the diaphragm or the intercostal muscles alone are sufficient for normal breathing

5 - If the phrenic nerve is damaged in an accident the diaphragm cannot function

6 - If the spinal injury is below the level of the phrenic nerve the diaphragm can still function

MECHANICS OF RESPIRATION

When the respiratory muscles contract they alter the pressures within the chest and therefore within the lungs and the conducting airways. Enlargement of the thoracic cavity by the action of the diaphragm and intercostal muscles reduces the pressure in the pleural cavity, which causes the lungs to enlarge and reduce their pressure. This allows the pressure of the atmosphere to force air in through the nose and mouth, occupying the additional volume created by expansion of the chest.

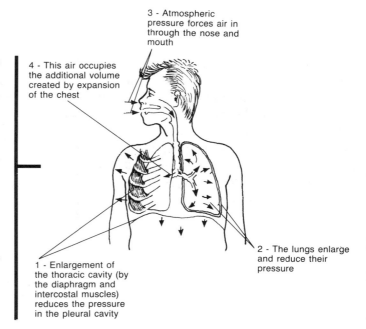

3 - Atmospheric pressure forces air in through the nose and mouth

4 - This air occupies the additional volume created by expansion of the chest

1 - Enlargement of the thoracic cavity (by the diaphragm and intercostal muscles) reduces the pressure in the pleural cavity

2 - The lungs enlarge and reduce their pressure

The ease with which the chest can be expanded by muscular effort is governed by the **stiffness** of the structures of the chest wall and the lung tissue. The reciprocal of stiffness is **compliance** (distensibility), which is defined as the volume change produced by a unit change in pressure, i.e. litres per kilopascal.

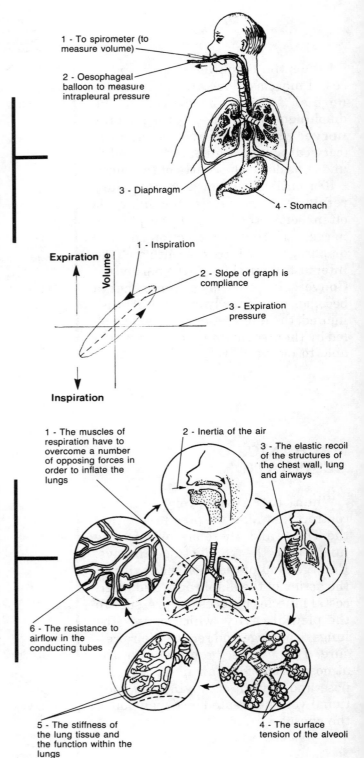

1 - To spirometer (to measure volume)

2 - Oesophageal balloon to measure intrapleural pressure

3 - Diaphragm

4 - Stomach

Expiration

Volume

1 - Inspiration

2 - Slope of graph is compliance

3 - Expiration pressure

Inspiration

The muscles of respiration have to overcome a number of opposing forces in order to inflate the lungs. These are: the inertia of the air (a small factor); the elastic recoil of the structures of the chest wall, lungs and airways; the surface tension of the alveoli; the stiffness of the lung tissue and the friction within the lungs; and the resistance to airflow in the conducting tubes.

1 - The muscles of respiration have to overcome a number of opposing forces in order to inflate the lungs

2 - Inertia of the air

3 - The elastic recoil of the structures of the chest wall, lung and airways

6 - The resistance to airflow in the conducting tubes

5 - The stiffness of the lung tissue and the function within the lungs

4 - The surface tension of the alveoli

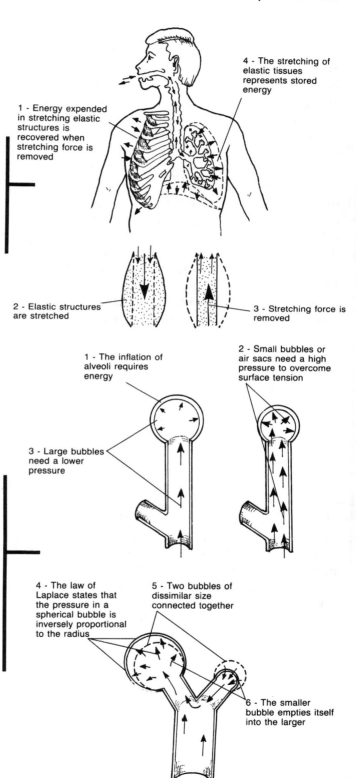

Elastic tissues

Energy expended in stretching elastic structures is recovered when the stretching force is removed, as the elastic structures return to their previous position; thus the stretching of elastic tissues represents stored energy.

Surface tension

The inflation of the alveoli requires energy, as small bubbles or air sacs need a high pressure to overcome surface tension, whereas large bubbles need a lower pressure. The law of Laplace states that the pressure in a spherical bubble is inversely proportional to the radius, and theoretically if two bubbles of dissimilar size are connected together, the smaller bubble should empty itself almost completely into the larger.

The fact that the interconnected alveoli do not develop such instability is explained by the presence of **surfactant** in the alveoli. This is a detergent secreted by cells in the alveolar wall, which substantially reduces the surface tension of the alveoli. There is a limited quantity in each alveolus and it has to spread itself over the whole surface area of that alveolus. It therefore becomes less effective as the alveoli become distended, so the surface tension is lowest in the smallest alveoli; this helps to stabilize the alveoli, and makes the onset of inspiration much easier than it would otherwise be.

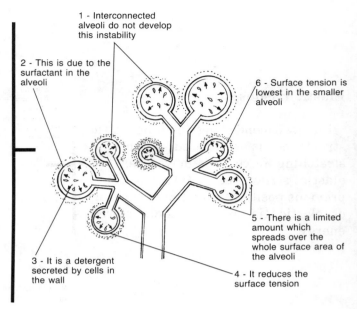

1 - Interconnected alveoli do not develop this instability

2 - This is due to the surfactant in the alveoli

6 - Surface tension is lowest in the smaller alveoli

3 - It is a detergent secreted by cells in the wall

5 - There is a limited amount which spreads over the whole surface area of the alveolus

4 - It reduces the surface tension

When a baby is born its lungs are full of fluid, and the first breath that it takes requires an enormous input of energy; there has never been any gas in its alveoli. Once the first breath has been taken, surfactant reduces surface tension and makes respiration much easier.

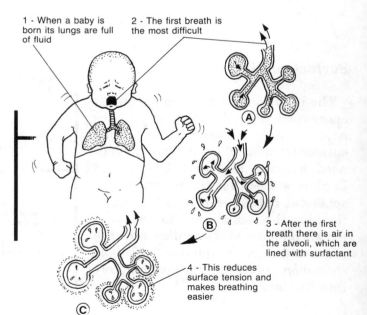

1 - When a baby is born its lungs are full of fluid

2 - The first breath is the most difficult

3 - After the first breath there is air in the alveoli, which are lined with surfactant

4 - This reduces surface tension and makes breathing easier

Babies that are born prematurely have a deficiency of surfactant, so every breath they take is as difficult as the first one, and they rapidly become exhausted (the **respiratory distress syndrome**).

Friction

Work is done in moving the various tissues of the lung and chest wall past each other; as the lungs expand, the various layers and structures rub against one another, creating frictional resistance and dissipating energy as heat. Friction between tissue layers occurs during both inspiration and expiration, so energy needs to be expended during both phases of respiration to overcome this resistance.

Airways resistance

The moving of gas through the airways is also subject to frictional resistance, and the rules governing airflow are exactly the same as those governing the flow of blood through blood vessels. The longer and narrower a tube is, the more frictional resistance it offers, and the points where tubes branch or get narrower are the places where turbulent airflow is likely to occur. As flow velocity increases, the likelihood of turbulence increases, and this is a very important factor in increasing the work of breathing at high rates of ventilation.

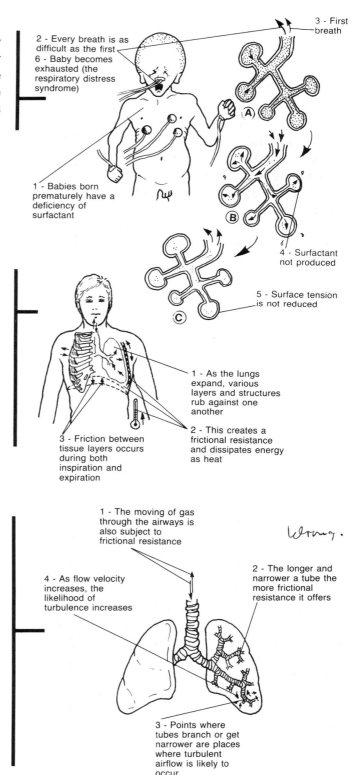

2 - Every breath is as difficult as the first
6 - Baby becomes exhausted (the respiratory distress syndrome)
1 - Babies born prematurely have a deficiency of surfactant
3 - First breath
4 - Surfactant not produced
5 - Surface tension is not reduced

1 - As the lungs expand, various layers and structures rub against one another
2 - This creates a frictional resistance and dissipates energy as heat
3 - Friction between tissue layers occurs during both inspiration and expiration

1 - The moving of gas through the airways is also subject to frictional resistance
2 - The longer and narrower a tube the more frictional resistance it offers
4 - As flow velocity increases, the likelihood of turbulence increases
3 - Points where tubes branch or get narrower are places where turbulent airflow is likely to occur

The friction of air moving through tubes represents lost energy (dissipated as heat) and this energy is lost during both phases of respiration. It follows that during inspiration the respiratory muscles need to exert enough force to stretch the elastic tissues and to overcome the tissue friction and the airways resistance; they must also store enough additional energy in the elastic tissues to overcome the frictional and resistive opposition during expiration.

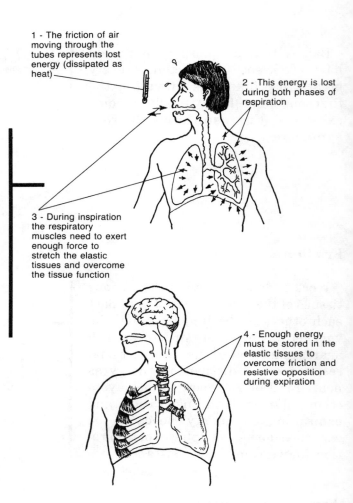

1 - The friction of air moving through the tubes represents lost energy (dissipated as heat)

2 - This energy is lost during both phases of respiration

3 - During inspiration the respiratory muscles need to exert enough force to stretch the elastic tissues and overcome the tissue function

4 - Enough energy must be stored in the elastic tissues to overcome friction and resistive opposition during expiration

Tissue compliance is reduced or tissue friction and stiffness are increased in many forms of lung disease. One of the commonest is pulmonary oedema, caused by lung infection or by disturbance of the pressures in the lung blood vessels (so that fluid is forced out of the capillaries and into the interstitial spaces or alveoli). Other conditions include the deposition of fibrous or inflammatory material in the lung tissue.

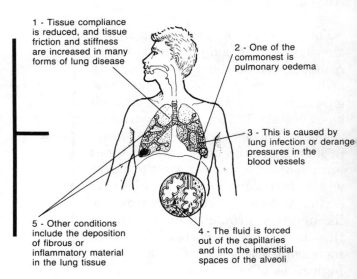

1 - Tissue compliance is reduced, and tissue friction and stiffness are increased in many forms of lung disease

2 - One of the commonest is pulmonary oedema

3 - This is caused by lung infection or derange pressures in the blood vessels

5 - Other conditions include the deposition of fibrous or inflammatory material in the lung tissue

4 - The fluid is forced out of the capillaries and into the interstitial spaces of the alveoli

The resistance to airflow is increased in several diseases, such as asthma and bronchitis. Typically a foreign antigen like pollen provokes an allergic reaction in the walls of the bronchi, with the release of histamine and other mediators from the mast cells, and the contraction of smooth muscle producing narrowing of the tubes.

Alternatively, infection with bacteria or viruses produces an inflammatory response in the airways. There is often oedema of the mucosal layer, which further narrows the airways. In this type of bronchospasm there is difficulty in moving air through the respiratory passages, but the most difficult phase is expiration, as the force attempting to deflate the lungs presses on the already narrowed airways and tends to narrow them still more.

The harder the patient tries to breathe out the more the tubes become narrowed and the harder it is to expire. Asthmatics are often seen to make full use of their accessory muscles of expiration, and can be intensely distressed by their inability to breathe out (air trapping).

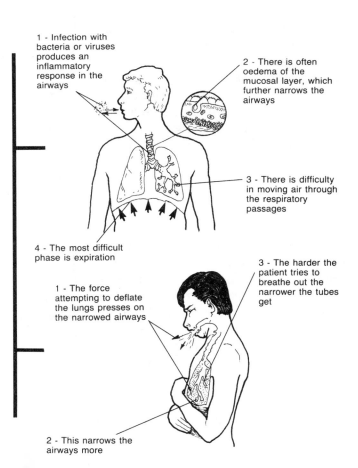

1 - The resistance to airflow is increased in several diseases, such as asthma and bronchitis

2 - A foreign antigen like pollen provokes an allergic reaction in the walls of the bronchi

4 - There is a contraction of smooth muscle, producing narrowing of the tubes

3 - There is a release in histamine and other mediators from mast cells

1 - Infection with bacteria or viruses produces an inflammatory response in the airways

2 - There is often oedema of the mucosal layer, which further narrows the airways

3 - There is difficulty in moving air through the respiratory passages

4 - The most difficult phase is expiration

1 - The force attempting to deflate the lungs presses on the narrowed airways

3 - The harder the patient tries to breathe out the narrower the tubes get

2 - This narrows the airways more

GAS EXCHANGE IN THE LUNGS

During inspiration the first portion of tidal air passes into the alveoli to take part in respiratory gas exchange. The last portion occupies the bronchi and other large airways, and cannot take part in gas exchange. This is the first portion of air to be breathed out of the mouth and nose, and is called **dead space air**.

A distinction is made between **anatomical** dead space which occupies recognizable structures where exchange cannot take place, and **physiological** or total dead space which includes the anatomical space as well as those areas of lung which are ventilated with gas but are poorly perfused with blood.

Dead space air has the same gaseous composition as the inspired atmospheric air, whereas later fractions of the expired air which come from the aveoli have a greatly modified gas composition. Pure **alveolar air** can be collected towards the end of a normal expiration, or during the later phases of a forced expiration.

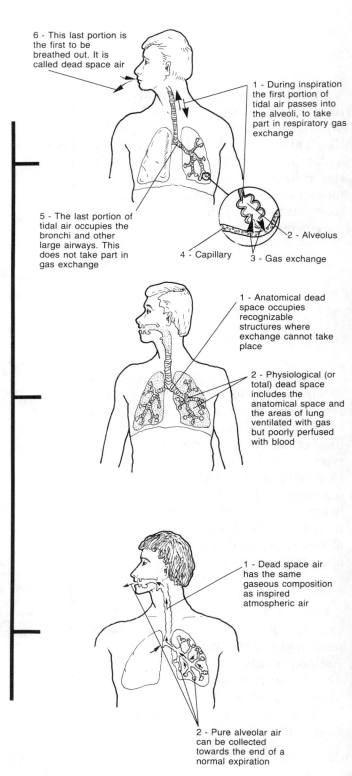

6 - This last portion is the first to be breathed out. It is called dead space air

1 - During inspiration the first portion of tidal air passes into the alveoli, to take part in respiratory gas exchange

5 - The last portion of tidal air occupies the bronchi and other large airways. This does not take part in gas exchange

2 - Alveolus

4 - Capillary

3 - Gas exchange

1 - Anatomical dead space occupies recognizable structures where exchange cannot take place

2 - Physiological (or total) dead space includes the anatomical space and the areas of lung ventilated with gas but poorly perfused with blood

1 - Dead space air has the same gaseous composition as inspired atmospheric air

2 - Pure alveolar air can be collected towards the end of a normal expiration

In the tidal volume of about 500 ml, the dead space air accounts for about 150 ml while the alveolar air is about 350 ml. The **ventilation** volume is the volume breathed in and out each minute; by analogy with the cardiac output, which is

stroke volume × heart rate

the ventilation volume is

tidal volume × respiratory rate

so with a tidal volume of 350 ml and a respiratory rate of about 16 per minute, the ventilation volume (minute volume) is 3600 ml/min. The alveolar ventilation is the proportion of the total which was alveolar air. If one collects the whole of the expired air, its composition is a mixture of alveolar and dead space air, and its gaseous content is intermediate between atmospheric and alveolar air.

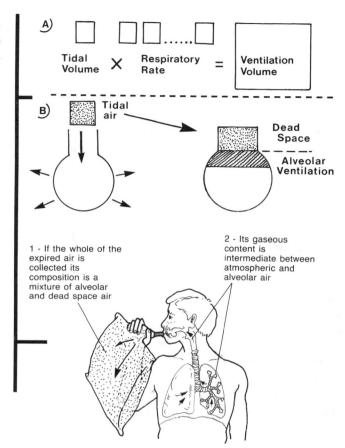

A) Tidal Volume × Respiratory Rate = Ventilation Volume

B) Tidal air — Dead Space — Alveolar Ventilation

1 - If the whole of the expired air is collected its composition is a mixture of alveolar and dead space air

2 - Its gaseous content is intermediate between atmospheric and alveolar air

The atmospheric air contains about 21% oxygen, with a small proportion of rare inert gases, while the majority of the volume is occupied by nitrogen; there is almost no carbon dioxide. The total atmospheric pressure at sea level is 101.3 kPa (1 bar, 760 mmHg), and the partial pressure of oxygen is around 19.9 kPa (150 mmHg).

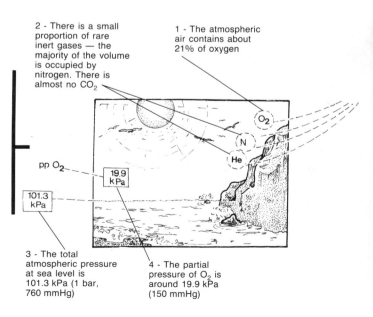

2 - There is a small proportion of rare inert gases — the majority of the volume is occupied by nitrogen. There is almost no CO_2

1 - The atmospheric air contains about 21% of oxygen

pp O_2

3 - The total atmospheric pressure at sea level is 101.3 kPa (1 bar, 760 mmHg)

4 - The partial pressure of O_2 is around 19.9 kPa (150 mmHg)

Alveolar air contains about 5% carbon dioxide, at a partial pressure of 5.3 kPa (40 mmHg) with 16% of oxygen at a tension of 13.8 kPa (104 mmHg); the proportion of nitrogen is slightly greater and the concentrations of other inert gases are largely unaltered.

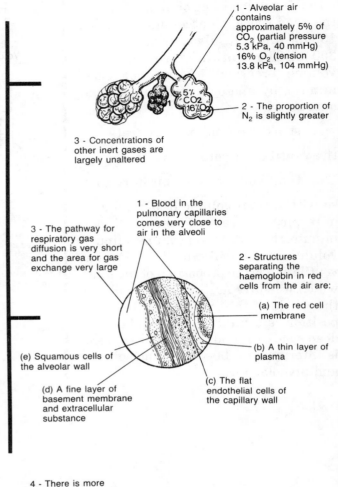

1 - Alveolar air contains approximately 5% of CO_2 (partial pressure 5.3 kPa, 40 mmHg) 16% O_2 (tension 13.8 kPa, 104 mmHg)

2 - The proportion of N_2 is slightly greater

3 - Concentrations of other inert gases are largely unaltered

Blood in the pulmonary capillaries comes very close to air in the alveoli. The structures separating the haemoglobin in red cells from the air are: the red cell membrane, a thin layer of plasma, the flat endothelial cells of the capillary wall, a fine layer of basement membrane and extracellular substance, and the squamous cells of the alveolar wall. The pathway for diffusion of respiratory gases is very short and the area for gas exchange is very large.

1 - Blood in the pulmonary capillaries comes very close to air in the alveoli

3 - The pathway for respiratory gas diffusion is very short and the area for gas exchange very large

2 - Structures separating the haemoglobin in red cells from the air are:

(a) The red cell membrane

(b) A thin layer of plasma

(c) The flat endothelial cells of the capillary wall

(d) A fine layer of basement membrane and extracellular substance

(e) Squamous cells of the alveolar wall

Gases move from alveoli to capillaries and vice versa by simple diffusion along concentration gradients: there is no active transport of oxygen or carbon dioxide. The gradients for gas transfer are usually expressed in terms of the partial pressures or tensions of the various gases. There is more oxygen in the air than in the capillaries and therefore this gas diffuses into the blood, whereas there is more carbon dioxide in the blood and this gas diffuses into the alveoli.

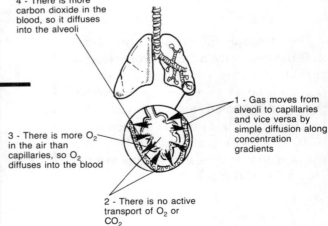

4 - There is more carbon dioxide in the blood, so it diffuses into the alveoli

1 - Gas moves from alveoli to capillaries and vice versa by simple diffusion along concentration gradients

3 - There is more O_2 in the air than capillaries, so O_2 diffuses into the blood

2 - There is no active transport of O_2 or CO_2

VENTILATION AND PERFUSION

Ideally the rate of blood flow in the capillaries supplying each alveolus should be just sufficient to allow the blood leaving the capillary to be saturated with oxygen, having given up the carbon dioxide which was transported from the peripheries.

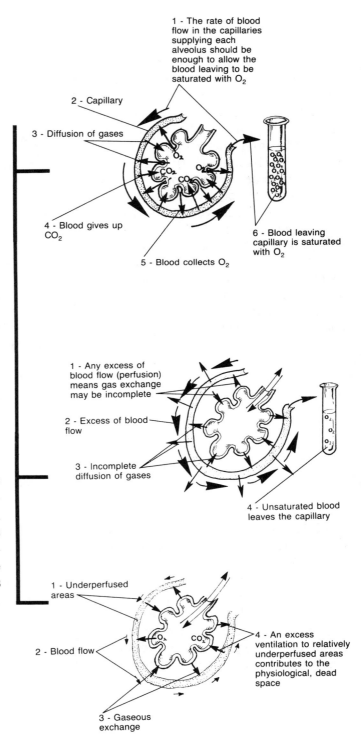

1 - The rate of blood flow in the capillaries supplying each alveolus should be enough to allow the blood leaving to be saturated with O_2

2 - Capillary

3 - Diffusion of gases

4 - Blood gives up CO_2

5 - Blood collects O_2

6 - Blood leaving capillary is saturated with O_2

1 - Any excess of blood flow (perfusion) means gas exchange may be incomplete

2 - Excess of blood flow

3 - Incomplete diffusion of gases

4 - Unsaturated blood leaves the capillary

1 - Underperfused areas

2 - Blood flow

3 - Gaseous exchange

4 - An excess ventilation to relatively underperfused areas contributes to the physiological, dead space

Any excess of blood flow (perfusion) means that gas exchange may be incomplete, with unsaturated blood leaving the capillary, while an excess of ventilation to relatively underperfused areas contributes to the physiological dead space, i.e. there is wasted ventilation.

Such imbalances in ventilation-to-perfusion ratio do occur in the lungs. A person standing upright has a higher blood flow through the base of the lungs than the apex, simply due to the effect of gravity, and there is a relatively higher ventilation of alveoli at the apex. If the person lies down, the most dependent part of the lungs, usually the back, becomes overperfused while the uppermost part becomes over-ventilated. The consequence of these imbalances in ventilation/perfusion ratio is that the blood returning to the left atrium is almost never fully saturated with oxygen, but is, at best, about 97% saturated.

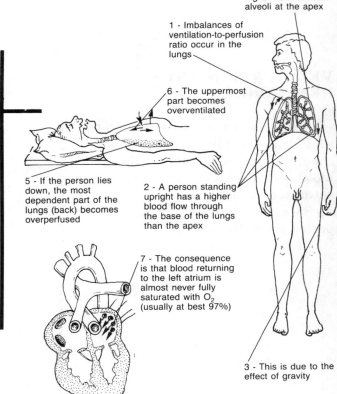

4 - There is relatively higher ventilation of alveoli at the apex

1 - Imbalances of ventilation-to-perfusion ratio occur in the lungs

6 - The uppermost part becomes overventilated

5 - If the person lies down, the most dependent part of the lungs (back) becomes overperfused

2 - A person standing upright has a higher blood flow through the base of the lungs than the apex

7 - The consequence is that blood returning to the left atrium is almost never fully saturated with O_2 (usually at best 97%)

3 - This is due to the effect of gravity

CARRIAGE OF OXYGEN AND CARBON DIOXIDE BY THE BLOOD

Oxygen diffuses into the plasma and dissolves in it. The concentration of any gas in simple physical solution is proportional to the partial pressure of the gas in the air mixture in the alveoli.

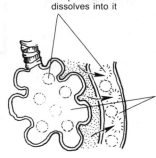

1 - O_2 diffuses into the plasma and dissolves into it

2 - The concentration in simple physical solution is proportional to the partial pressure of the gas in the air mixture in the alveoli

Gases differ in their solubility in water, so that carbon dioxide is much more soluble than oxygen; thus the amount of each gas dissolved depends upon both the partial pressure (or tension) of that gas and its solubility. A partial pressure of 50 mmHg for oxygen represents a considerably smaller **quantity** of dissolved gas than the same partial pressure of carbon dioxide, but it has been conventional to refer to dissolved gases in terms of the partial pressure or tension they would exert in a gas phase in equilibrium with the fluid phase in which they are dissolved.

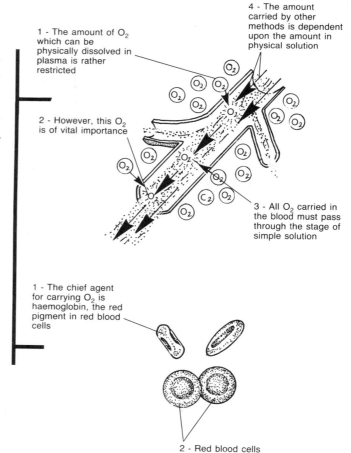

3 - Gases differ in their solubility in water

4 - CO_2 is very soluble in water

5 - O_2 is not as soluble in water as CO_2

The amount of oxygen which can be physically dissolved in plasma is rather restricted, but this fraction of oxygen in the blood is of vital importance, because all of the oxygen carried in the blood must pass through the stage of simple solution, and the amount which can be carried by other methods is dependent upon the amount in physical solution in the plasma.

1 - The amount of O_2 which can be physically dissolved in plasma is rather restricted

4 - The amount carried by other methods is dependent upon the amount in physical solution

2 - However, this O_2 is of vital importance

3 - All O_2 carried in the blood must pass through the stage of simple solution

The chief agent for carrying oxygen is haemoglobin, the red pigment found in the red blood cells (erythrocytes).

1 - The chief agent for carrying O_2 is haemoglobin, the red pigment in red blood cells

2 - Red blood cells (erythrocytes)

This complex substance consists of a globular protein part (globin) and a porphyrin ring portion (haem) which contains an iron atom.

The functional unit of haemoglobin is made of four haem and four globin subunits; the globin units are often different from one another, with two alpha-chains and two beta-chains.

There are many genetic variants such as the type of globin found in carriers of and sufferers from sickle-cell anaemia, thalassaemia and other rarer defects, as well as the slightly different haemoglobin found in the fetus.

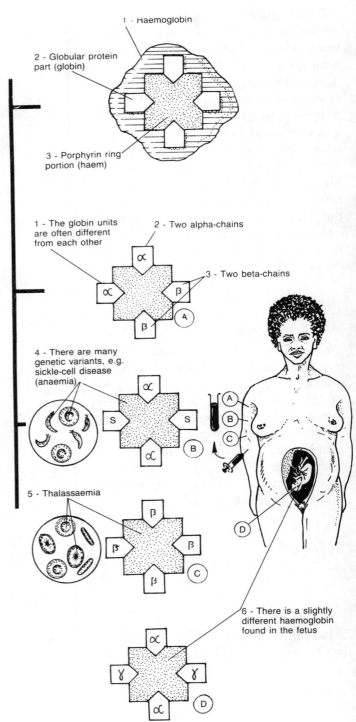

1 - Haemoglobin

2 - Globular protein part (globin)

3 - Porphyrin ring portion (haem)

1 - The globin units are often different from each other

2 - Two alpha-chains

3 - Two beta-chains

4 - There are many genetic variants, e.g. sickle-cell disease (anaemia)

5 - Thalassaemia

6 - There is a slightly different haemoglobin found in the fetus

The haemoglobin molecule has an enormous affinity for oxygen, binding it to a specific site in the molecule. Each mole of haemoglobin can carry four moles of oxygen, or each gram of haemoglobin can combine with 1.34 ml. The total amount of oxygen carried in the blood is about 20 ml per 100 ml, of which about 19.4 ml is bound to haemoglobin. This binding is not an active process, in the sense that no metabolic energy is expended in forming or breaking the link between haemoglobin and oxygen, but the amount of oxygen which can be bound to haemoglobin is substantially more than the amount carried in simple solution (about 0.6 ml/100 ml).

The binding of oxygen to haemoglobin is cooperative; that is, it is easier for oxygen to become bound if there is already some oxygen bound to the molecule.

There are four binding sites in haemoglobin, and the most difficult oxygen molecule to bind is the first one. Once it is bound, the second and third molecules are bound much more easily. The fourth molecule becomes a little more difficult to bind as the haemoglobin molecule approaches saturation.

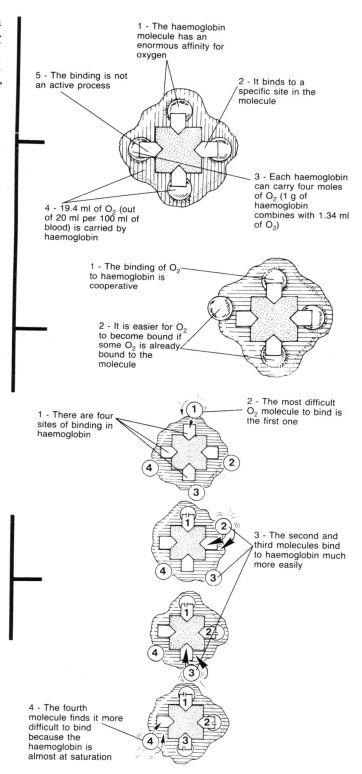

1 - The haemoglobin molecule has an enormous affinity for oxygen

5 - The binding is not an active process

2 - It binds to a specific site in the molecule

3 - Each haemoglobin can carry four moles of O_2 (1 g of haemoglobin combines with 1.34 ml of O_2)

4 - 19.4 ml of O_2 (out of 20 ml per 100 ml of blood) is carried by haemoglobin

1 - The binding of O_2 to haemoglobin is cooperative

2 - It is easier for O_2 to become bound if some O_2 is already bound to the molecule

1 - There are four sites of binding in haemoglobin

2 - The most difficult O_2 molecule to bind is the first one

3 - The second and third molecules bind to haemoglobin much more easily

4 - The fourth molecule finds it more difficult to bind because the haemoglobin is almost at saturation

If the amount of oxygen bound (expressed as percentage saturation, or a proportion of the maximum amount that could be bound) is plotted against the partial pressure of oxygen in physical solution (or in the alveolar gas) then a sigmoid (S-shaped) curve is drawn.

The shallow slope at the left represents the difficult binding of the first oxygen molecule; the steeper part in the middle represents the enhanced cooperative binding of the second and third molecules, and the curve flattens at the top as full saturation is approached.

This curve is called the **oxygen dissociation curve** (it could just as well be called the association curve, but it is usually constructed by equilibrating blood with various gas mixtures and then measuring how much oxygen can be released from the blood).

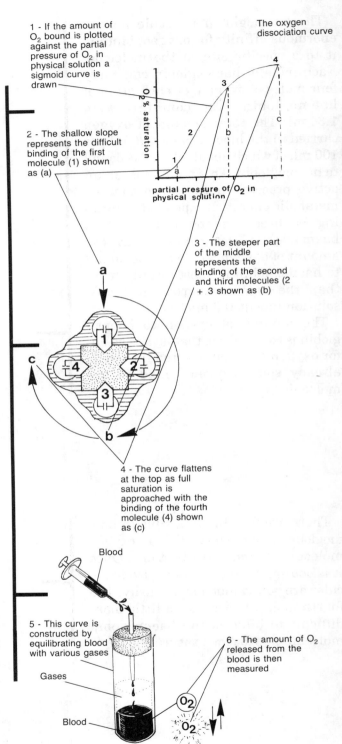

1 - If the amount of O$_2$ bound is plotted against the partial pressure of O$_2$ in physical solution a sigmoid curve is drawn

The oxygen dissociation curve

2 - The shallow slope represents the difficult binding of the first molecule (1) shown as (a)

3 - The steeper part of the middle represents the binding of the second and third molecules (2 + 3 shown as (b)

4 - The curve flattens at the top as full saturation is approached with the binding of the fourth molecule (4) shown as (c)

5 - This curve is constructed by equilibrating blood with various gases

6 - The amount of O$_2$ released from the blood is then measured

Oxygen diffuses from the alveoli into the plasma and becomes dissolved there, then diffuses across the erythrocyte membrane and becomes bound to intracellular haemoglobin.

The amount becoming bound is determined by the partial pressure of oxygen, but it is not a linear function (unlike the simple solution in plasma).

The blood leaving the pulmonary capillaries is laden with oxygen, the haemoglobin in the erythrocytes being almost completely saturated. When the blood reaches the tissue capillaries it enters an environment much less rich in oxygen, as the tissues have been using it up in their metabolism. This lowered concentration corresponds to a lower oxygen tension, and some of the oxygen carried by haemoglobin becomes dissociated, allowing molecular oxygen to leave the red cells, pass through the plasma and enter the tissues. The amount of oxygen still bound to haemoglobin is determined by the oxygen tension in the peripheral tissues.

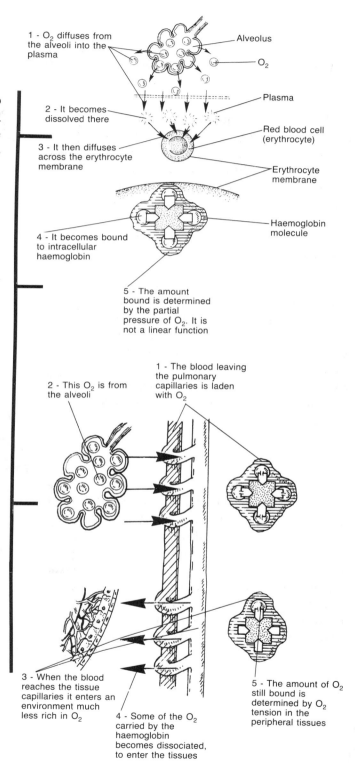

1 - O_2 diffuses from the alveoli into the plasma

Alveolus

O_2

2 - It becomes dissolved there

Plasma

3 - It then diffuses across the erythrocyte membrane

Red blood cell (erythrocyte)

Erythrocyte membrane

4 - It becomes bound to intracellular haemoglobin

Haemoglobin molecule

5 - The amount bound is determined by the partial pressure of O_2. It is not a linear function

2 - This O_2 is from the alveoli

1 - The blood leaving the pulmonary capillaries is laden with O_2

3 - When the blood reaches the tissue capillaries it enters an environment much less rich in O_2

4 - Some of the O_2 carried by the haemoglobin becomes dissociated, to enter the tissues

5 - The amount of O_2 still bound is determined by O_2 tension in the peripheral tissues

The range of oxygen tensions usually encountered in active tissues falls on the steep part of the oxygen dissociation curve, so that a small change in oxygen tension can cause a large change in the oxygen released from binding.

There is another important factor in the tissues which enhances the ability of haemoglobin to release its oxygen — the presence of carbon dioxide. This gas also binds to the haemoglobin molecule, and its presence there reduces haemoglobin's affinity for oxygen, so that at any given oxygen tension the amount carried is reduced. This can be expressed by shifting the oxygen dissociation curve to the right, the **Bohr effect**.

Another factor which causes a rightward shift in the dissociation curve is the presence of 2,3-diphosphoglycerate (2,3-DPG), an intermediate substance in the glycolytic pathway for metabolism of glucose. Active tissues produce 2,3-DPG in large quantities, and binding of this molecule to haemoglobin reduces its affinity for oxygen.

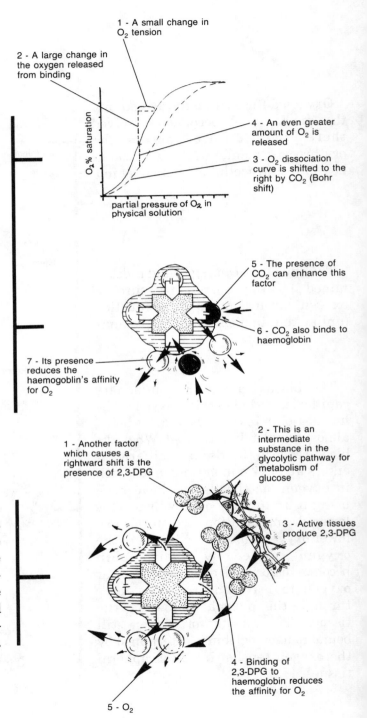

1 - A small change in O_2 tension

2 - A large change in the oxygen released from binding

4 - An even greater amount of O_2 is released

3 - O_2 dissociation curve is shifted to the right by CO_2 (Bohr shift)

O_2 % saturation

partial pressure of O_2 in physical solution

5 - The presence of CO_2 can enhance this factor

6 - CO_2 also binds to haemoglobin

7 - Its presence reduces the haemogoblin's affinity for O_2

2 - This is an intermediate substance in the glycolytic pathway for metabolism of glucose

1 - Another factor which causes a rightward shift is the presence of 2,3-DPG

3 - Active tissues produce 2,3-DPG

4 - Binding of 2,3-DPG to haemoglobin reduces the affinity for O_2

5 - O_2

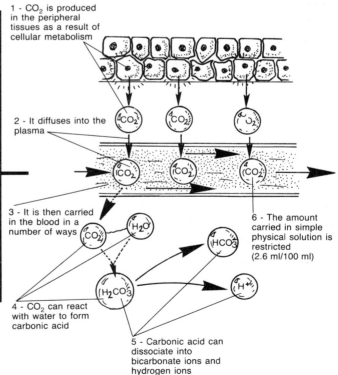

3 - The ability of blood to give up O_2 is greatly enhanced

An increase in temperature and a decrease in pH (greater acidity) also shift the dissociation curve to the right. Both these factors as well as carbon dioxide are present in active tissues; the ability of the blood to give up its oxygen is greatly enhanced, so oxygen is delivered to the tissues just where it is needed.

2 - Both these factors and CO_2 are present in active tissues

4 - O_2 is then delivered to the tissues exactly where needed

1 - An increase in temperature and a decrease in pH also shift the curve to the right

Carbon dioxide, too, is carried by the blood in a number of different ways. It is produced in the peripheral tissues as a result of cellular metabolism, and diffuses into the plasma. The amount which can be carried in simple physical solution is rather restricted (up to about 2.6 ml/100 ml), and is directly proportional to the partial pressure or tension of the gas. Carbon dioxide can also react with water to form carbonic acid, a reaction which occurs rather slowly in normal solutions. Carbonic acid can further dissociate into bicarbonate ions and hydrogen ions: the whole reaction is

$$CO_2 + H_2O \rightleftharpoons H_2CO_3 \rightleftharpoons H^+ + HCO_3^-$$

1 - CO_2 is produced in the peripheral tissues as a result of cellular metabolism

2 - It diffuses into the plasma

3 - It is then carried in the blood in a number of ways

4 - CO_2 can react with water to form carbonic acid

5 - Carbonic acid can dissociate into bicarbonate ions and hydrogen ions

6 - The amount carried in simple physical solution is restricted (2.6 ml/100 ml)

This series of reactions proceeds much more rapidly (around 13 000 times faster) in the presence of an enzyme called **carbonic anhydrase**; the enzyme is absent from plasma, but is present in large quantities inside the red cells. The carbon dioxide diffusing into plasma from the active tissues moves into the red cells (by passive diffusion down a concentration gradient), where it is converted by the action of carbonic anhydrase into carbonic acid and thence into bicarbonate and hydrogen ions.

The excess H^+ ions bind to haemoglobin, reducing its affinity for oxygen and helping to release some more for the tissues' needs.

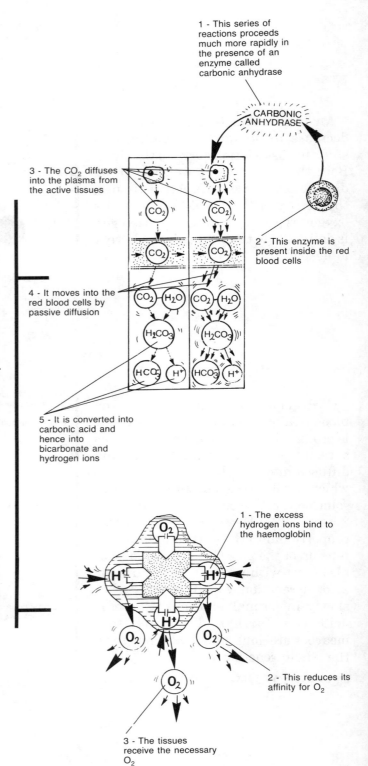

1 - This series of reactions proceeds much more rapidly in the presence of an enzyme called carbonic anhydrase

CARBONIC ANHYDRASE

3 - The CO_2 diffuses into the plasma from the active tissues

2 - This enzyme is present inside the red blood cells

4 - It moves into the red blood cells by passive diffusion

5 - It is converted into carbonic acid and hence into bicarbonate and hydrogen ions

1 - The excess hydrogen ions bind to the haemoglobin

2 - This reduces its affinity for O_2

3 - The tissues receive the necessary O_2

There is an excess of bicarbonate ions inside the cell, but these cannot easily diffuse out because cell membranes are relatively impermeable to bicarbonate. However, there is a facilitated diffusion mechanism involving a specific carrier which binds intracellular bicarbonate ions, carries them across the membrane to the outside, releases them and binds chloride ions from the plasma, carrying them into the cell. This process, known as the **chloride shift**, results in the exchange of one chloride ion for one bicarbonate ion, and maintains electro-neutrality within the cell.

Carbon dioxide has to enter the red cell in order to be converted to bicarbonate; this moves out of the cell into the plasma, leaving room for more molecules of carbon dioxide to enter the cell for conversion. A very much larger amount of carbon dioxide can be carried as bicarbonate than as molecular carbon dioxide in simple solution, and the red cells play a key part in making possible this additional means of transport.

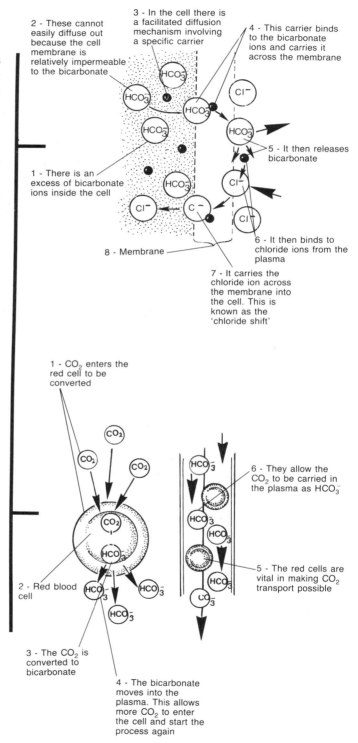

2 - These cannot easily diffuse out because the cell membrane is relatively impermeable to the bicarbonate

3 - In the cell there is a facilitated diffusion mechanism involving a specific carrier

4 - This carrier binds to the bicarbonate ions and carries it across the membrane

1 - There is an excess of bicarbonate ions inside the cell

5 - It then releases bicarbonate

6 - It then binds to chloride ions from the plasma

7 - It carries the chloride ion across the membrane into the cell. This is known as the 'chloride shift'

8 - Membrane

1 - CO_2 enters the red cell to be converted

2 - Red blood cell

3 - The CO_2 is converted to bicarbonate

4 - The bicarbonate moves into the plasma. This allows more CO_2 to enter the cell and start the process again

5 - The red cells are vital in making CO_2 transport possible

6 - They allow the CO_2 to be carried in the plasma as HCO_3^-

There is a third means of carbon dioxide transport; carbon dioxide can react with protein molecules both inside and outside the cells to form **carbamino** compounds. The proportion of the total carried in this way is rather small: about 23% compared to 70% as bicarbonate and only 7% in simple solution. The total amount of carbon dioxide carried in the blood is about 50–60 ml/100 ml.

When venous blood laden with carbon dioxide and its derivatives reaches the alveoli of the lungs, the driving forces for diffusion and binding of carbon dioxide are in the opposite direction to those in the tissues. Dissolved carbon dioxide in the plasma diffuses into the alveoli, lowering the concentration in the plasma. Carbon dioxide in the red cells diffuses out into the plasma, leaving room for the conversion of bicarbonate and hydrogen ions into carbonic acid and thence into carbon dioxide.

As the bicarbonate ions already inside the cell get used up in this process, more bicarbonate ions enter the cell from the plasma, in exchange for chloride ions from inside the red cell. Thus the whole mechanism, including the chloride shift, is thrown into reverse, allowing the blood to yield up its store of carbon dioxide for expiration out of the lungs.

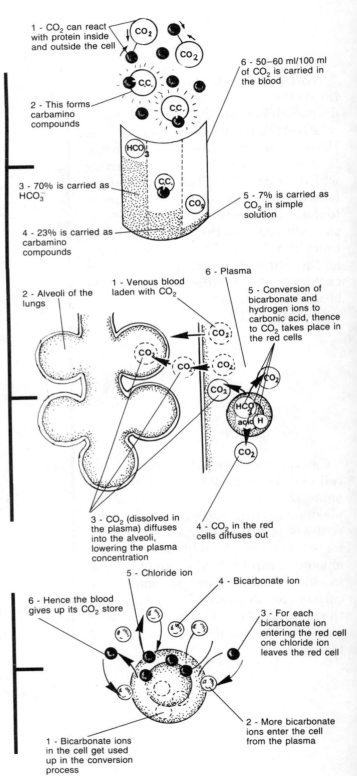

1 - CO_2 can react with protein inside and outside the cell

2 - This forms carbamino compounds

3 - 70% is carried as HCO_3^-

4 - 23% is carried as carbamino compounds

6 - 50–60 ml/100 ml of CO_2 is carried in the blood

5 - 7% is carried as CO_2 in simple solution

2 - Alveoli of the lungs

1 - Venous blood laden with CO_2

6 - Plasma

5 - Conversion of bicarbonate and hydrogen ions to carbonic acid, thence to CO_2 takes place in the red cells

3 - CO_2 (dissolved in the plasma) diffuses into the alveoli, lowering the plasma concentration

4 - CO_2 in the red cells diffuses out

5 - Chloride ion

4 - Bicarbonate ion

6 - Hence the blood gives up its CO_2 store

3 - For each bicarbonate ion entering the red cell one chloride ion leaves the red cell

2 - More bicarbonate ions enter the cell from the plasma

1 - Bicarbonate ions in the cell get used up in the conversion process

The ability of the lungs to eliminate large quantities of carbon dioxide makes the carbon dioxide/carbonic acid mechanism very important in regulating the pH of plasma. The equilibrium reaction for formation of carbonic acid and bicarbonate from carbon dioxide can be expressed as

$$pH = pK + \log \frac{[HCO_3^-]}{[CO_2]}$$

This is called the Henderson—Hesselbach equation, where pK is the negative logarithm of the dissociation constant, and has a value for blood of 6.1.

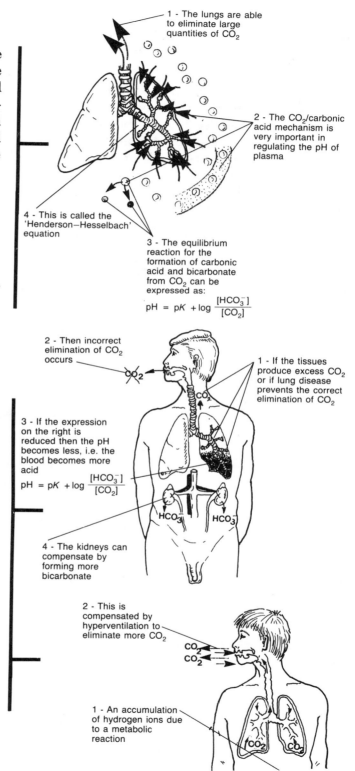

1 - The lungs are able to eliminate large quantities of CO_2

2 - The CO_2/carbonic acid mechanism is very important in regulating the pH of plasma

4 - This is called the 'Henderson—Hesselbach' equation

3 - The equilibrium reaction for the formation of carbonic acid and bicarbonate from CO_2 can be expressed as:

$$pH = pK + \log \frac{[HCO_3^-]}{[CO_2]}$$

If the tissues produce excess carbon dioxide or there is lung disease which prevents the correct elimination of carbon dioxide then the expression on the right is reduced and the pH becomes less (the blood becomes more acid). This can be compensated by the formation of more bicarbonate in the kidneys (see the chapter on the kidney).

2 - Then incorrect elimination of CO_2 occurs

1 - If the tissues produce excess CO_2 or if lung disease prevents the correct elimination of CO_2

3 - If the expression on the right is reduced then the pH becomes less, i.e. the blood becomes more acid

$$pH = pK + \log \frac{[HCO_3^-]}{[CO_2]}$$

4 - The kidneys can compensate by forming more bicarbonate

HCO_3^- HCO_3^-

On the other hand, if there is an accumulation of hydrogen ions due to some metabolic reaction, this can be compensated by hyperventilation to eliminate more CO_2 through the lungs.

2 - This is compensated by hyperventilation to eliminate more CO_2

CO_2
CO_2

1 - An accumulation of hydrogen ions due to a metabolic reaction

CO_2 CO_2

TISSUE RESPIRATION: METABOLISM

The oxygen transported to the tissues is used for the biochemical reactions occurring within each cell. Many of the reactions require the supply of energy, usually derived from the breakdown of carbohydrate, protein or fat. The breakdown of carbohydrate can be summarized as follows:

$$C_6H_{12}O_6 + 6O_2 = 6CO_2 + 6H_2O$$

In other words each molecule of oxygen gives rise to one molecule of carbon dioxide.

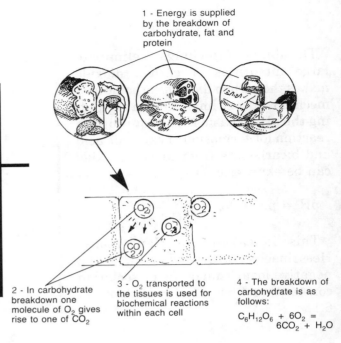

1 - Energy is supplied by the breakdown of carbohydrate, fat and protein

2 - In carbohydrate breakdown one molecule of O_2 gives rise to one of CO_2

3 - O_2 transported to the tissues is used for biochemical reactions within each cell

4 - The breakdown of carbohydrate is as follows:

$$C_6H_{12}O_6 + 6O_2 = 6CO_2 + H_2O$$

The equation is, of course, a gross oversimplification of the myriad biochemical reactions taking place; complex molecules are broken down in a stepwise manner, with transfer of the released energy along complicated pathways in the mitochondria, and other molecules are built up from their simpler building blocks, with the input of energy to drive the synthesis.

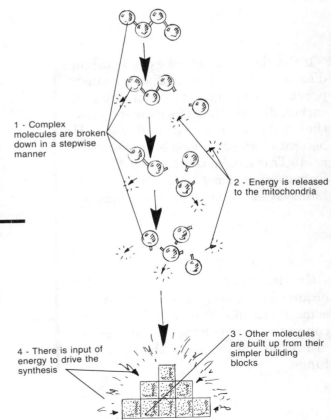

1 - Complex molecules are broken down in a stepwise manner

2 - Energy is released to the mitochondria

3 - Other molecules are built up from their simpler building blocks

4 - There is input of energy to drive the synthesis

The ratio of oxygen uptake to carbon dioxide production is called the **respiratory exchange ratio** or respiratory quotient (RQ) and for the metabolism of carbohydrate is equal to 1. For lipid metabolisms the RQ is 0.7, and for protein it is 0.8. Since most cells throughout the body metabolize a mixture of energy sources, the average RQ for a person on a normal mixed diet is about 0.85. The combination of oxygen with the various foodstuffs releases different amounts of energy: carbohydrate metabolism produces 21.1 kJ of energy per litre of oxygen, fat metabolism produces 20 kJ per litre of oxygen, and the breakdown of protein releases 18.7 kJ per litre of oxygen. On a normal mixed diet each litre of oxygen consumed releases about 20.2 kJ.

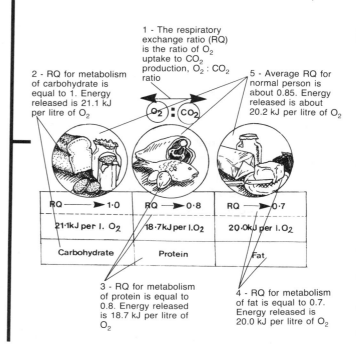

1 - The respiratory exchange ratio (RQ) is the ratio of O_2 uptake to CO_2 production, $O_2 : CO_2$ ratio

2 - RQ for metabolism of carbohydrate is equal to 1. Energy released is 21.1 kJ per litre of O_2

5 - Average RQ for normal person is about 0.85. Energy released is about 20.2 kJ per litre of O_2

3 - RQ for metabolism of protein is equal to 0.8. Energy released is 18.7 kJ per litre of O_2

4 - RQ for metabolism of fat is equal to 0.7. Energy released is 20.0 kJ per litre of O_2

RQ ⟶ 1·0	RQ ⟶ 0·8	RQ ⟶ 0·7
21·1 kJ per l. O_2	18·7 kJ per l. O_2	20·0 kJ per l. O_2
Carbohydrate	Protein	Fat

The normal utilization of oxygen for metabolic processes is called **aerobic** activity. It is possible, if the oxygen supply is inadequate, to perform **anaerobic** activity for short periods. Alternative metabolic pathways are used; for example, instead of the complete combustion of glucose with oxygen to carbon dioxide and water, the glucose can be converted, without oxygen, into lactic acid and carbon dioxide.

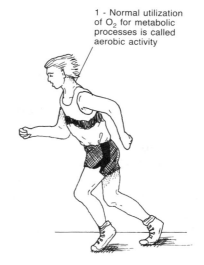

1 - Normal utilization of O_2 for metabolic processes is called aerobic activity

There is a limit to how much lactic acid can be allowed to build up, as acidosis inhibits many other metabolic processes, but a transient 'oxygen debt' can be built up during bursts of strenuous activity (such as sprinting or lifting heavy weights), and this debt is later 'repaid' by using oxygen to convert the lactic acid to carbon dioxide.

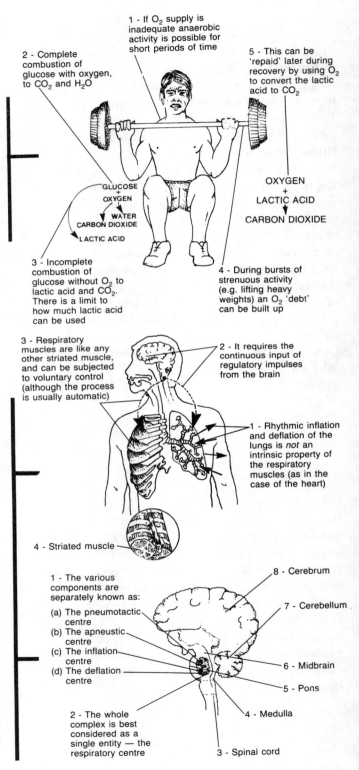

1 - If O_2 supply is inadequate anaerobic activity is possible for short periods of time

2 - Complete combustion of glucose with oxygen, to CO_2 and H_2O

5 - This can be 'repaid' later during recovery by using O_2 to convert the lactic acid to CO_2

GLUCOSE + OXYGEN
WATER CARBON DIOXIDE
LACTIC ACID

OXYGEN + LACTIC ACID
CARBON DIOXIDE

3 - Incomplete combustion of glucose without O_2 to lactic acid and CO_2. There is a limit to how much lactic acid can be used

4 - During bursts of strenuous activity (e.g. lifting heavy weights) an O_2 'debt' can be built up

CONTROL OF VENTILATION

The rhythmic inflation and deflation of the lungs is not an intrinsic property of the respiratory muscles, but (unlike the heart) requires the continuous input of regulatory impulses from the brain. The respiratory muscles are just like any other striated voluntary muscle and can be subjected to voluntary control, though their function usually proceeds automatically. The spinal motor neurones which activate the respiratory muscles are controlled by a number of areas in the medulla oblongata of the brain stem, collectively known as the **respiratory centre**. The various components are separately known as the **pneumotactic** centre, the **apneustic** centre, and the **inflation** and **deflation** centres, but the centres are best considered as a single functional entity.

3 - Respiratory muscles are like any other striated muscle, and can be subjected to voluntary control (although the process is usually automatic)

2 - It requires the continuous input of regulatory impulses from the brain

1 - Rhythmic inflation and deflation of the lungs is *not* an intrinsic property of the respiratory muscles (as in the case of the heart)

4 - Striated muscle

1 - The various components are separately known as:
(a) The pneumotactic centre
(b) The apneustic centre
(c) The inflation centre
(d) The deflation centre

8 - Cerebrum

7 - Cerebellum

6 - Midbrain

5 - Pons

4 - Medulla

3 - Spinal cord

2 - The whole complex is best considered as a single entity — the respiratory centre

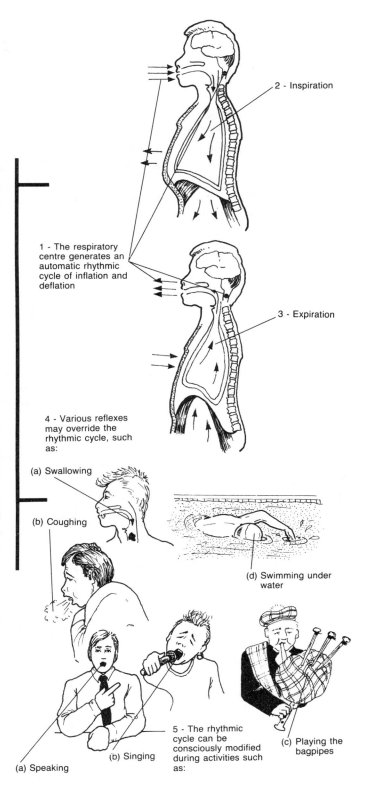

The respiratory centre generates an automatic rhythmic cycle of inflation and deflation which is subject to a number of modifying influences.

The first influence is from higher centres in the brain, and the rhythm of breathing may be overriden in various reflexes such as swallowing or coughing, or may be consciously modified during such diverse activities as speech, singing, playing the bagpipes, voluntary breath-holding for a bet or swimming under water.

2 - Inspiration

1 - The respiratory centre generates an automatic rhythmic cycle of inflation and deflation

3 - Expiration

4 - Various reflexes may override the rhythmic cycle, such as:

(a) Swallowing

(b) Coughing

(d) Swimming under water

5 - The rhythmic cycle can be consciously modified during activities such as:

(a) Speaking

(b) Singing

(c) Playing the bagpipes

Another modifying influence comes from stretch receptors within the lung and chest wall. Inflation of the lungs stimulates the receptors and signals are transferred to the brain, mainly up the vagus nerve but also along the somatic sensory pathways from the chest wall. These impulses inhibit inspiration and stimulate expiration, and hence modify the basic rhythm of respiration. The reflexes arising from pulmonary stretch receptors and mediated via the vagus are called **Hering–Breuer** reflexes.

Impulses reaching the brain from proprioceptors in other parts of the body can also affect respiration; movements of muscles and joints in the arms and legs stimulate ventilation, and this may be important in the ventilatory response to exercise. The mechanism whereby proprioceptors influence ventilation is called the 'J-reflex'.

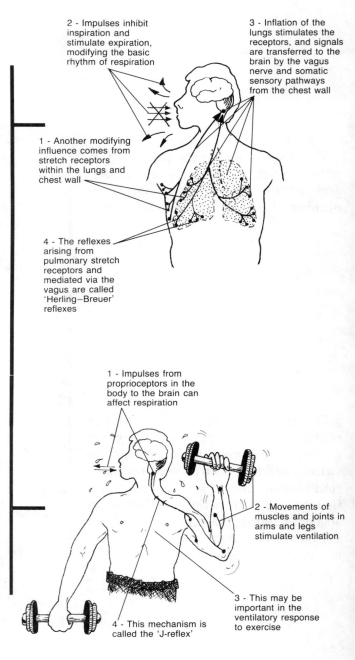

2 - Impulses inhibit inspiration and stimulate expiration, modifying the basic rhythm of respiration

3 - Inflation of the lungs stimulates the receptors, and signals are transferred to the brain by the vagus nerve and somatic sensory pathways from the chest wall

1 - Another modifying influence comes from stretch receptors within the lungs and chest wall

4 - The reflexes arising from pulmonary stretch receptors and mediated via the vagus are called 'Herling–Breuer' reflexes

1 - Impulses from proprioceptors in the body to the brain can affect respiration

2 - Movements of muscles and joints in arms and legs stimulate ventilation

3 - This may be important in the ventilatory response to exercise

4 - This mechanism is called the 'J-reflex'

The most important modifying influence on the basic respiratory rhythm is the input from peripheral and central **chemoreceptors**. These sense the content of oxygen and carbon dioxide in the blood and alter the ventilation rate in order to try to maintain normal levels. The peripheral chemoreceptors are the carotid body (situated near the carotid bifurcation) and the aortic body (on the arch of the aorta), and these are essentially oxygen receptors. The primary stimulus is a fall in the partial pressure of oxygen, and this causes a rapid discharge of impulses up the sensory nerve (a branch of the glossopharyngeal nerve — cranial nerve IX). The impulse frequency in the nerve fibres is an inverse function of the oxygen partial pressure.

The sensitivity of the chemoreceptors to hypoxia is modified by the amount of carbon dioxide in the blood; if there is more carbon dioxide then a given degree of hypoxia will produce a more rapid discharge. This has led some students to think that the carotid and aortic bodies are carbon dioxide receptors, but all that carbon dioxide does is to modify the response to hypoxia, shifting the curve of frequency/partial pressure of oxygen to a different place along the pressure axis.

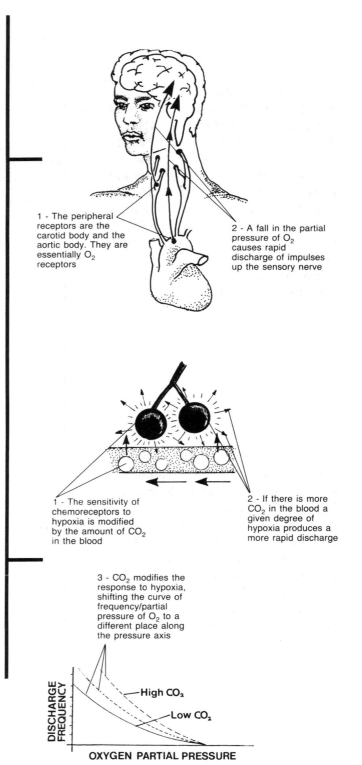

1 - The peripheral receptors are the carotid body and the aortic body. They are essentially O_2 receptors

2 - A fall in the partial pressure of O_2 causes rapid discharge of impulses up the sensory nerve

1 - The sensitivity of chemoreceptors to hypoxia is modified by the amount of CO_2 in the blood

2 - If there is more CO_2 in the blood a given degree of hypoxia produces a more rapid discharge

3 - CO_2 modifies the response to hypoxia, shifting the curve of frequency/partial pressure of O_2 to a different place along the pressure axis

DISCHARGE FREQUENCY

High CO_2

Low CO_2

OXYGEN PARTIAL PRESSURE

The true receptors for carbon dioxide are the **central** chemoreceptors, found in the medulla oblongata of the brain, in the floor of the fourth ventricle. Carbon dioxide itself is probably not the primary stimulus, but the partial pressure of carbon dioxide in the plasma affects the carbon dioxide level in the cerebrospinal fluid (CSF), and this in turn affects the pH of the CSF. It is the hydrogen ions in the CSF that stimulate the receptors and cause increased ventilation.

The central pH-sensitive chemoreceptors are the most important in regulating ventilation. If one tries to hold one's breath for as long as possible, the factor which makes one give up and take another breath is the build up of carbon dioxide in the blood rather than the lack of oxygen; in fact one cannot hold the breath any longer by breathing pure oxygen, as the level of carbon dioxide still builds up at the same rate.

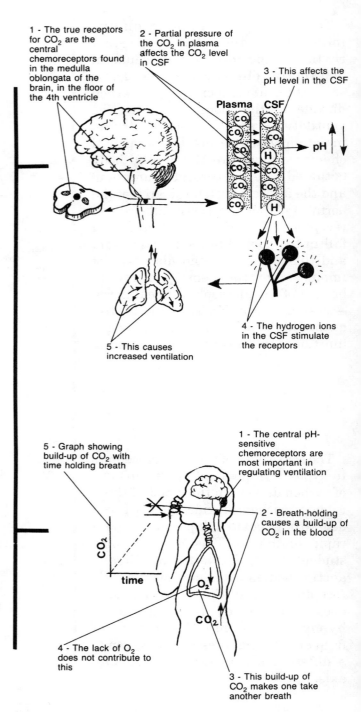

1 - The true receptors for CO_2 are the central chemoreceptors found in the medulla oblongata of the brain, in the floor of the 4th ventricle

2 - Partial pressure of the CO_2 in plasma affects the CO_2 level in CSF

3 - This affects the pH level in the CSF

4 - The hydrogen ions in the CSF stimulate the receptors

5 - This causes increased ventilation

5 - Graph showing build-up of CO_2 with time holding breath

1 - The central pH-sensitive chemoreceptors are most important in regulating ventilation

2 - Breath-holding causes a build-up of CO_2 in the blood

3 - This build-up of CO_2 makes one take another breath

4 - The lack of O_2 does not contribute to this

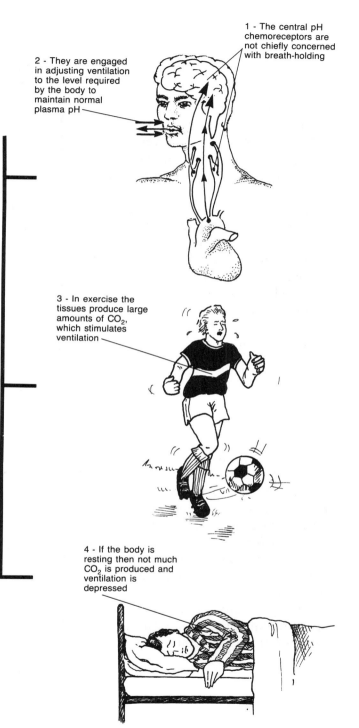

1 - The central pH chemoreceptors are not chiefly concerned with breath-holding

2 - They are engaged in adjusting ventilation to the level required by the body to maintain normal plasma pH

3 - In exercise the tissues produce large amounts of CO_2, which stimulates ventilation

4 - If the body is resting then not much CO_2 is produced and ventilation is depressed

The chemoreceptors are not, of course, chiefly concerned with breath-holding, but are engaged in adjusting ventilation to the level required by the body.

If the tissues are working hard and producing large amounts of carbon dioxide then ventilation is stimulated, while if the body is resting and not much carbon dioxide is being produced then ventilation is depressed. Ventilation is adjusted to meet the body's needs and prevent the build-up of carbon dioxide, keeping the plasma pH within narrow limits (normally 7.38−7.42). This is a fine example of a homeostatic mechanism.

While the main chemical control of ventilation is performed by the central carbon dioxide chemoreceptors, the peripheral oxygen receptors become important when one breathes a gas mixture which is deficient in oxygen. This occurs, for instance, at high altitude where the partial pressure of oxygen is reduced; hypoxia stimulates the carotid body even though the production of carbon dioxide is not increased, and in fact the hypoxic hyperventilation results in the loss of carbon dioxide through the lungs and alkalinization of the blood.

1 - The peripheral O_2 receptors become important when a gas mixture deficient in O_2 is breathed (e.g. at high altitude)

2 - The partial pressure of O_2 is reduced

3 - Hypoxic hyperventilation results in the loss of CO_2 through lungs and alkalinization of the blood

O_2 CO_2

The oxygen receptors become important in chronic lung disease where there is retention of carbon dioxide and the central carbon dioxide receptors become desensitized because of a persistently high level. In these circumstances the main stimulus to respiration becomes hypoxia rather than hypercapnia, and if the patient is given too much oxygen to breathe his respiration may become depressed.

3 - The main stimulus to respiration becomes hypoxia, and if the patient is given too much O_2 to breathe respiration may become depressed

2 - Central CO_2 receptors become desensitized because of the persistently high CO_2 level

1 - The O_2 receptors (carotid and aortic bodies) become important in chronic lung disease, where there is retention of CO_2

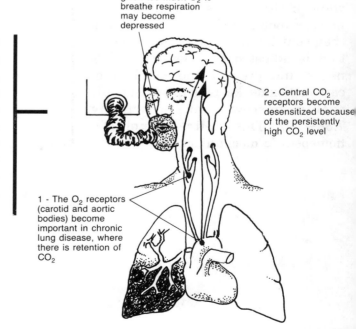

Another chemical influence which stimulates the respiratory centre is adrenaline circulating in the blood. This may be the most important factor in the ventilatory response to exercise: the anticipation of activity causes the release of hormone from the adrenal gland and this has a direct effect on the respiratory centre.

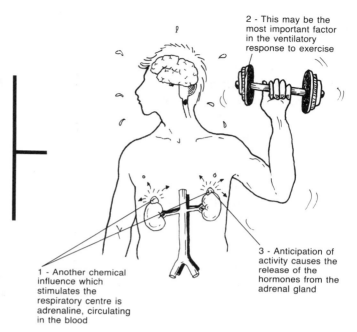

2 - This may be the most important factor in the ventilatory response to exercise

3 - Anticipation of activity causes the release of the hormones from the adrenal gland

1 - Another chemical influence which stimulates the respiratory centre is adrenaline, circulating in the blood

Other factors are the returning carbon dioxide from the exercising muscles, the movement of muscles and joints in active limbs, and the interaction between cardiac, vasomotor and respiratory centres. During exercise the cardiac output can increase fivefold, and in parallel the ventilation volume can increase from about 5.6 l/min to well over 25 l/min.

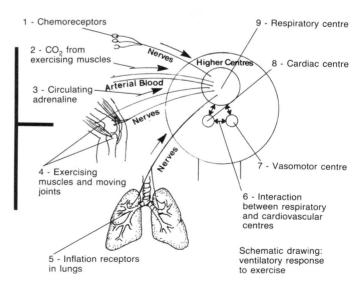

1 - Chemoreceptors

2 - CO_2 from exercising muscles

3 - Circulating adrenaline

4 - Exercising muscles and moving joints

5 - Inflation receptors in lungs

6 - Interaction between respiratory and cardiovascular centres

7 - Vasomotor centre

8 - Cardiac centre

9 - Respiratory centre

Higher Centres

Nerves

Arterial Blood

Schematic drawing: ventilatory response to exercise

RESPIRATORY FUNCTION TESTS

The assessment of respiratory function is very important in clinical medicine. Simple tests of respiratory adequacy include attempting to blow out a lighted match, or measuring the distance which a patient can walk.

It is fairly easy to measure the lung volumes with a spirometer, and one of the commonest tests is measurement of vital capacity and FEV_1; this can help to distinguish between obstructive and restrictive forms of lung disease, but is dependent upon the motivation, experience and cooperation of the patient.

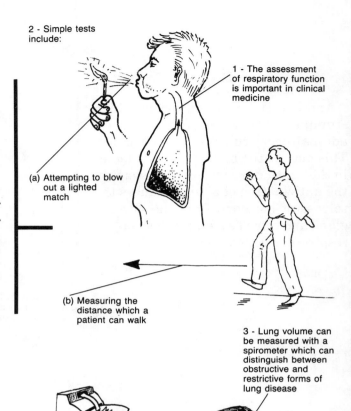

2 - Simple tests include:

1 - The assessment of respiratory function is important in clinical medicine

(a) Attempting to blow out a lighted match

(b) Measuring the distance which a patient can walk

3 - Lung volume can be measured with a spirometer which can distinguish between obstructive and restrictive forms of lung disease

The **peak flow meter** can be used to measure the maximal expiratory flow rate in the assessment of airways resistance, but its use is subject to the same limitations.

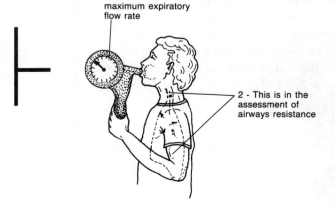

1 - The peak flow meter can be used to measure the maximum expiratory flow rate

2 - This is in the assessment of airways resistance

A test which is less dependent upon motivation is the construction of flow—volume curves. A **pneumotachograph** (a device for measuring the rate of gas flow) is connected to a mouthpiece through which the subject breathes, and the rate of flow is plotted against the total volume of air breathed out so far. The flat part of the curve during forceful expiration gives information about the elasticity of the lungs and the resistance to flow in the airways, but if accurate information is needed about pulmonary compliance or airways resistance then more complex measurement techniques have to be used.

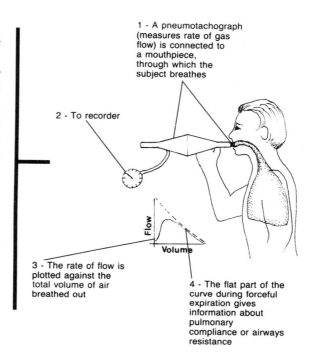

1 - A pneumotachograph (measures rate of gas flow) is connected to a mouthpiece, through which the subject breathes

2 - To recorder

3 - The rate of flow is plotted against the total volume of air breathed out

4 - The flat part of the curve during forceful expiration gives information about pulmonary compliance or airways resistance

In the measurement of compliance it is necessary to know accurately the pressure gradient between the pleura and alveoli; an estimate of intrapleural pressure is obtained by passing a balloon into the oesophagus and allowing it to come into equilibrium with the pleural cavity. Transpulmonary pressure and volume of air breathed are plotted to calculate the compliance of the lungs and chest.

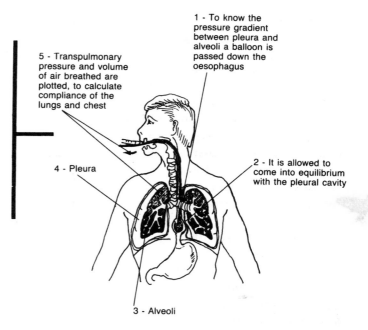

1 - To know the pressure gradient between pleura and alveoli a balloon is passed down the oesophagus

5 - Transpulmonary pressure and volume of air breathed are plotted, to calculate compliance of the lungs and chest

4 - Pleura

2 - It is allowed to come into equilibrium with the pleural cavity

3 - Alveoli

Airways resistance is usually measured in the **body plethysmograph**, an airtight box into which the subject is placed and allowed to breathe while his airflow is measured. As he breathes in he lowers the intra-pulmonary pressure, which makes the volume of gas already in the alveoli expand; the total pressure in the box therefore increases and can be measured with a very sensitive manometer. During expiration the air in the lungs is compressed and therefore the box pressure falls. From the measurement of these tiny pressure fluctuations the alveolar pressures can be calculated, and if the rate of airflow is plotted against pressure the slope of the line indicates the resistance of the airways.

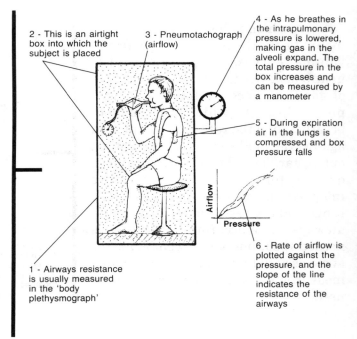

2 - This is an airtight box into which the subject is placed

3 - Pneumotachograph (airflow)

4 - As he breathes in the intrapulmonary pressure is lowered, making gas in the alveoli expand. The total pressure in the box increases and can be measured by a manometer

5 - During expiration air in the lungs is compressed and box pressure falls

6 - Rate of airflow is plotted against the pressure, and the slope of the line indicates the resistance of the airways

1 - Airways resistance is usually measured in the 'body plethysmograph'

Measurements of compliance and airways resistance are difficult. They require elaborate apparatus and are therefore performed only in large centres, often in association with extensive research programmes.

Other tests of respiratory function include the measurement of blood gas concentrations (e.g. oxygen and carbon dioxide in the arterial blood), and estimation of the diffusing capacity of the lung membrane by studying the uptake of a marker gas such as carbon monoxide.

The simplest respiratory function tests are probably those which give the most useful clinical information; they are certainly cheaper than the more elaborate ones, which may give little additional information that would influence clinical decisions.

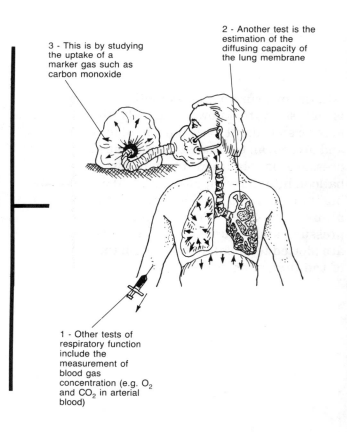

3 - This is by studying the uptake of a marker gas such as carbon monoxide

2 - Another test is the estimation of the diffusing capacity of the lung membrane

1 - Other tests of respiratory function include the measurement of blood gas concentration (e.g. O_2 and CO_2 in arterial blood)

The Digestive System

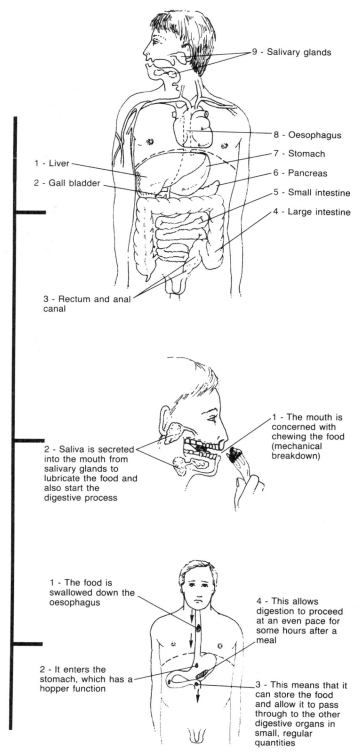

ANATOMY AND GENERAL ORGANIZATION

The digestive system is a set of organs concerned with taking in food, breaking it down mechanically and chemically, and absorbing the products into the bloodstream for transport to other parts of the body where they are built up again into the complex chemicals which the body needs.

9 - Salivary glands
8 - Oesophagus
7 - Stomach
6 - Pancreas
5 - Small intestine
4 - Large intestine
1 - Liver
2 - Gall bladder
3 - Rectum and anal canal

The **mouth** is concerned with **chewing** the food (mechanical breakdown), and **secreting** saliva which lubricates the food and starts some of the digestive process.

1 - The mouth is concerned with chewing the food (mechanical breakdown)

2 - Saliva is secreted into the mouth from salivary glands to lubricate the food and also start the digestive process

The food is **swallowed** down the **oesophagus** — a conduit — and enters the **stomach**, which has a **hopper** function, storing the food and allowing it to be passed to the other digestive organs in small regular quantities, so that digestion can proceed at an even pace for some hours after a meal.

1 - The food is swallowed down the oesophagus

2 - It enters the stomach, which has a hopper function

3 - This means that it can store the food and allow it to pass through to the other digestive organs in small, regular quantities

4 - This allows digestion to proceed at an even pace for some hours after a meal

There is also some **mixing** and **digestive** function in the stomach. The **small intestine** is the main site of **digestion** (breakdown) and **absorption**; the **large intestine** is concerned mainly with **absorption** of water and salts, and with **storage** of the waste produces of digestion (faeces) until their **elimination** at the **anus**.

The structure of the digestive tract (alimentary canal, gut, gastrointestinal tract) follows the same basic pattern from lower oesophagus to rectum; there may be individual variations in detail in the various parts. The wall is arranged as a number of layers. The innermost is the mucous membrane, which typically consists of columnar or cuboidal epithelial cells; the layer is often thrown into folds, may have flask-like invaginations forming secretory glands, particularly mucus glands, and may also have finger-like projections or **villi** which are concerned with absorption of digested food.

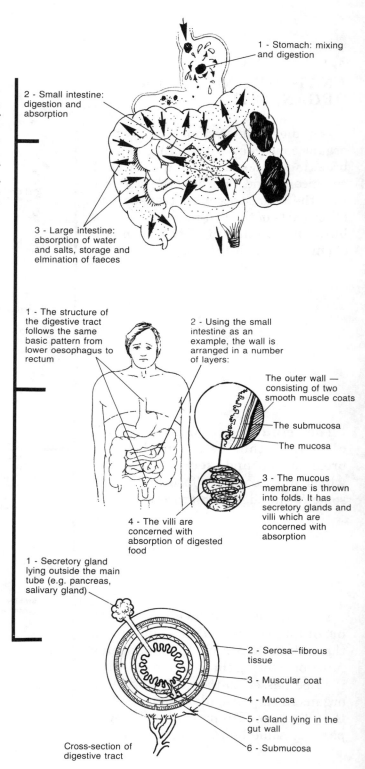

1 - Stomach: mixing and digestion

2 - Small intestine: digestion and absorption

3 - Large intestine: absorption of water and salts, storage and elmination of faeces

1 - The structure of the digestive tract follows the same basic pattern from lower oesophagus to rectum

2 - Using the small intestine as an example, the wall is arranged in a number of layers:

The outer wall — consisting of two smooth muscle coats

The submucosa

The mucosa

3 - The mucous membrane is thrown into folds. It has secretory glands and villi which are concerned with absorption

4 - The villi are concerned with absorption of digested food

1 - Secretory gland lying outside the main tube (e.g. pancreas, salivary gland)

2 - Serosa—fibrous tissue

3 - Muscular coat

4 - Mucosa

5 - Gland lying in the gut wall

6 - Submucosa

Cross-section of digestive tract

Under the mucous layer is the **sub-mucosa**, consisting of connective tissue in which run the nerves and blood vessels that supply the mucous membrane; there may be a small amount of smooth muscle in this layer, and some small localized glands which open by ducts into the **lumen** (cavity) of the gut.

The **muscle layer** may consist of several coats of smooth muscle, arranged circularly, longitudinally and sometimes obliquely. In the muscle layer are found the nerves and ganglia of the **myenteric plexus**, a network of nerves which control the function of the gut muscle.

The **serosal** layer is the outermost layer, consisting typically of some connective tissue and a layer of squamous epithelium which forms the lining of the **peritoneal** cavity. The blood vessels and nerves reach each segment of the gut through the **mesentery**, a reflection of the serosal layers to form a pedicle of attachment of the gut to the body wall.

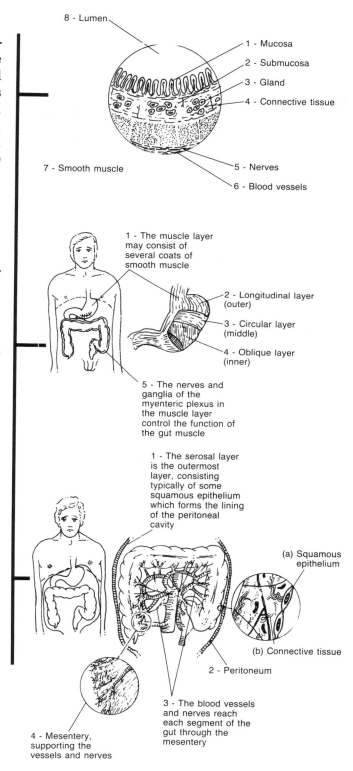

8 - Lumen

1 - Mucosa
2 - Submucosa
3 - Gland
4 - Connective tissue

7 - Smooth muscle

5 - Nerves
6 - Blood vessels

1 - The muscle layer may consist of several coats of smooth muscle

2 - Longitudinal layer (outer)
3 - Circular layer (middle)
4 - Oblique layer (inner)

5 - The nerves and ganglia of the myenteric plexus in the muscle layer control the function of the gut muscle

1 - The serosal layer is the outermost layer, consisting typically of some squamous epithelium which forms the lining of the peritoneal cavity

(a) Squamous epithelium

(b) Connective tissue

2 - Peritoneum

3 - The blood vessels and nerves reach each segment of the gut through the mesentery

4 - Mesentery, supporting the vessels and nerves

There are several accessory secretory glands such as the liver, salivary glands and pancreas, which lie outside the main part of the alimentary canal, but communicate with its lumen through major **ducts** which pierce the gut wall.

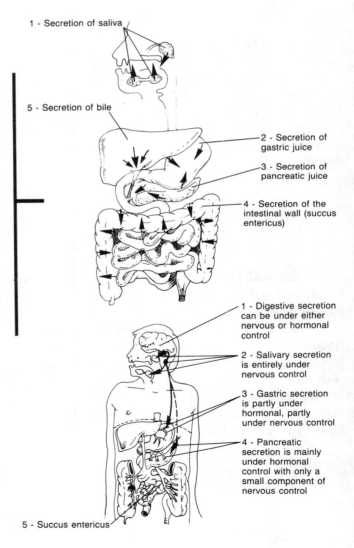

1 - There are several accessory secretory glands to the alimentary system:

2 - The salivary glands

3 - The liver

4 - The pancreas

5 - They lie outside the main part of the alimentary canal but communicate with its lumen through major ducts which pierce the gut wall

SECRETIONS OF THE DIGESTIVE SYSTEM

The main secretions of the gut are saliva, gastric juice, bile, pancreatic juice and the secretion of the intestinal wall (succus entericus). Digestive secretion can be under either nervous or hormonal control. Salivary secretion is entirely under nervous control with no influence from hormones, gastric secretion is partly under nervous and partly under hormonal control, and pancreatic secretion is chiefly under hormonal control, with only a small component of nervous control. Succus entericus is not strictly speaking a controlled secretion at all, consisting as it does of cellular debris.

1 - Secretion of saliva

5 - Secretion of bile

2 - Secretion of gastric juice

3 - Secretion of pancreatic juice

4 - Secretion of the intestinal wall (succus entericus)

1 - Digestive secretion can be under either nervous or hormonal control

2 - Salivary secretion is entirely under nervous control

3 - Gastric secretion is partly under hormonal, partly under nervous control

4 - Pancreatic secretion is mainly under hormonal control with only a small component of nervous control

5 - Succus entericus

Saliva is secreted by the salivary glands, whose ducts open into the mouth. There are three pairs of main glands — the parotid, submandibular and sublingual glands — as well as a number of small groups of gland cells on the surface of the tongue and the palate. About 750 ml of saliva is secreted per day; about 70% is from the submandibular, 20% from the parotids and 5% from the sublingual. During maximal secretory activity, a gland can produce its own weight of saliva in one minute.

Saliva is a watery fluid with an electrolyte content similar to plasma and a slightly alkaline pH. Its major enzyme is **ptyalin**, an alpha-amylase: i.e. it breaks down starch to maltose. It also contains **lysozyme**, a non-specific enzyme which has a protective function, breaking down bacteria in the mouth; this enzyme is also found in tears, nasal secretions and other body fluids.

The salivary glands are controlled by the autonomic nervous system; stimulation of the parasympathetic nerves causes the flow of a watery fluid rich in enzymes, while the sympathetic nerves cause the flow of a watery fluid rich in enzymes, while the sympathetic nerves cause the secretion of a more viscous fluid rich in mucus. Both types of nerves cause an increase in blood flow through the glands, but this is probably an indirect effect rather than a specific influence of any neurotransmitter on the blood vessels.

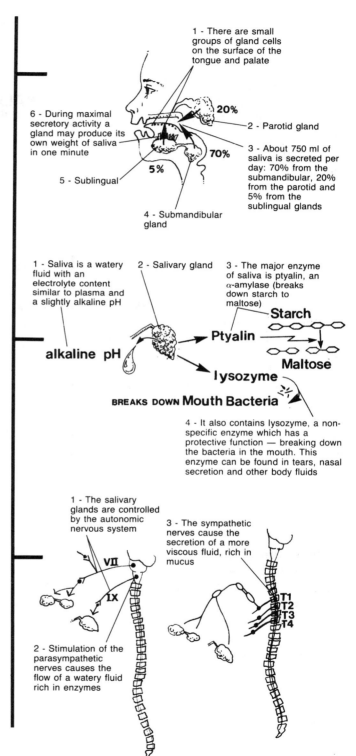

1 - There are small groups of gland cells on the surface of the tongue and palate

6 - During maximal secretory activity a gland may produce its own weight of saliva in one minute

20%

2 - Parotid gland

3 - About 750 ml of saliva is secreted per day: 70% from the submandibular, 20% from the parotid and 5% from the sublingual glands

70%

5%

5 - Sublingual

4 - Submandibular gland

1 - Saliva is a watery fluid with an electrolyte content similar to plasma and a slightly alkaline pH

2 - Salivary gland

3 - The major enzyme of saliva is ptyalin, an α-amylase (breaks down starch to maltose)

Starch

alkaline pH

Ptyalin

Maltose

lysozyme

BREAKS DOWN Mouth Bacteria

4 - It also contains lysozyme, a non-specific enzyme which has a protective function — breaking down the bacteria in the mouth. This enzyme can be found in tears, nasal secretion and other body fluids

1 - The salivary glands are controlled by the autonomic nervous system

VII

3 - The sympathetic nerves cause the secretion of a more viscous fluid, rich in mucus

V

IX

T1
T2
T3
T4

2 - Stimulation of the parasympathetic nerves causes the flow of a watery fluid rich in enzymes

Secretory activity in the glands, under autonomic control, causes the release of **kallikrein,** an enzyme which converts tissue alpha-globulins into **bradykinin**, a peptide with strong vasodilator properties.

Salivary secretion is initiated in a number of reflexes; the sight, smell or even the thought of food can cause salivation, though only to a small extent, and the presence of food in the mouth, stimulation of taste receptors and the act of chewing are very powerful stimuli to secretion. One of the most powerful stimuli is chewing candle wax!

The **stomach** produces about three litres of juice per day. There are two main types of secretion from the glands present in the mucosa of the fundus and body regions: **hydrochloric acid** from the **parietal** or oxyntic cells, around the necks of the glands, and **pepsinogen** from the **chief** cells in the depths of the glands.

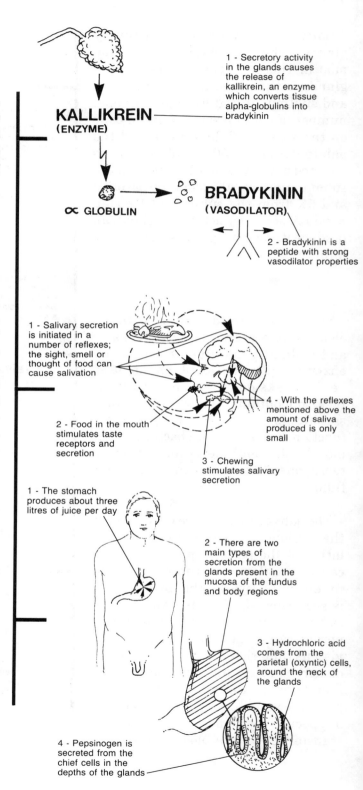

KALLIKREIN (ENZYME)

∝ GLOBULIN

BRADYKININ (VASODILATOR)

1 - Secretory activity in the glands causes the release of kallikrein, an enzyme which converts tissue alpha-globulins into bradykinin

2 - Bradykinin is a peptide with strong vasodilator properties

1 - Salivary secretion is initiated in a number of reflexes; the sight, smell or thought of food can cause salivation

2 - Food in the mouth stimulates taste receptors and secretion

3 - Chewing stimulates salivary secretion

4 - With the reflexes mentioned above the amount of saliva produced is only small

1 - The stomach produces about three litres of juice per day

2 - There are two main types of secretion from the glands present in the mucosa of the fundus and body regions

3 - Hydrochloric acid comes from the parietal (oxyntic) cells, around the neck of the glands

4 - Pepsinogen is secreted from the chief cells in the depths of the glands

Pepsinogen is the inactive precursor of the enzyme **pepsin**, a protease which breaks down proteins to short chains of amino acids (polypeptides). Most studies of gastric secretory control have concentrated on acid production, as this is so much easier to measure (because of the acid, the pH of the gastric juice is low, around 1.0), but the control of pepsinogen secretion is essentially similar.

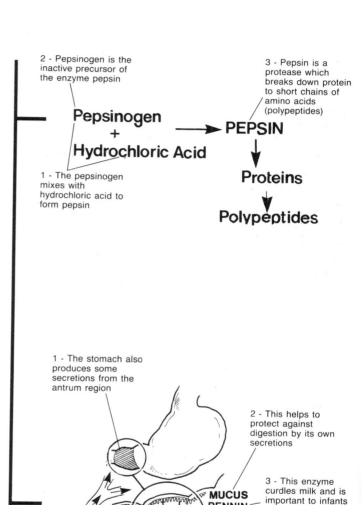

2 - Pepsinogen is the inactive precursor of the enzyme pepsin

3 - Pepsin is a protease which breaks down protein to short chains of amino acids (polypeptides)

Pepsinogen + Hydrochloric Acid → PEPSIN

1 - The pepsinogen mixes with hydrochloric acid to form pepsin

Proteins

Polypeptides

The stomach also produces some secretions from the antrum region: these include mucus (which helps to protect against digestion by its own secretions), rennin (an enzyme which curdles milk and is important in infants) and intrinsic factor, which is essential to the absorption of vitamin B$_{12}$ (see Chapter 3). The antrum also releases a hormone — **gastrin** which is important in the control of gastric secretion.

1 - The stomach also produces some secretions from the antrum region

2 - This helps to protect against digestion by its own secretions

3 - This enzyme curdles milk and is important to infants

MUCUS RENNIN GASTRIN INTRINSIC FACTOR

4 - Intrinsic factor is essential to the absorption of vitamin B$_{12}$

5 - This hormone is important in the control of gastric secretion and enters the blood

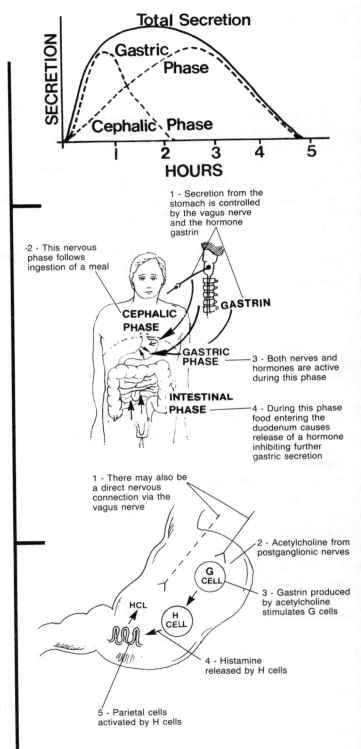

Secretion from the stomach is controlled by the vagus nerve (parasympathetic) and by the hormone gastrin. Following the ingestion of a meal the control of secretion has a **cephalic** phase (nervous) lasting about half an hour, followed by **gastric** phase in which both nerves and hormones are active, and which lasts several hours. There is also an **intestinal** phase of control in which food entering the duodenum causes the release of a hormone which **inhibits** further gastric secretion. This helps to protect the small intestine from being assaulted with too much acid.

During the **cephalic** phase of gastric secretion, the anticipation, ingestion, chewing, tasting and swallowing of food cause impulses to be sent down the vagus nerve; acetylcholine is released from postganglionic nerve endings near the parietal cells, and this causes the cells to secrete hydrochloric acid. This may be partly a direct effect of the transmitter on the parietal cells, but acetylcholine also stimulates an intermediate group of cells, the G cells, which liberate the hormone gastrin and this stimulates the secretory cells. It has been suggested that both of these mechanisms use a final common pathway, the stimulation of yet another intermediate cell, the H cell, which releases **histamine**; it is the histamine which actually activates the parietal cell.

1 - Secretion from the stomach is controlled by the vagus nerve and the hormone gastrin

2 - This nervous phase follows ingestion of a meal

CEPHALIC PHASE

GASTRIN

GASTRIC PHASE

3 - Both nerves and hormones are active during this phase

INTESTINAL PHASE

4 - During this phase food entering the duodenum causes release of a hormone inhibiting further gastric secretion

1 - There may also be a direct nervous connection via the vagus nerve

2 - Acetylcholine from postganglionic nerves

3 - Gastrin produced by acetylcholine stimulates G cells

G CELL

HCL

H CELL

4 - Histamine released by H cells

5 - Parietal cells activated by H cells

Once food is present in the stomach, it initiates the **gastric** phase of secretion. The presence of food can stimulate local nerve nets in the stomach wall; there may be mechanical distension of the wall of the gastric antrum; there may be chemical stimulation of the antral mucosa. Of these stimuli, the most powerful is the chemical; the presence of protein or protein breakdown products in the antrum stimulates the specialized G cells, which are particularly numerous in this region, to produce the hormone **gastrin**. This is secreted into the bloodstream and is eventually carried to the fundus and body of the stomach, where it causes secretion of gastric juice.

In the **intestinal** phase of gastric secretory control, food entering the small intestine stimulates the mucosa to produce the hormones **secretin** and **pancreozymin**, whose chief functions are the control of the pancreas and gall bladder, but which also inhibit gastric secretion and slow gastric emptying. They thus form part of a negative feedback loop, controlling the rate of digestion. Some earlier texts refer to an intestinal hormone 'enterogastrone'; it is now almost certain that this is identical to secretin or pancreozymin or both.

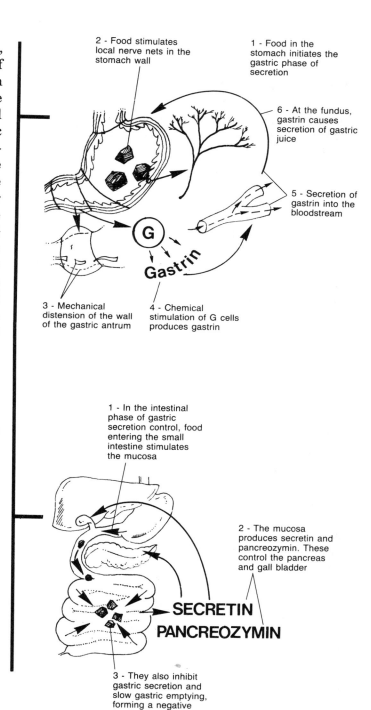

2 - Food stimulates local nerve nets in the stomach wall

1 - Food in the stomach initiates the gastric phase of secretion

6 - At the fundus, gastrin causes secretion of gastric juice

5 - Secretion of gastrin into the bloodstream

G

Gastrin

3 - Mechanical distension of the wall of the gastric antrum

4 - Chemical stimulation of G cells produces gastrin

1 - In the intestinal phase of gastric secretion control, food entering the small intestine stimulates the mucosa

2 - The mucosa produces secretin and pancreozymin. These control the pancreas and gall bladder

SECRETIN
PANCREOZYMIN

3 - They also inhibit gastric secretion and slow gastric emptying, forming a negative feedback

Gastric secretion can be investigated in humans by persuading the subject to swallow a tube (Ryle's tube) which is used to aspirate the gastric fluid for analysis of acid content. A standardized test meal can be given, and the rate of acid secretion is measured at intervals after the meal is ingested.

Other techniques include the use of radio pills, whose broadcast frequency is a function of the local pH; and fibre-optic gastroscopy, where a highly flexible telescope is introduced into the stomach, to allow the mucosa to be examined, and to permit biopsy specimens to be taken for pathological or biochemical analysis.

The **pancreas** (from a Greek word meaning all-secreting) has both endocrine secretions (which are dealt with in another chapter) and exocrine secretions, which are important in digestion.

From the acini it produces a number of inactive precursors of enzymes, including trypsinogen, chymotrypsinogen and procarboxypeptidase, which can form proteolytic enzymes; deoxyribonuclease and ribonuclease which break down nucleic acids; alpha-amylase which digests starch, and lipase which breaks down fats. It also produces in its ducts an aqueous fluid containing electrolytes including bicarbonate, which helps to neutralize the acid produced by the stomach.

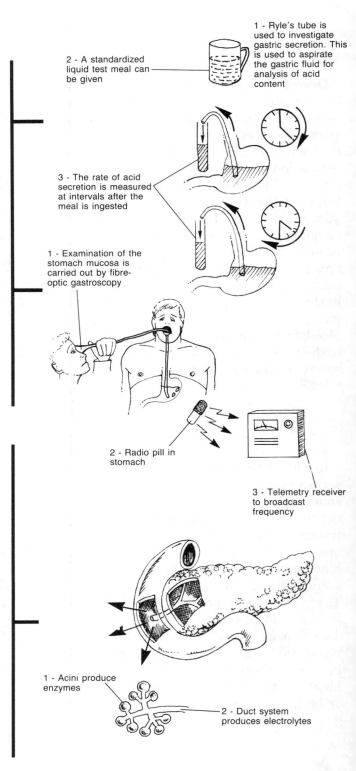

1 - Ryle's tube is used to investigate gastric secretion. This is used to aspirate the gastric fluid for analysis of acid content

2 - A standardized liquid test meal can be given

3 - The rate of acid secretion is measured at intervals after the meal is ingested

1 - Examination of the stomach mucosa is carried out by fibre-optic gastroscopy

2 - Radio pill in stomach

3 - Telemetry receiver to broadcast frequency

1 - Acini produce enzymes

2 - Duct system produces electrolytes

Pancreatic secretion has a small cephalic phase, in which entry of food to higher levels of the system stimulates the vagus and initiates secretion of a watery enzyme-rich fluid. (This represents stimulation of the acini.) However, the most important part of pancreatic control is by **hormones** produced by the duodenal mucosa.

1 - Pancreatic secretion has a small cephalic phase in which entry of food to higher levels of the system stimulates the vagus

2 - This initiates secretion of a watery enzyme-rich fluid

Pancreozymin (which is identical to the hormone **cholecystokinin** controlling the gall bladder, and is sometimes referred to as Cck-Pz) is produced in response to the arrival of fat and protein products in the duodenum, and acts on the pancreatic acini, causing them to secrete enzymes; it also makes the gall bladder contract. The other hormone is **secretin** (the first hormone ever described), which is released from the upper small intestine in response to the entry of acid into the duodenum. It stimulates the pancreatic ducts to secrete copious quantities of alkaline fluid containing bicarbonate, which effectively neutralizes the acid.

2 - It also makes the gall bladder contract

PANCREOZYMIN

1 - This hormone, produced in response to fat and protein products in the duodenum, causes the pancreatic acini to secrete enzymes

3 - Secretin stimulates secretion of alkaline fluid in the pancreas. This neutralizes acid

SECRETIN

4 - Secretin is released in the upper small intestine in response to acid in the duodenum

While secretin and pancreozymin have separate actions, they also potentiate each other so that the presence of secretin enables pancreozymin to exert a greater stimulant effect on the acini and vice versa.

1 - Pancreozymin stimulates the acini

2 - Secretin stimulates the ducts

PANCREOZYMIN SECRETIN

The **small intestine** has very few anatomically distinct glands, but does produce a number of important secretions. The Brunner's glands in the duodenum produce alkaline mucus, as do the goblet cells scattered throughout the mucosa of the whole small intestine.

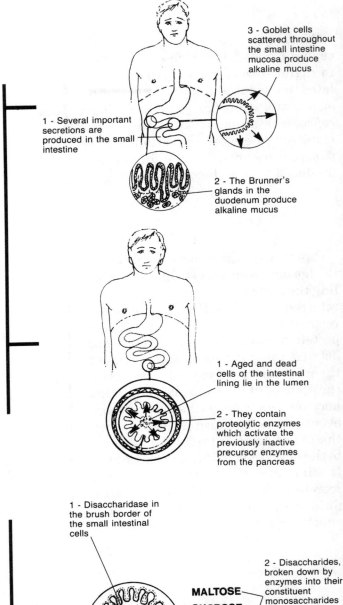

The aged and dead cells of the intestinal lining which become detached from the wall and lie in the lumen contain proteolytic enzymes ('enterokinase') which activate the previously inactive precursor enzymes produced by the pancreas.

The cells lining the small intestine have a brush border in which are incorporated molecules of disaccharidase enzymes, which break down disaccharides such as maltose and sucrose (cane sugar) into their constituent monosaccharides such as glucose and fructose. This action occurs as the intestinal contents come into contact with the intestinal wall; the enzymes are not really secreted at all, but remain attached to their cells.

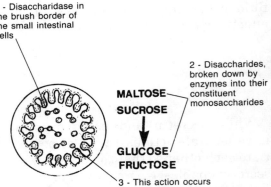

MECHANISMS OF SECRETION

Protein is secreted by the salivary glands and the pancreas. These glands are arranged in **acini** (meaning bunches of grapes) in which a group of cells surrounds a central lumen into which they secrete their products. The nuclei of these cells are placed either centrally or towards the base (away from the lumen) and the apices of the cells (nearest to the lumen) are packed with granules visible with the light microscope, known as **zymogen** granules.

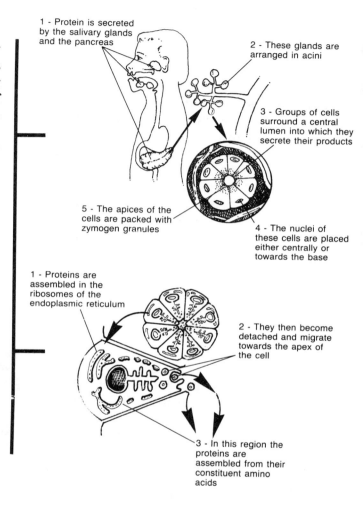

1 - Protein is secreted by the salivary glands and the pancreas

2 - These glands are arranged in acini

3 - Groups of cells surround a central lumen into which they secrete their products

5 - The apices of the cells are packed with zymogen granules

4 - The nuclei of these cells are placed either centrally or towards the base

Under the electron microscope the region of the cell nearest the basement membrane is seen to contain large amounts of endoplasmic reticulum with numerous ribosomes; this is the region in which the proteins are assembled from their constituent amino acids, and pieces of endoplasmic reticulum then become detached and migrate towards the apex of the cell.

1 - Proteins are assembled in the ribosomes of the endoplasmic reticulum

2 - They then become detached and migrate towards the apex of the cell

3 - In this region the proteins are assembled from their constituent amino acids

Near the nucleus is a very well-developed Golgi apparatus, whose function is to package the proteins into membrane-lined granules which correspond to the zymogen ('enzyme-creating') granules seen with the light microscope. The granules are extruded from the cells by a process of **exocytosis** similar to the way in which transmitter vesicles are released from nerve terminals (see Chapter 2).

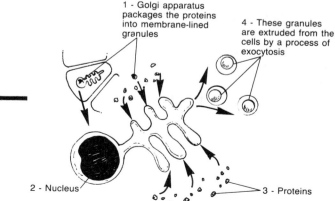

1 - Golgi apparatus packages the proteins into membrane-lined granules

4 - These granules are extruded from the cells by a process of exocytosis

2 - Nucleus

3 - Proteins

Electrolytes are secreted by the ducts of acinar glands such as the salivary glands and the pancreas. Sodium and potassium are secreted in about the same concentrations as plasma, but this is not a simple process of ultrafiltration; rather it is a poorly understood process of active transport.

Water is secreted passively as an osmotic response to the secretion of ions. **Bicarbonate** ions are secreted by a process involving the cellular enzyme carbonic anhydrase. Carbon dioxide in the blood diffuses into the duct cell, where it combines with water to form carbonic acid, which dissociates into hydrogen and bicarbonate ions. The hydrogen ions are returned to the blood by an active transport process in exchange for sodium ions; the bicarbonate and sodium ions are then pumped into the lumen of the gland.

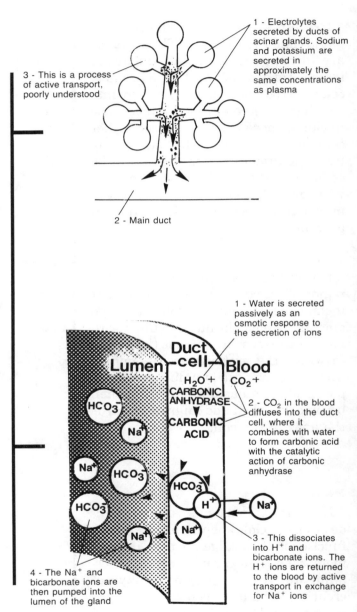

1 - Electrolytes secreted by ducts of acinar glands. Sodium and potassium are secreted in approximately the same concentrations as plasma

3 - This is a process of active transport, poorly understood

2 - Main duct

1 - Water is secreted passively as an osmotic response to the secretion of ions

2 - CO_2 in the blood diffuses into the duct cell, where it combines with water to form carbonic acid with the catalytic action of carbonic anhydrase

3 - This dissociates into H^+ and bicarbonate ions. The H^+ ions are returned to the blood by active transport in exchange for Na^+ ions

4 - The Na^+ and bicarbonate ions are then pumped into the lumen of the gland

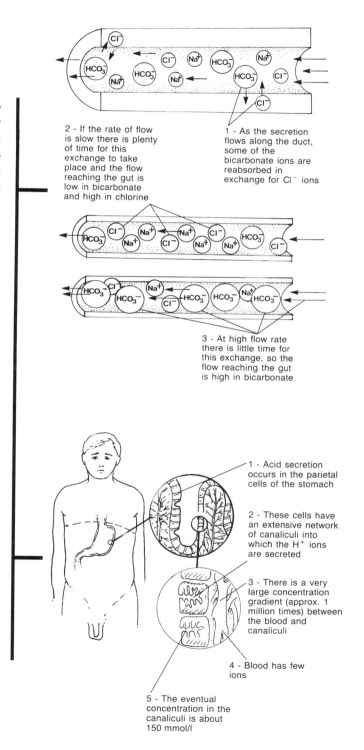

As the secretion flows along the duct, some of the bicarbonate ions are reabsorbed in exchange for chloride ions; if the rate of flow is slow, then there is plenty of time for this exchange to take place and the flow reaching the gut is low in bicarbonate and high in chloride, but at high flow rates the duct cells have not enough time to perform the exchange and the resulting fluid is rich in bicarbonate.

2 - If the rate of flow is slow there is plenty of time for this exchange to take place and the flow reaching the gut is low in bicarbonate and high in chlorine

1 - As the secretion flows along the duct, some of the bicarbonate ions are reabsorbed in exchange for Cl^- ions

3 - At high flow rate there is little time for this exchange, so the flow reaching the gut is high in bicarbonate

Acid secretion occurs in the parietal cells of the stomach, which have an extensive network of **canaliculi** into which the hydrogen ions are secreted. There is a very large concentration gradient (about one million times) between the blood and the contents of the canaliculi; blood has relatively few hydrogen ions, and the eventual concentration in the canaliculi is about 150 mmol/l.

1 - Acid secretion occurs in the parietal cells of the stomach

2 - These cells have an extensive network of canaliculi into which the H^+ ions are secreted

3 - There is a very large concentration gradient (approx. 1 million times) between the blood and canaliculi

4 - Blood has few ions

5 - The eventual concentration in the canaliculi is about 150 mmol/l

The acid is formed by dissociation of cellular water into hydroxyl and hydrogen ions; the hydroxyl ions are removed by combination with carbonic acid (formed by the solution of carbon dioxide in water) to form bicarbonate ions; these pass into the blood flowing through the stomach, and after a meal the blood leaving the stomach exhibits an 'alkaline tide'. The hydrogen ions and chloride ions (which enter the cell passively from the blood) are secreted into the canaliculi by a process of active transport, which requires a very large expenditure of metabolic energy.

Mucus is produced by goblet cells, whose nucleus is pushed and flattened to the basal part of the cell by the central part, which becomes gradually filled with a single enormous vesicle containing mucus. When the whole of the cell is filled with mucus it bursts, releasing the mucus into the lumen and leaving an empty, flaccid cell.

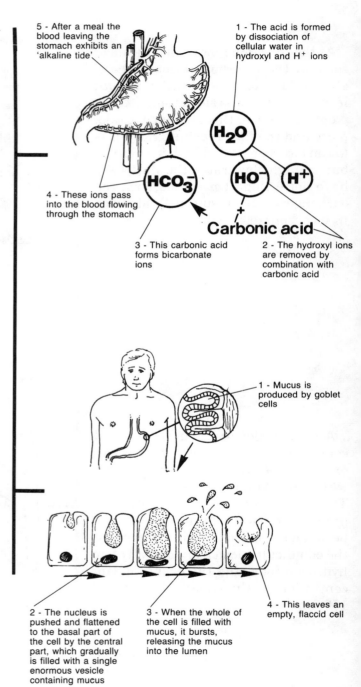

5 - After a meal the blood leaving the stomach exhibits an 'alkaline tide'

1 - The acid is formed by dissociation of cellular water in hydroxyl and H^+ ions

4 - These ions pass into the blood flowing through the stomach

3 - This carbonic acid forms bicarbonate ions

2 - The hydroxyl ions are removed by combination with carbonic acid

Carbonic acid

1 - Mucus is produced by goblet cells

2 - The nucleus is pushed and flattened to the basal part of the cell by the central part, which gradually is filled with a single enormous vesicle containing mucus

3 - When the whole of the cell is filled with mucus, it bursts, releasing the mucus into the lumen

4 - This leaves an empty, flaccid cell

THE LIVER

The liver is a large organ situated in the upper right part of the abdomen; its functions are only partly secretory. It produces **bile**, a watery electrolyte-rich fluid which has no enzymes, but contains bile salts which are important in emulsifying fats, and bile pigments which are essentially an excretory product.

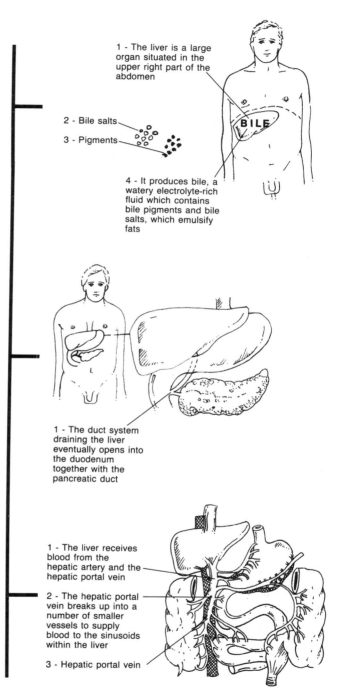

1 - The liver is a large organ situated in the upper right part of the abdomen

2 - Bile salts

3 - Pigments

4 - It produces bile, a watery electrolyte-rich fluid which contains bile pigments and bile salts, which emulsify fats

The duct system draining the liver eventually opens into the duodenum together with the pancreatic duct.

1 - The duct system draining the liver eventually opens into the duodenum together with the pancreatic duct

The blood supply to the liver is unique; not only does it receive arterial blood through the hepatic artery, but also it receives almost all of the venous blood draining the stomach and intestines through the hepatic portal vein, which breaks up into a number of smaller vessels to supply blood to the sinusoids or blood-filled cavities within the liver.

1 - The liver receives blood from the hepatic artery and the hepatic portal vein

2 - The hepatic portal vein breaks up into a number of smaller vessels to supply blood to the sinusoids within the liver

3 - Hepatic portal vein

The presence of sinusoids rather than capillaries is another unusual feature of the liver's structure. The sinusoids run close to columns of liver cells (**hepatocytes**) forming the lining to small channels or bile canaliculi which carry bile to the duct system.

The major function of the liver is the chemical processing of almost all of the foodstuffs which are absorbed from the gut; it is uniquely placed to perform this function, because most of the venous blood draining the gut flows into the **portal** vein. Thus the food absorbed from the gut is taken directly to the liver for processing.

The main processing functions performed by the liver are **storage**, **synthesis** and **detoxication**. The liver is one of the most important storage sites in the body for carbohydrate; glucose absorbed from the intestine is built up in the liver to **glycogen**, a complex polysaccharide which is sometimes called 'animal starch'.

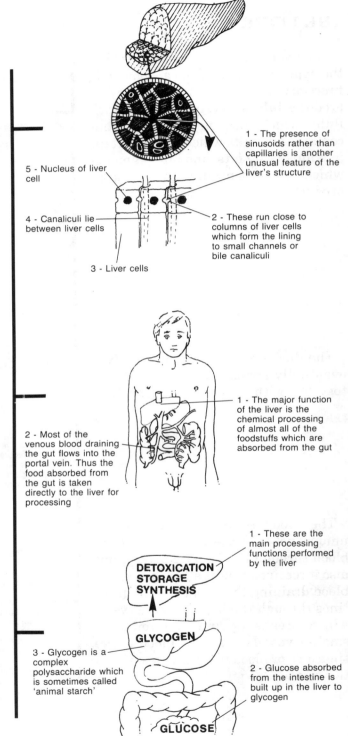

5 - Nucleus of liver cell

4 - Canaliculi lie between liver cells

3 - Liver cells

1 - The presence of sinusoids rather than capillaries is another unusual feature of the liver's structure

2 - These run close to columns of liver cells which form the lining to small channels or bile canaliculi

2 - Most of the venous blood draining the gut flows into the portal vein. Thus the food absorbed from the gut is taken directly to the liver for processing

1 - The major function of the liver is the chemical processing of almost all of the foodstuffs which are absorbed from the gut

1 - These are the main processing functions performed by the liver

DETOXICATION
STORAGE
SYNTHESIS

GLYCOGEN

3 - Glycogen is a complex polysaccharide which is sometimes called 'animal starch'

2 - Glucose absorbed from the intestine is built up in the liver to glycogen

GLUCOSE

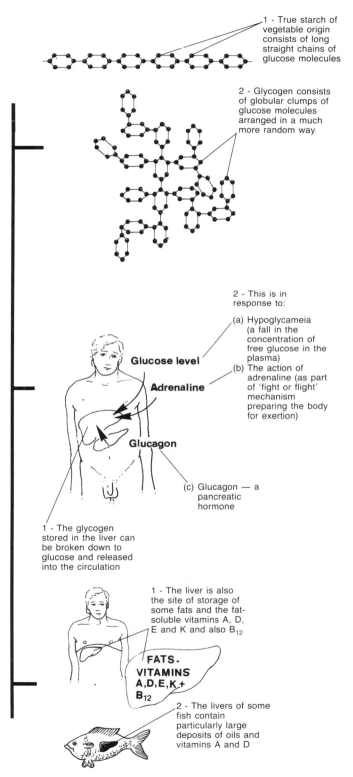

1 - True starch of vegetable origin consists of long straight chains of glucose molecules

2 - Glycogen consists of globular clumps of glucose molecules arranged in a much more random way

While true starch of vegetable origin consists of long straight chains of glucose molecules joined end to end, glycogen consists of globular clumps of glucose molecules arranged in a much more random way.

The glycogen stored in the liver can be broken down to glucose and released into the circulation in response to hypoglycaemia (a fall in the concentration of free glucose in the plasma), or by the action of the hormones adrenaline (as part of the 'fight or flight' mechanism, preparing the body for exertion) and glucagon, a pancreatic hormone.

Glucose level

Adrenaline

Glucagon

2 - This is in response to:

(a) Hypoglycameia (a fall in the concentration of free glucose in the plasma)
(b) The action of adrenaline (as part of 'fight or flight' mechanism preparing the body for exertion)

(c) Glucagon — a pancreatic hormone

1 - The glycogen stored in the liver can be broken down to glucose and released into the circulation

The liver is also the site of storage of some fats and the fat-soluble vitamins **A, D, E** and **K**; vitamin B_{12} is also stored there. The livers of some fish contain particularly large deposits of oils and vitamins **A** and **D**.

1 - The liver is also the site of storage of some fats and the fat-soluble vitamins A, D, E and K and also B_{12}

FATS. VITAMINS A,D,E,K+ B_{12}

2 - The livers of some fish contain particularly large deposits of oils and vitamins A and D

In some human disease states, large quantities of fat become stored in the liver. The liver is also an important storage site for several minerals, particularly iron, which is important for haemopoiesis.

The liver is the most important site of **synthesis** of plasma proteins, especially albumin. Some of the globulins, fibrinogen and the other blood clotting factors, and some of the specific transport and binding proteins such as transferrin (for iron) and caeruloplasmin (for copper) are also manufactured there. The liver receives a rich supply of amino acids from the breakdown of protein in the gut, and uses these to assemble the complex molecules which the body needs.

Detoxication is the process of rendering harmless the poisons ingested by the body or produced as a result of the body's metabolism. A closely related activity is the conversion of one particular molecule into another form, for example the conversion of one type of amino acid (present in excess) into another (required by the body) — the process of transamination, carried out by the enzyme **transaminase**. Any excess amino groups are converted to urea, a relatively harmless substance which is easily excreted by the kidneys.

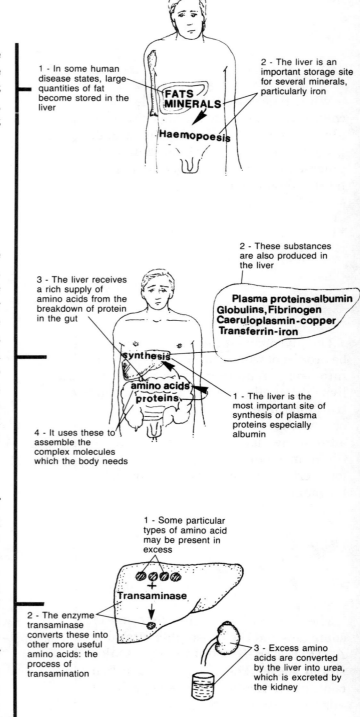

1 - In some human disease states, large quantities of fat become stored in the liver

2 - The liver is an important storage site for several minerals, particularly iron

FATS MINERALS

Haemopoesis

2 - These substances are also produced in the liver

3 - The liver receives a rich supply of amino acids from the breakdown of protein in the gut

Plasma proteins-albumin Globulins, Fibrinogen Caeruloplasmin-copper Transferrin-iron

synthesis

amino acids proteins

1 - The liver is the most important site of synthesis of plasma proteins especially albumin

4 - It uses these to assemble the complex molecules which the body needs

1 - Some particular types of amino acid may be present in excess

Transaminase

2 - The enzyme transaminase converts these into other more useful amino acids: the process of transamination

3 - Excess amino acids are converted by the liver into urea, which is excreted by the kidney

The liver has two main pathways for detoxication: there may be specific enzymes for breaking down particular substances, such as **ethanol dehydrogenase**, which breaks down alcohol, or the liver may use a non-specific process of **conjugation**, in which a potentially toxic molecule becomes joined onto a glucose molecule by the enzyme **glucuronyl transferase** to form a **glucuronide**.

This is the pathway followed by the breakdown products of **haemoglobin**. The protein part of the molecule is recovered for the body's amino acid pool.

The haem ring is split to form a straight chain of porphyrins. This product is insoluble in water but circulates bound to a protein; it cannot be excreted in the urine in this form. The liver cells take up the molecule, called bilirubin (unconjugated), and form the water-soluble product **bilirubin glucuronide**, which is then actively secreted into the bile canaliculi.

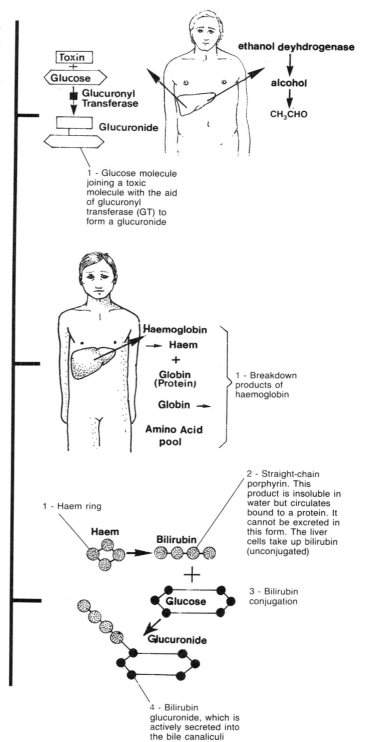

1 - Glucose molecule joining a toxic molecule with the aid of glucuronyl transferase (GT) to form a glucuronide

1 - Breakdown products of haemoglobin

2 - Straight-chain porphyrin. This product is insoluble in water but circulates bound to a protein. It cannot be excreted in this form. The liver cells take up bilirubin (unconjugated)

3 - Bilirubin conjugation

4 - Bilirubin glucuronide, which is actively secreted into the bile canaliculi

Some of this conjugated bilirubin escapes into the blood and can be excreted by the kidney; some of the bilirubin appearing in the bile is reabsorbed by the intestine, travels in the portal blood and is resecreted by the liver (the enterohepatic recirculation); and some of the conjugated bilirubin in the gut is broken down by bacteria to **urobilinogen**, which is reabsorbed and appears in the urine. Any bilirubin products remaining in the faeces (giving them their characteristic colour) are called **stercobilinogen**.

The main secretory product of the liver is **bile**, which contains bile pigments such as bilirubin and its derivatives. These have no digestive purpose but use the bile as a convenient excretory route. Bile also contains the bile salts **taurocholate** and **glycocholate**, which have an important function as emulsifiers of fat and as activators of lipase, the pancreatic hormone which breaks down fat, and electrolytes such as bicarbonate.

The bile from the liver canaliculi is collected into the bile duct system; the opening into the duodenum (**sphincter of Oddi**) is usually closed, so the bile flows into the gall bladder — a storage sac which also absorbs water, concentrating the bile about five- or tenfold. When food is eaten, a **nervous** reflex causes relaxation of the sphincter of Oddi. The entry of food, especially fats, into the duodenum causes the release of the hormone **cholecystokinin**, a cholagogue (literally a 'bile leader'). This hormone causes contraction of the gall bladder and the flow of bile into the duodenum.

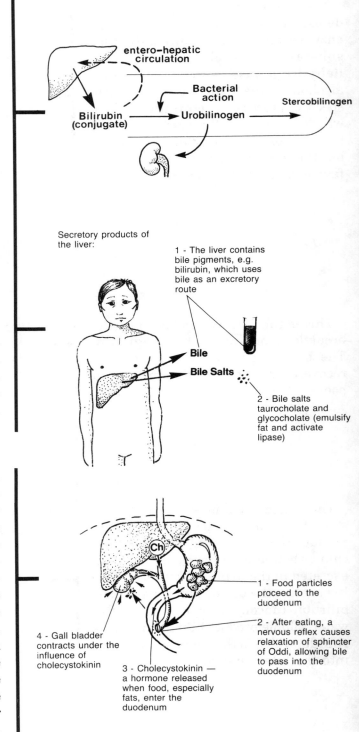

entero–hepatic circulation

Bilirubin (conjugate) → Urobilinogen → Stercobilinogen

Bacterial action

Secretory products of the liver:

1 - The liver contains bile pigments, e.g. bilirubin, which uses bile as an excretory route

Bile

Bile Salts

2 - Bile salts taurocholate and glycocholate (emulsify fat and activate lipase)

1 - Food particles proceed to the duodenum

2 - After eating, a nervous reflex causes relaxation of sphincter of Oddi, allowing bile to pass into the duodenum

3 - Cholecystokinin — a hormone released when food, especially fats, enter the duodenum

4 - Gall bladder contracts under the influence of cholecystokinin

Sometimes gall stones form within the gall bladder or bile ducts. These are usually precipitates of either cholesterol or bilirubin salts, and require the presence of a focus such as bacteria or other foreign substances to trigger their formation.

1 - Infected gall bladder helps stone formation

3 - Bile duct

2 - Varying types of gall stones may form in gall bladder or bile ducts, either of cholesterol or bilirubin salts

They can cause pain, particularly after fatty meals when the gall bladder contracts, or blockage of the biliary ducts, causing jaundice.

3 - Contraction of gall bladder

2 - Pain in gall bladder after contraction

1 - Fatty meal

4 - Blockage of duct, causing jaundice

If the gall bladder is surgically removed (**cholecystectomy**) the common bile duct becomes slightly dilated, and there is an almost continuous stream of dilute bile into the duodenum. These patients seem to suffer no digestive harm as a result of removal of the gall bladder.

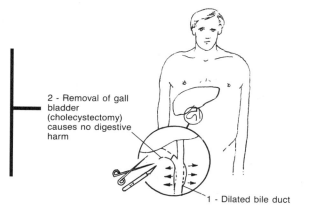

2 - Removal of gall bladder (cholecystectomy) causes no digestive harm

1 - Dilated bile duct

As well as its biochemical, excretory and secretory functions, the liver forms part of the reticuloendothelial system. Large phagocytic cells — **Kupffer** cells — are found in the walls of the sinusoids and have a protective role.

2 - The liver forms part of the reticuloendothelial system as well as its other functions

1 - Large Kupffer cells are found in the walls of the sinusoids and have a protective role

At some times in life including the fetal stage and in cases of severe anaemia the liver also produces red and white blood cells.

1 - Red and white cells may be produced in the liver at certain times

2 - In fetal life

(Low haematocrit and low haemoglobin)

3 - During severe anaemia

DIGESTION AND ABSORPTION

Absorption is the most important function of the gut; all of the other functions simply exist so that it can occur. Some substances, including the drug nicotine, are absorbed through the mucosa of the mouth, and water, ethanol and some drugs are absorbed through the wall of the stomach, but the most important site of absorption is the small intestine. The majority of foodstuffs can be absorbed by any part of the small intestine, but only the terminal portion is able to absorb vitamin B_{12}. Water and sodium are the only substances to be absorbed in the large intestine.

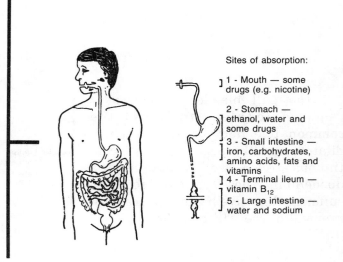

Sites of absorption:

1 - Mouth — some drugs (e.g. nicotine)

2 - Stomach — ethanol, water and some drugs

3 - Small intestine — iron, carbohydrates, amino acids, fats and vitamins

4 - Terminal ileum — vitamin B_{12}

5 - Large intestine — water and sodium

Mechanisms of absorption

A number of different mechanisms exist for the transport of substances across the intestinal wall, and indeed for the transport of substances in general. The simplest is **diffusion**, where molecules move down a concentration gradient from regions of high to low concentration. The rate of diffusion depends on the size of the molecule, its relative solubility in water and in the substance of the cell membrane, and its electric charge and potential gradient, if any.

A closely related phenomenon is **bulk diffusion** — the mass movement of water and its solutes through a leaky membrane, due to hydrostatic or osmotic forces. There may or may not be filtration of certain molecules; this depends on the size of the particles and the size of the leaks.

Facilitated diffusion is a mechanism whereby molecules move through a membrane at a much higher rate than would be predicted by the laws of diffusion, given their particle size and solubility. The movement is still passive, down a concentration gradient, but there is a specific carrier molecule in the membrane to which the diffusing molecule can become attached, and the complex molecule can then move rapidly through the membrane. No input of metabolic energy is required for this process.

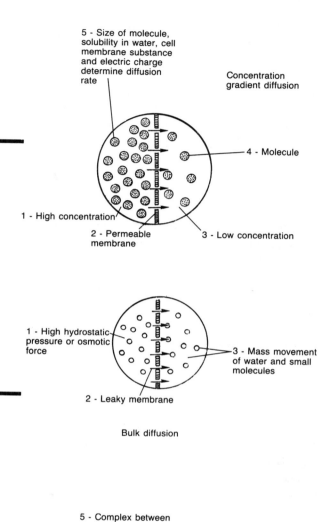

5 - Size of molecule, solubility in water, cell membrane substance and electric charge determine diffusion rate

Concentration gradient diffusion

4 - Molecule

1 - High concentration

2 - Permeable membrane

3 - Low concentration

1 - High hydrostatic pressure or osmotic force

3 - Mass movement of water and small molecules

2 - Leaky membrane

Bulk diffusion

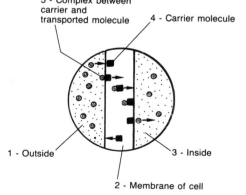

5 - Complex between carrier and transported molecule

4 - Carrier molecule

1 - Outside

3 - Inside

2 - Membrane of cell

Facilitated diffusion

Active transport is the movement of molecules against a concentration or electrochemical gradient. It requires the expenditure of cellular energy to move highly specific carrier molecules through cell membranes. The sodium–potassium pump at the cell membrane of nerves and red cells is an example.

1 - Molecule

2 - Cellular energy

3 - Carrier molecule

4 - Movement of molecules against a concentration gradient

Active transport

Other types of transport include **pinocytosis**, in which tiny vesicles filled with water and solutes become pinched off from one surface of the cell and migrate to the opposite surface. Little is known about the mechanism of this phenomenon, except that is requires cellular energy.

1 - Tiny vesicles pinched off from surface of another cell

2 - Pinocytosis

3 - Surface of penetrated cell

4 - Vesicle filled with water and solutes

5 - Migration involves cellular energy

Pinocytosis

Phagocytosis, the behaviour typical of white blood cells, involves the active engulfing of whole particules by the pseudopodia of a cell, and their incorporation into the cell's substance.

1 - Foreign body

2 - Fusion in pseudopodia

3 - Body is engulfed in cell

Phagocytosis

Exocytosis is the reverse phenomenon, where products of the cell are packaged into membrane-lined vesicles which are then extruded through the cell membrane; the process is described elsewhere in connection with transmitter release from nerves and secretion from exocrine glands.

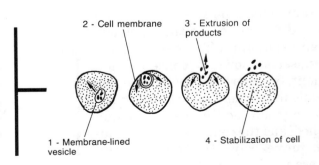

2 - Cell membrane

3 - Extrusion of products

1 - Membrane-lined vesicle

4 - Stabilization of cell

Exocytosis

Intestinal absorption can readily be studied by removing a segment of intestine from an animal, and placing it in an artificial nutrient medium. While test substances could be introduced into the lumen and their appearance outside the gut could be detected, it is actually much more convenient to turn the gut inside-out (everted sac preparation), so that the mucosa can be in contact with a large volume of test solution and only a small volume within the sac need be analysed for the substance transported.

Intestinal absorption can be studied in man by swallowing a tube whose tip lies in the intestine, and repeatedly sampling the intestinal juice; alternatively one could measure the rate of appearance of ingested marker substances in the blood or urine.

The area of intestinal surface available for absorption is very large. This is the result, firstly, of the extreme length of the organ itself; secondly, the wall is thrown into a number of longitudinal folds which increase the surface area. Thirdly, the mucosal surface has vast numbers of **villi** — finger-like projections into the lumen; and fourthly, the individual epithelial cells have a **brush border**, in other words the cell membrane is thrown into countless folds which further increase the absorptive area.

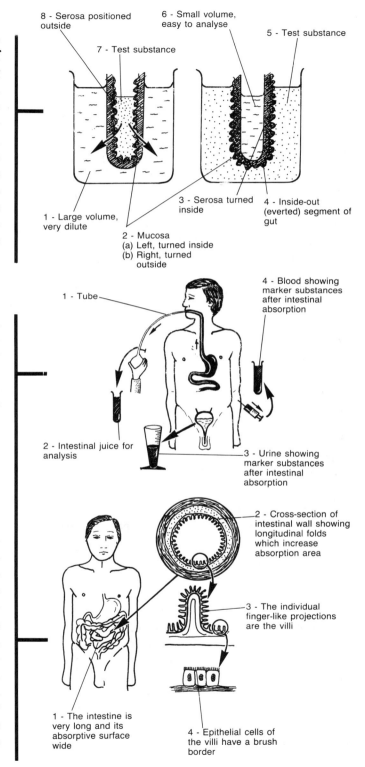

8 - Serosa positioned outside

7 - Test substance

6 - Small volume, easy to analyse

5 - Test substance

3 - Serosa turned inside

4 - Inside-out (everted) segment of gut

1 - Large volume, very dilute

2 - Mucosa
(a) Left, turned inside
(b) Right, turned outside

1 - Tube

4 - Blood showing marker substances after intestinal absorption

2 - Intestinal juice for analysis

3 - Urine showing marker substances after intestinal absorption

2 - Cross-section of intestinal wall showing longitudinal folds which increase absorption area

3 - The individual finger-like projections are the villi

1 - The intestine is very long and its absorptive surface wide

4 - Epithelial cells of the villi have a brush border

Digestion and absorption of carbohydrates

This occurs in stages. Starch is broken down to the disaccharide **maltose** by the enzyme alpha-amylase, in saliva and pancreatic juice; maltose and the other disaccharides sucrose and lactose are broken down to their constituent monosaccharides by specific **disaccharidases** which exist on the brush border of the epithelial cells rather than free in the intestinal lumen. The disaccharides are thus broken down close to the site for uptake of sugars into the epithelial cells.

Monosaccharides are transported into the cells by facilitated diffusion. A carrier molecule in the membrane combines with sugar and a sodium ion in the lumen to form a ternary complex which diffuses across the membrane driven by the inward concentration gradient for sodium. At the inner surface of the membrane the complex dissociates, releasing the sodium ion and glucose molecule into the cell. The cell thus accumulates glucose, which diffuses passively into the blood. This process is not called active transport, although sugars are accumulated in the cell against a concentration gradient, because the driving energy comes from the concentration gradient for sodium. Entry of sodium into the cell would eventually abolish the sodium gradient, so metabolic energy is expended in the sodium−potassium pump to remove this sodium. However, this occurs at a different site from the sugar transport; no metabolic energy is expended directly in transporting the monosaccharides. The carrier is highly specific, and can distinguish between D- and L-forms of the monosaccharides.

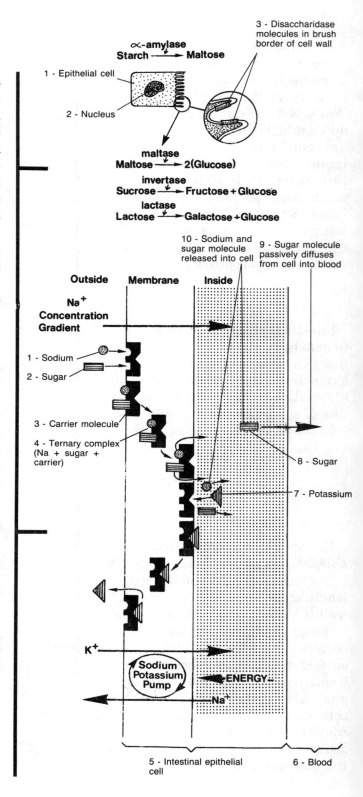

Digestion and absorption of proteins

Proteins are digested by a number of enzymes; pepsin in the stomach starts the process by cleaving large molecules at internal sites into shorter chains of amino acids, called polypeptides. The process is continued by the pancreatic hormones trypsin and chymotrypsin, which successively remove amino acids from the terminal regions of the polypeptide molecule, until we are left with a mixture of separate amino acids.

The amino acids are transported across the gut wall by a process of facilitated diffusion, rather similar to sugar transport. There are three separate carriers for different groups of amino acids; the transport is linked to the sodium concentration gradient, and the carriers can distinguish between L-amino acids, whose transport is facilitated, and the D-forms, which simply diffuse passively. Once the amino acids enter the intestinal epithelial cell, they diffuse passively into the blood.

In infants, some undigested proteins are absorbed intact into the circulation. These include the antibodies from the mother's milk, which confer passive immunity until the child's own immune system becomes fully developed; it is believed that this absorption occurs by pinocytosis.

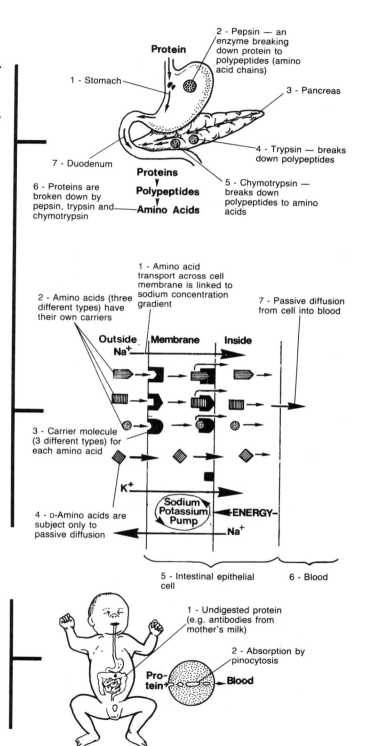

Digestion and absorption of fats

Fats are ingested in the form of triglycerides, and are broken down by lipase into diglycerides, then monogylcerides, and finally into fatty acids and glycerol.

The process of fat digestion is greatly assisted by the emulsifying or detergent effect of the bile salts, which prevent all the lipids from clumping together into huge globules, and instead aggregate into smaller units called **micelles.** The bile salts combine with the slightly hydrophilic ends of some molecules, making them more attracted to water. The more hydrophobic parts of the molecules clump together at the centres of the micelles.

The contents of the micelles are taken up by the epithelial cells, probably by passive diffusion. Bile salts are removed and returned to the portal blood, making their way back to the liver for an enterohepatic recirculation. The short-chain fatty acids are passed into the portal blood and thence to the liver, but the long-chain fatty acids are re-esterified with glycerol into fats which are packaged into little globules called **chylomicrons**; these are covered with beta-lipoproteins which the intestinal cells supply from their endoplasmic reticulum. The chylomicrons are secreted into the **lacteals** — small capillary-like vessels present in each of the villi, which unite to form lymphatic vessels.

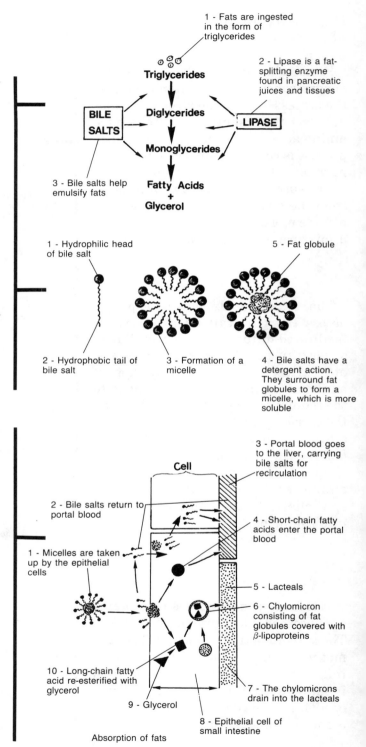

1 - Fats are ingested in the form of triglycerides

2 - Lipase is a fat-splitting enzyme found in pancreatic juices and tissues

Triglycerides

BILE SALTS

Diglycerides

LIPASE

Monoglycerides

3 - Bile salts help emulsify fats

Fatty Acids + Glycerol

1 - Hydrophilic head of bile salt

5 - Fat globule

2 - Hydrophobic tail of bile salt

3 - Formation of a micelle

4 - Bile salts have a detergent action. They surround fat globules to form a micelle, which is more soluble

Cell

3 - Portal blood goes to the liver, carrying bile salts for recirculation

2 - Bile salts return to portal blood

4 - Short-chain fatty acids enter the portal blood

1 - Micelles are taken up by the epithelial cells

5 - Lacteals

6 - Chylomicron consisting of fat globules covered with β-lipoproteins

10 - Long-chain fatty acid re-esterified with glycerol

9 - Glycerol

7 - The chylomicrons drain into the lacteals

8 - Epithelial cell of small intestine

Absorption of fats

The lacteals eventually combine to form the **thoracic duct**, a major lymph trunk which eventually drains into the venous system in the neck. Thus many of the lipids do not go directly to the liver, but bypass it through the lymphatic system.

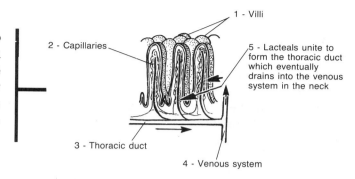

1 - Villi

2 - Capillaries

5 - Lacteals unite to form the thoracic duct which eventually drains into the venous system in the neck

3 - Thoracic duct

4 - Venous system

Absorption of vitamins and minerals

The mode of absorption of vitamins depends upon their type. The water-soluble vitamins, B and C are absorbed by passive diffusion.

2 - Mucosal cell

3 - Bloodstream

1 - Lumen

4 - The water-soluble Vitamins B and C are absorbed into the blood by passive diffusion

B

C

The fat-soluble vitamins A, D, E and K are absorbed along with the lipids and cholesterol, in the micelles.

1 - These fat-soluble vitamins are absorbed in micelles

A,D,E,K →

Vitamin B_{12} is a special case; it requires the presence of **intrinsic factor**, secreted by the stomach. The complex of intrinsic factor and vitamin is absorbed in the terminal part of the ileum, by a process of **pinocytosis**.

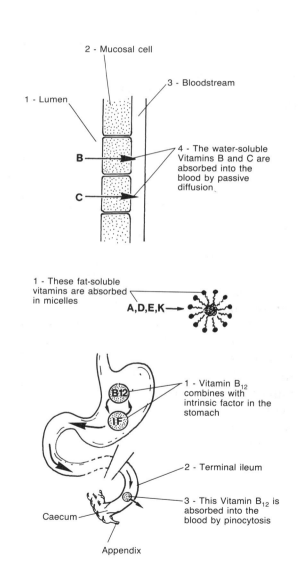

B12

IF

1 - Vitamin B_{12} combines with intrinsic factor in the stomach

2 - Terminal ileum

3 - This Vitamin B_{12} is absorbed into the blood by pinocytosis

Caecum

Appendix

Transport of **minerals** occurs all along the small intestine. The movement of water and sodium occurs passively, into or out of the lumen, depending on the osmotic strength of the intestinal contents. In the colon there is active transport of sodium, which is followed passively by water, so that the contents of the colon become progressively dried out. Chloride and potassium ions are absorbed passively. Calcium ions are actively absorbed throughout the small intestine; the process is aided by the presence of vitamin D, and is under the control of the parathyroid hormone.

Iron is an important component of the diet; any ferric (Fe^{3+}) ions must be converted to ferrous (Fe^{2+}) ions, and this is performed by reducing agents like vitamin C, once the iron has dissolved in the gastric acid. There is active uptake of ferrous iron in the upper jejunum; in the cells it becomes bound to the small protein **apoferritin** to form **ferritin**, which is transported in the plasma attached to the much bigger protein **transferrin**. This is eventually carried to the bone marrow, where the iron is incorporated into haemoglobin.

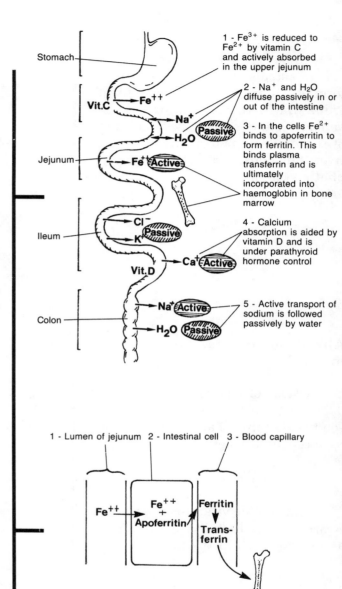

1 - Fe^{3+} is reduced to Fe^{2+} by vitamin C and actively absorbed in the upper jejunum

2 - Na^+ and H_2O diffuse passively in or out of the intestine

3 - In the cells Fe^{2+} binds to apoferritin to form ferritin. This binds plasma transferrin and is ultimately incorporated into haemoglobin in bone marrow

4 - Calcium absorption is aided by vitamin D and is under parathyroid hormone control

5 - Active transport of sodium is followed passively by water

Stomach

Vit.C Fe^{++}

Na^+

Passive

H_2O

Jejunum Fe^{++} Active

Ileum Cl^-
Passive
K^+

Ca^+ Active

Vit.D

Colon Na^+ Active

H_2O Passive

1 - Lumen of jejunum   2 - Intestinal cell   3 - Blood capillary

Fe^{++} Fe^{++} + Apoferritin   Ferritin

Transferrin

4 - Hb of bone marrow utilizes transferrin

MOVEMENTS OF THE DIGESTIVE ORGANS

The organs comprising the alimentary canal have smooth muscle in their walls. One of the most obvious properties of this smooth muscle is its spontaneous, rhythmic contractions; if a piece of gut is removed from an animal and suspended in a bath of physiological saline solution at body temperature, it will exhibit rhythmic contractions and relaxations which can be recorded by attaching a writing level to the end of the piece of gut.

The spontaneous ('**myogenic**') activity will persist even in the presence of neurotoxins, local anaesthetics or ganglion blockers, and is thus an intrinsic property of the muscle itself, not requiring any nervous influence to initiate it. There are 'pacemaker' areas scattered through the muscle layer.

Despite the fact that nerves are not required to **initiate** rhythmic contractions, the activity of smooth muscle is very strongly influenced by autonomic nerves, which can **modify** its behaviour. Even an isolated segment of gut can exhibit reflex activity: if a loop of gut is closed at one end and connected at the other end to a manometer, the sudden distension of the gut segment can initiate a complex sequence of events known as the **peristaltic reflex**.

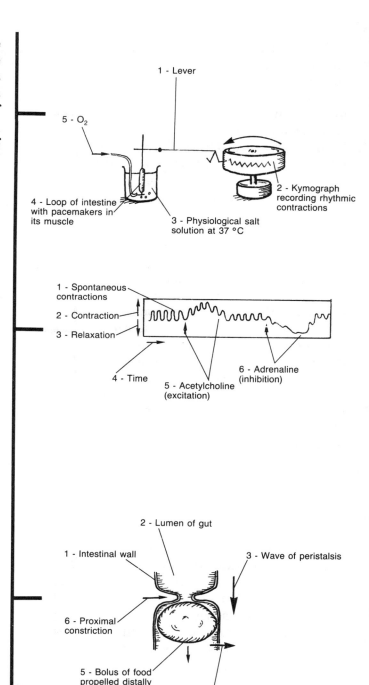

1 - Lever
5 - O_2
4 - Loop of intestine with pacemakers in its muscle
3 - Physiological salt solution at 37 °C
2 - Kymograph recording rhythmic contractions

1 - Spontaneous contractions
2 - Contraction
3 - Relaxation
4 - Time
5 - Acetylcholine (excitation)
6 - Adrenaline (inhibition)

2 - Lumen of gut
1 - Intestinal wall
3 - Wave of peristalsis
6 - Proximal constriction
5 - Bolus of food propelled distally
4 - Distal relaxation

There is, first, contraction of the longitudinal muscle layer, causing shortening of the segment, followed by relaxation of the longitudinal muscle and simultaneous contraction of circular muscle, causing a rise in intraluminal pressure. This reflex depends upon the presence of nerves within the gut wall, and is abolished by nerve blockers and anaesthetics.

The autonomic nerves in the gut wall are arranged as a number of plexuses including Meissner's, Auerbach's and the submucous plexus. The neurones can interact in a complex way, producing stimulation and inhibition of the smooth muscle, without any reference to the central nervous system. The intrinsic nervous plexuses of the gut are known collectively as the **myenteric plexus**.

It is possible to record the electrical activity of individual myenteric plexus neurones in isolated segments of gut; one of the most dramatic findings is that distension of a proximal part of the gut produces inhibitory activity in more distal neurones: this is called 'descending inhibition'.

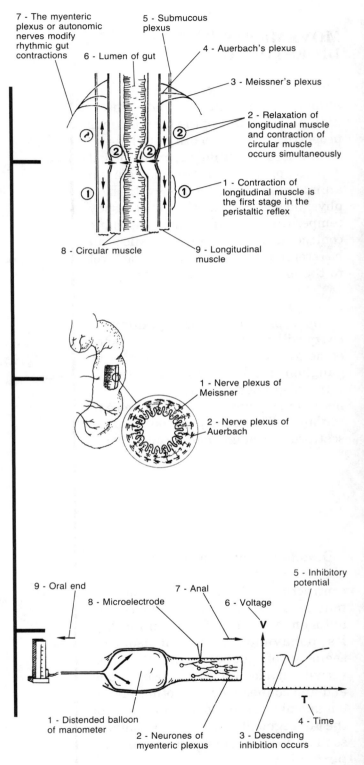

7 - The myenteric plexus or autonomic nerves modify rhythmic gut contractions

5 - Submucous plexus

6 - Lumen of gut

4 - Auerbach's plexus

3 - Meissner's plexus

2 - Relaxation of longitudinal muscle and contraction of circular muscle occurs simultaneously

1 - Contraction of longitudinal muscle is the first stage in the peristaltic reflex

8 - Circular muscle

9 - Longitudinal muscle

1 - Nerve plexus of Meissner

2 - Nerve plexus of Auerbach

9 - Oral end

8 - Microelectrode

7 - Anal

6 - Voltage

5 - Inhibitory potential

V

T

4 - Time

1 - Distended balloon of manometer

2 - Neurones of myenteric plexus

3 - Descending inhibition occurs

Although the myenteric plexus has a certain amount of autonomy, it is subject to influences from the more central parts of the autonomic nervous system. Both the vagus and the sympathetic nerves have extensive branches supplying the gut, and they can modify both the myogenic activity and the intrinsic nervous reflexes. In general, the parasympathetic nerves and their transmitter acetylcholine cause stimulation of gut contractions, while the sympathetic nerves and their transmitters noradrenaline and adrenaline cause inhibition of gut motility.

In the mouth, the main movement is chewing, which is entirely under voluntary control, and serves to break the food into smaller pieces, mixing it with saliva and allowing the food to be tasted. The muscles of the jaws, the cheeks and the tongue are all involved.

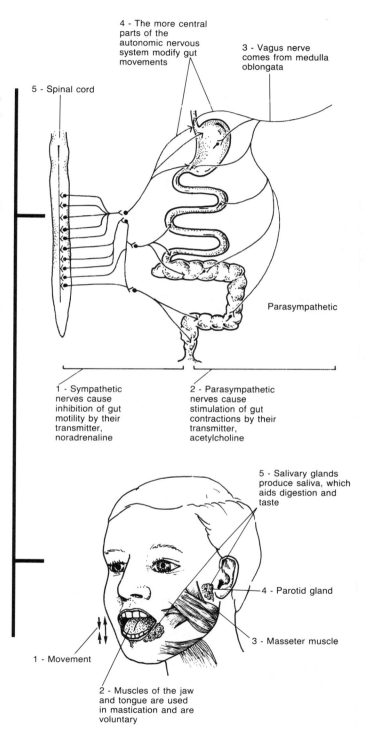

4 - The more central parts of the autonomic nervous system modify gut movements

3 - Vagus nerve comes from medulla oblongata

5 - Spinal cord

Parasympathetic

1 - Sympathetic nerves cause inhibition of gut motility by their transmitter, noradrenaline

2 - Parasympathetic nerves cause stimulation of gut contractions by their transmitter, acetylcholine

5 - Salivary glands produce saliva, which aids digestion and taste

4 - Parotid gland

3 - Masseter muscle

1 - Movement

2 - Muscles of the jaw and tongue are used in mastication and are voluntary

The next phase is **swallowing**, which is initially under voluntary control; the muscles of the cheeks and tongue manipulate the 'bolus' of food into the back of the mouth, and when the bolus makes contact with the posterior wall of the pharynx, the automatic reflex stages of swallowing are initiated.

There is a cessation of respiratory movements and a closure of the glottis so that food is not inhaled into the lungs; the larynx and epiglottis are elevated and the large pharyngeal constrictor muscles begin to contract. All of these muscles are striated voluntary muscles, but their control is entirely automatic.

Next, a peristaltic wave passes down the oesophagus; there is a ring of contraction proximal to the bolus, with relaxation of the muscle distal to the bolus. The wave of relaxation migrates in a distal direction, followed by the ring of contraction, and the net result is propulsion of the bolus towards the stomach.

About one-third of the way down the oesophagus, the striated muscle becomes replaced by smooth muscle, but the control of swallowing and peristalsis is no different. As the bolus reaches the lower end of the oesophagus, the oesophageal sphincter relaxes to permit the food to enter the stomach.

The act of swallowing does not require the help of gravity; it is quite possible to swallow while standing on one's head, and astronauts in space have no difficulty in swallowing.

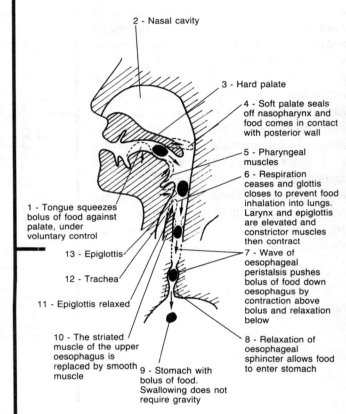

2 - Nasal cavity

3 - Hard palate

4 - Soft palate seals off nasopharynx and food comes in contact with posterior wall

5 - Pharyngeal muscles

6 - Respiration ceases and glottis closes to prevent food inhalation into lungs. Larynx and epiglottis are elevated and constrictor muscles then contract

7 - Wave of oesophageal peristalsis pushes bolus of food down oesophagus by contraction above bolus and relaxation below

8 - Relaxation of oesophageal sphincter allows food to enter stomach

9 - Stomach with bolus of food. Swallowing does not require gravity

10 - The striated muscle of the upper oesophagus is replaced by smooth muscle

11 - Epiglottis relaxed

12 - Trachea

13 - Epiglottis

1 - Tongue squeezes bolus of food against palate, under voluntary control

As food reaches the bottom of the oesophagus, the muscle of the stomach relaxes reflexly in order to receive the food — 'receptive relaxation'. The food in the stomach is usually a semi-solid gruel, which is subjected to a variety of mixing and churning movements by the smooth muscle in the stomach wall, which is arranged in longitudinal, circular and oblique layers.

As well as the weak alternate contractions and relaxations characteristic of almost all gut muscles, the stomach is subject to extremely regular waves of constriction, about three per minute, which start at the fundus and move towards the pylorus, getting stronger as they go. The function of these waves is to 'milk' the food towards the pylorus. The pyloric sphincter is normally open, and only closes when the constriction wave reaches it. At this time some food is forced through the sphincter into the duodenum, but most of it is forced back into the body and fundus of the stomach, producing very thorough mixing.

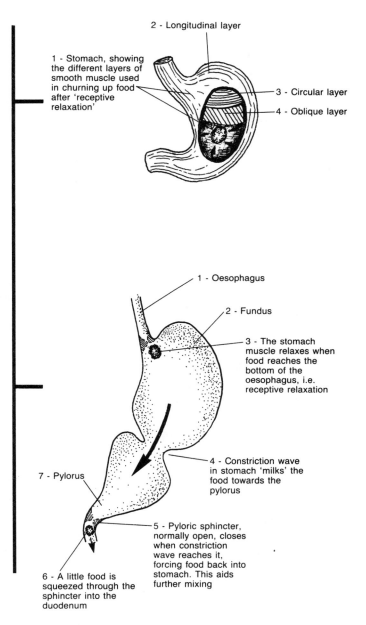

2 - Longitudinal layer

1 - Stomach, showing the different layers of smooth muscle used in churning up food after 'receptive relaxation'

3 - Circular layer

4 - Oblique layer

1 - Oesophagus

2 - Fundus

3 - The stomach muscle relaxes when food reaches the bottom of the oesophagus, i.e. receptive relaxation

4 - Constriction wave in stomach 'milks' the food towards the pylorus

7 - Pylorus

5 - Pyloric sphincter, normally open, closes when constriction wave reaches it, forcing food back into stomach. This aids further mixing

6 - A little food is squeezed through the sphincter into the duodenum

The rate of gastric emptying is regulated by the duodenal hormones secretin and pancreozymin; when food from the stomach enters the duodenum, these hormones not only modify gastric secretion but also reduce gastric motility. Gastric emptying can be studied by giving a test meal and performing serial aspirations of stomach contents through a Ryle's tube, or by giving a test meal containing a radioactive substance, and monitoring the disappearance of radioactivity from the region over the stomach.

Vomiting is an unusual but physiological aspect of gastric function; it is essentially a protective reflex, ridding the body of noxious substances ingested by mouth. There is an **emetic** centre in the brain stem, which can be influenced by a number of trigger factors which include mechanical irritation of the pharynx, and mechanical or chemical irritation of the gastric mucosa. Unpleasant tastes, especially bitter ones, can initiate vomiting, and this is fortunate because many of the poisonous alkaloids found in plants are very bitter. Intense emotions or unpleasant sights, such as open wounds or accidents, and severe pain can induce vomiting. Many drugs can stimulate emesis, either by irritating the stomach or by a central effect on the emetic centre; the most notable are morphine and ethanol. Mechanical obstruction to lower parts of the gut, and in particular to the pylorus, can cause severe vomiting.

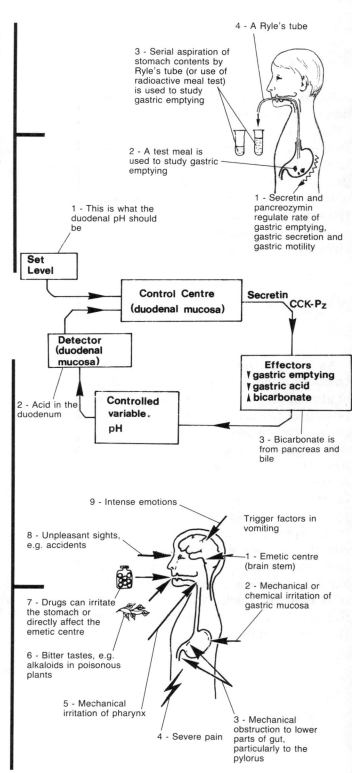

4 - A Ryle's tube

3 - Serial aspiration of stomach contents by Ryle's tube (or use of radioactive meal test) is used to study gastric emptying

2 - A test meal is used to study gastric emptying

1 - Secretin and pancreozymin regulate rate of gastric emptying, gastric secretion and gastric motility

1 - This is what the duodenal pH should be

Set Level

Control Centre (duodenal mucosa)

Secretin CCK-Pz

Detector (duodenal mucosa)

2 - Acid in the duodenum

Controlled variable. pH

Effectors
▼ gastric emptying
▼ gastric acid
▲ bicarbonate

3 - Bicarbonate is from pancreas and bile

9 - Intense emotions

8 - Unpleasant sights, e.g. accidents

Trigger factors in vomiting

1 - Emetic centre (brain stem)

2 - Mechanical or chemical irritation of gastric mucosa

7 - Drugs can irritate the stomach or directly affect the emetic centre

6 - Bitter tastes, e.g. alkaloids in poisonous plants

5 - Mechanical irritation of pharynx

4 - Severe pain

3 - Mechanical obstruction to lower parts of gut, particularly to the pylorus

The process of vomiting is preceded by a feeling of intense nausea, usually accompanied by hyperventilation and salivation. Then there is closure of the glottis and elevation of the soft palate, closure of the pylorus and opening of the oesophagus. The main propulsive effort comes from intense contraction of the abdominal muscles and descent of the diaphragm; this is possibly helped partially by a reverse peristalsis of the gastric muscles. The net result is forcible ejection of the gastric contents.

The **small intestine** undergoes all of the types of activity mentioned earlier; as well as peristaltic movements which propel the food onwards there are pendular shortening and lengthening movements which produce little propulsion but good mixing. There are **segmentation** movements, in which the semi-solid food in a section of intestine is subjected to repeated pinching at alternate sites along its length; these movements also produce good mixing.

There are also slow electrical waves in the smooth muscle and nerves (the **migratory myoelectrical complex**) which migrate from the duodenum towards the caecum, gradually decelerating from 12 per minute in the duodenum to nine per minute in the ileum. These electrical waves are associated with changes in the tone of the smooth muscle.

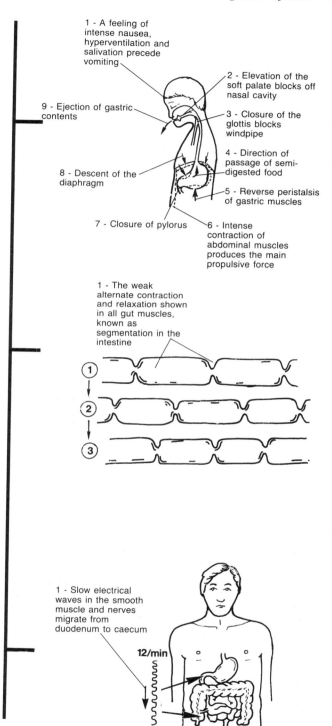

1 - A feeling of intense nausea, hyperventilation and salivation precede vomiting

2 - Elevation of the soft palate blocks off nasal cavity

9 - Ejection of gastric contents

3 - Closure of the glottis blocks windpipe

4 - Direction of passage of semi-digested food

8 - Descent of the diaphragm

5 - Reverse peristalsis of gastric muscles

7 - Closure of pylorus

6 - Intense contraction of abdominal muscles produces the main propulsive force

1 - The weak alternate contraction and relaxation shown in all gut muscles, known as segmentation in the intestine

1 - Slow electrical waves in the smooth muscle and nerves migrate from duodenum to caecum

12/min

9/min

The junction of the small and large intestines has a valve — the ileocaecal valve — which is usually closed but opens when a paristaltic wave reaches it, allowing small intestinal contents to enter the colon. There is also a vagally mediated gastro-ileal reflex in which food entering the stomach provokes opening of the ileocaecal valve.

The **colon** has its longitudinal smooth muscle arranged as three ribbon-like bands, the **taeniae coli**. The circular smooth muscle undergoes localized contractions, dimpling the semi-solid contents and producing the appearance of **haustra**.

The colon has mixing and propulsive contractile activity very like the small intestine, but this activity is much less effective than in the small intestine, as the colonic contents are much more solid. There are colonic slow waves which have a frequency of two per minute at the caecum but build up to six per minute at the sigmoid colon. The colon also undergoes mass contractions of its muscles about three times per day; these contractions are unrelated to the times of defaecation, but serve to move the faeces along the colon. All of these movements require the presence of the myenteric plexus.

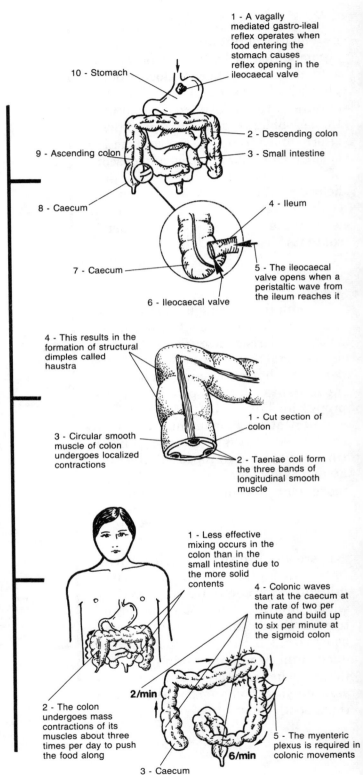

10 - Stomach

1 - A vagally mediated gastro-ileal reflex operates when food entering the stomach causes reflex opening in the ileocaecal valve

2 - Descending colon

9 - Ascending colon

3 - Small intestine

8 - Caecum

4 - Ileum

7 - Caecum

5 - The ileocaecal valve opens when a peristaltic wave from the ileum reaches it

6 - Ileocaecal valve

4 - This results in the formation of structural dimples called haustra

1 - Cut section of colon

3 - Circular smooth muscle of colon undergoes localized contractions

2 - Taeniae coli form the three bands of longitudinal smooth muscle

1 - Less effective mixing occurs in the colon than in the small intestine due to the more solid contents

4 - Colonic waves start at the caecum at the rate of two per minute and build up to six per minute at the sigmoid colon

2/min

2 - The colon undergoes mass contractions of its muscles about three times per day to push the food along

5 - The myenteric plexus is required in colonic movements

6/min

3 - Caecum

Defaecation is a spinal reflex involving both autonomic and somatic components. The rectum is normally empty, but when faecal material distends the rectum there is a reflex contraction of the whole muscle mass of the colon, together with a contraction of the muscles of the abdominal wall and a relaxation of the anal sphincter, with resultant expulsion of faeces through the anus. This very powerful reflex can be inhibited by voluntary control, so that defaecation can be delayed until a more socially convenient time.

The entry of food into the stomach initiates the **gastrocolic** reflex, causing contraction of the colon; this often leads to the entry of faeces into the rectum, and explains why many people defaecate after breakfast as a matter of habit.

The frequency of defaecation varies widely; while one bowel motion per day is the norm, the individual comes to no harm from a considerably lower or higher frequency. It is usually incorrect to think of 'poisons building up in the system' if one fails to visit the lavatory for a bowel motion every day, although a **change** in one's normal bowel habit may signify the presence of disease.

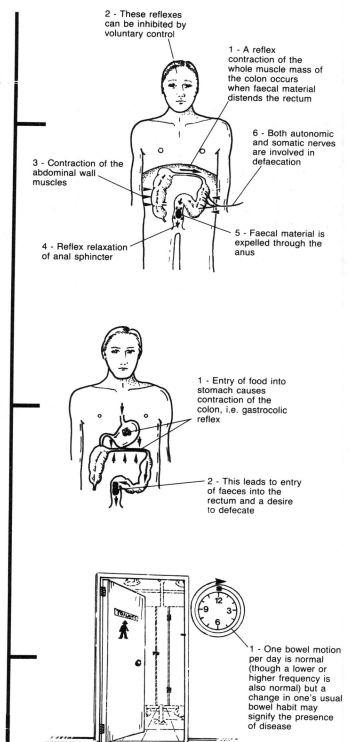

2 - These reflexes can be inhibited by voluntary control

1 - A reflex contraction of the whole muscle mass of the colon occurs when faecal material distends the rectum

6 - Both autonomic and somatic nerves are involved in defaecation

3 - Contraction of the abdominal wall muscles

5 - Faecal material is expelled through the anus

4 - Reflex relaxation of anal sphincter

1 - Entry of food into stomach causes contraction of the colon, i.e. gastrocolic reflex

2 - This leads to entry of faeces into the rectum and a desire to defecate

1 - One bowel motion per day is normal (though a lower or higher frequency is also normal) but a change in one's usual bowel habit may signify the presence of disease

The stomach, small intestine and colon contain quantities of gas, the movement of which can often be heard as 'borborygmi' by one's companions and which can easily be detected by a stethoscope on the abdominal wall. Most of the gas is atmospheric air which has been swallowed during eating or speech, but some of it is produced by bacteria in the colon which make methane and hydrogen sulphide, which is largely responsible for its repellent smell.

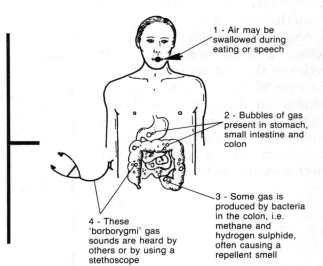

1 - Air may be swallowed during eating or speech

2 - Bubbles of gas present in stomach, small intestine and colon

3 - Some gas is produced by bacteria in the colon, i.e. methane and hydrogen sulphide, often causing a repellent smell

4 - These 'borborygmi' gas sounds are heard by others or by using a stethoscope

The Kidney and Urinary System

The kidneys modify and regulate the composition of the blood, and eliminate several of the waste products of metabolism. Almost a quarter of the cardiac output flows through the kidneys, which together weigh about 200 g; this blood flow is far in excess of the kidneys' own metabolic needs, and reflects the importance of the functions these organs perform in the homeostasis of plasma composition.

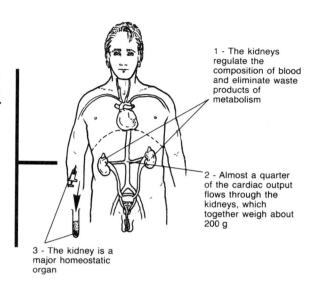

1 - The kidneys regulate the composition of blood and eliminate waste products of metabolism

2 - Almost a quarter of the cardiac output flows through the kidneys, which together weigh about 200 g

3 - The kidney is a major homeostatic organ

ANATOMICAL AND FUNCTIONAL OVERVIEW

Each kidney has a fibrous **capsule**, a compact and vascular **cortex**, and a **medulla** which on a cut surface of the kidney appears radially striped (the medullary rays). The medulla is arranged as a series of peg-like **pyramids** projecting into a cavity called the **pelvis** of the kidney, which is continuous with the **ureter**, a tube that drains the urine away into the **bladder**.

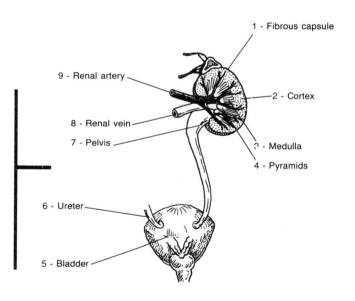

1 - Fibrous capsule

9 - Renal artery

2 - Cortex

8 - Renal vein

7 - Pelvis

3 - Medulla

4 - Pyramids

6 - Ureter

5 - Bladder

Posterior view of the kidney and bladder

The fundamental structural element of the kidney is the **nephron**, of which there are several million almost identical units in parallel. Each nephron is derived from a simple straight tube, whose component parts become progressively more convoluted and looped during development, while still retaining their proximity to one another. The blood vessels of each nephron develop in parallel with it, retaining their intimate relationship to the various constituent parts.

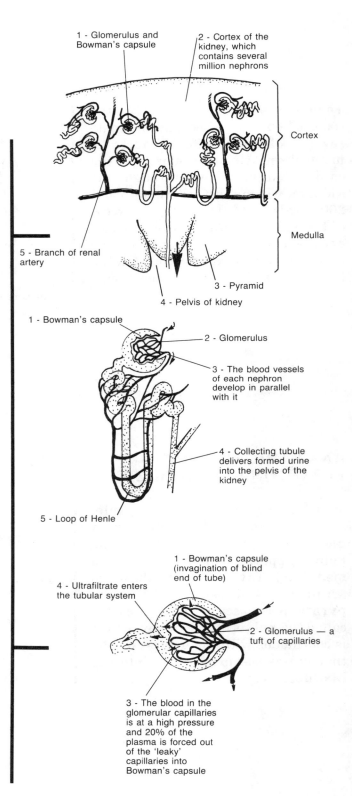

1 - Glomerulus and Bowman's capsule

2 - Cortex of the kidney, which contains several million nephrons

Cortex

Medulla

5 - Branch of renal artery

3 - Pyramid

4 - Pelvis of kidney

1 - Bowman's capsule

2 - Glomerulus

3 - The blood vessels of each nephron develop in parallel with it

4 - Collecting tubule delivers formed urine into the pelvis of the kidney

5 - Loop of Henle

1 - Bowman's capsule (invagination of blind end of tube)

4 - Ultrafiltrate enters the tubular system

2 - Glomerulus — a tuft of capillaries

3 - The blood in the glomerular capillaries is at a high pressure and 20% of the plasma is forced out of the 'leaky' capillaries into Bowman's capsule

The first part of the nephron is **Bowman's capsule**, an invagination of the blind end of the tube into which protrudes the **glomerulus**, a highly branching and recombining tuft of capillaries. The blood in the glomerular capillaries is at a much higher pressure than in most systemic capillaries, and a proportion of the plasma (about 20%) is forced out of the capillaries and into Bowman's capsule through the rather leaky walls of the blood vessels. This is a process of high-pressure filtration, and the **ultrafiltrate** so formed enters the tubular system.

The glomerular filtration rate of an average adult male is about 125 ml/min, or about one-tenth of the blood flowing through the kidneys; this amounts to about 180 litres per day. If there were no reabsorption by the kidney tubules, the body would very rapidly become depleted of all its fluid!

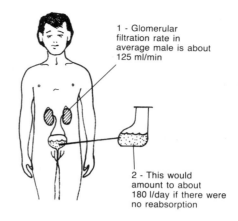

1 - Glomerular filtration rate in average male is about 125 ml/min

2 - This would amount to about 180 l/day if there were no reabsorption

The next part of the nephron is the **proximal convoluted tubule**, where about 75% of the material in the filtrate is reabsorbed into the blood, and some substances are actively secreted into the tubular fluid. The proximal tubule performs a relatively crude 'bulk transport' function.

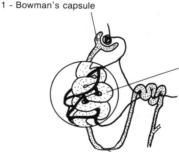

1 - Bowman's capsule

2 - Proximal convoluted tubule, where approximately 75% of the material in the filtrate is reabsorbed into the blood, but also where substances are secreted into the tubular fluid

3 - Loop of Henle

The final fine regulation of what is excreted is provided by the **distal convoluted tubule**, which adjusts its rate of reabsorption or secretion according to the body's requirements: it is a powerful agent for controlling the composition of plasma.

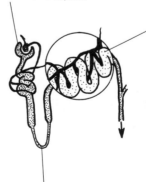

1 - Bowman's capsule

2 - Distal convoluted tubule, which adjusts its rate of reabsorption or secretion according to the body's requirements. It powerfully adjusts plasma composition

3 - Loop of Henle

The epithelial cells lining the renal tubules are structurally adapted for transport and exchange. The cells of the proximal tubule have an extensive **brush border** on their luminal surface, which greatly increases the area in contact with the tubular fluid; at the surface furthest away from the lumen there are numerous **basal channels** which increase the surface area in this region.

There are large numbers of mitochondria in the basal region of these cells, providing energy for the active transport which is occurring. The individual epithelial cells are separated by deep **intercellular clefts**, but have regions of contact at the **tight junctions** which bridge the gaps near the luminal surface and maintain the continuity of the epithelium as a sheet of cells.

The cells of the distal tubule have a rather similar structure, but they lack the brush border.

Between the proximal and distal tubules is the **loop of Henle**, which extends deep into the medulla of the kidney and then returns to the cortex close to the proximal tubule of the same nephron. Its function is to create a concentration gradient within the renal medulla, so that when the urine finally passes down the collecting duct its osmotic composition can be modified by passage through these areas of altered osmolality.

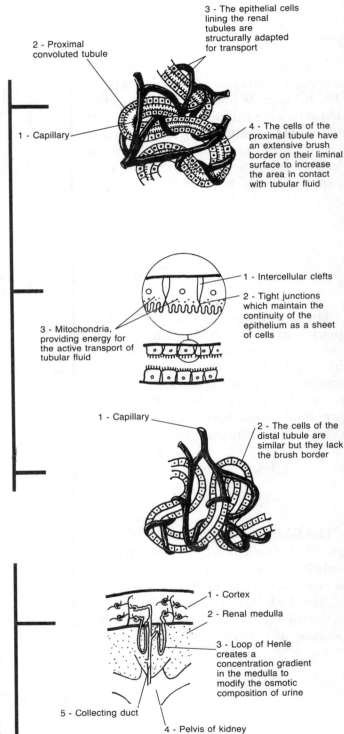

2 - Proximal convoluted tubule

3 - The epithelial cells lining the renal tubules are structurally adapted for transport

1 - Capillary

4 - The cells of the proximal tubule have an extensive brush border on their liminal surface to increase the area in contact with tubular fluid

3 - Mitochondria, providing energy for the active transport of tubular fluid

1 - Intercellular clefts

2 - Tight junctions which maintain the continuity of the epithelium as a sheet of cells

1 - Capillary

2 - The cells of the distal tubule are similar but they lack the brush border

1 - Cortex

2 - Renal medulla

3 - Loop of Henle creates a concentration gradient in the medulla to modify the osmotic composition of urine

5 - Collecting duct

4 - Pelvis of kidney

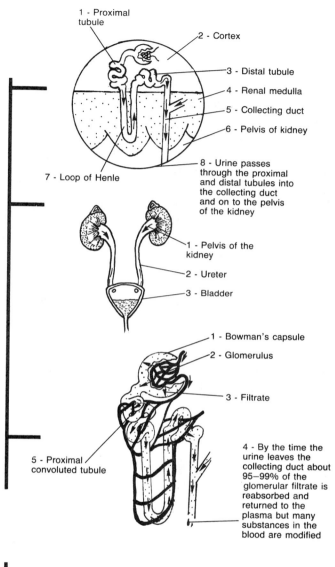

1 - Proximal tubule

2 - Cortex

3 - Distal tubule

4 - Renal medulla

5 - Collecting duct

6 - Pelvis of kidney

7 - Loop of Henle

8 - Urine passes through the proximal and distal tubules into the collecting duct and on to the pelvis of the kidney

1 - Pelvis of the kidney

2 - Ureter

3 - Bladder

1 - Bowman's capsule

2 - Glomerulus

3 - Filtrate

5 - Proximal convoluted tubule

4 - By the time the urine leaves the collecting duct about 95—99% of the glomerular filtrate is reabsorbed and returned to the plasma but many substances in the blood are modified

After passage through the proximal tubule, the loop of Henle and the distal convoluted tubule, the urine flows into the **collecting duct** which passes through the renal medulla to drain into the pelvis of the kidney. This is connected to the ureter — the tube that conveys urine to the bladder.

By the time the urine leaves the collecting duct, about 95—99% of the material filtered in the glomerulus has been reabsorbed and returned to the plasma, but the concentrations of many substances in the blood have been substantially modified and controlled.

GLOMERULAR FILTRATION

The blood vessels supplying the kidney are arranged in a unique fashion. The capillaries of the glomerulus are supplied by **afferent** arterioles, and are drained by another set of arterioles, the **efferent** arterioles. The blood then flows through another set of capillaries, supplying either the proximal or distal convoluted tubules or the loop of Henle (the **vasa recta**) before returning via conventional venules and veins to the renal vein.

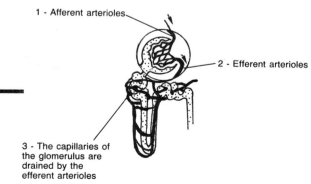

1 - Afferent arterioles

2 - Efferent arterioles

3 - The capillaries of the glomerulus are drained by the efferent arterioles

The presence of two sets of arterioles means that the blood in the glomerular capillaries is at a higher pressure than the blood in most systemic capillaries, and the outward hydrostatic force on the fluid is correspondingly greater. This is the driving force producing **glomerular filtration**, and the filtration pressure is a function of the smooth muscle tone in the afferent and efferent arterioles.

If the afferents are relaxed and the efferents constricted, then there is a high filtration pressure.

If the afferents constrict and the efferents dilate then the filtration pressure is low.

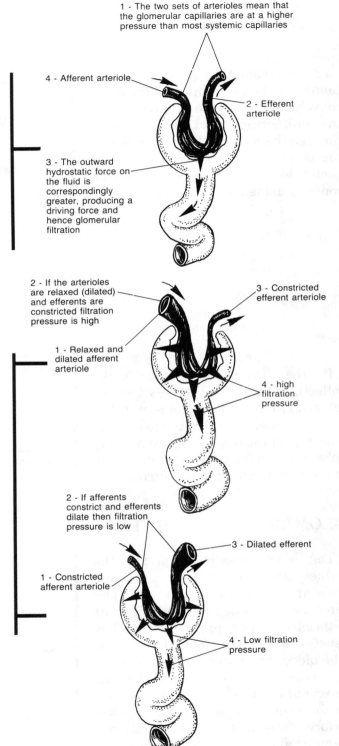

1 - The two sets of arterioles mean that the glomerular capillaries are at a higher pressure than most systemic capillaries

4 - Afferent arteriole

2 - Efferent arteriole

3 - The outward hydrostatic force on the fluid is correspondingly greater, producing a driving force and hence glomerular filtration

2 - If the arterioles are relaxed (dilated) and efferents are constricted filtration pressure is high

3 - Constricted efferent arteriole

1 - Relaxed and dilated afferent arteriole

4 - high filtration pressure

2 - If afferents constrict and efferents dilate then filtration pressure is low

3 - Dilated efferent

1 - Constricted afferent arteriole

4 - Low filtration pressure

The hydrostatic pressure in the capillaries (about 50 mmHg) is opposed by the intracapsular or tissue pressure in the kidney (about 10 mmHg), giving a net filtration pressure of 40 mmHg. The proteins are retained in the capillaries, so the colloid osmotic pressure rises to around 30 mmHg, producing an inward attractive force for fluid and leaving a net pressure of 10 mmHg to force fluid through the filtration barrier of the glomerulus.

1 - The intracapsular pressure (or tissue pressure in kidney) is about 10 mmHg

2 - Capillary hydrostatic pressure is about 50 mmHg, so net filtration pressure is about 40 mmHg

3 - Proteins are retained in capillaries, producing a colloidal osmotic pressure of about 30 mmHg

4 - Net outward driving force is:

50 mmHg (capillary hydrostatic pressure)
−10 mmHg (renal tissue pressure)
−30 mmHg (colloid osmotic pressure)
_____
= 10 mmHg

The endothelial cells of the glomerular capillaries are fenestrated ('windowed'), i.e. they are perforated by large numbers of holes. The cells which form the lining of Bowman's capsule are also extensively perforated; they are called **podocytes** because they have many foot-like processes which are placed against the capillary wall, and there are holes passing completely through the podocytes between the foot-processes.

1 - The endothelial cells of the glomerular capillaries are fenestrated ('windowed'), i.e. they are perforated by large numbers of holes

2 - Basement membrane

3 - The cells which form the lining of Bowman's capsule are perforated; they are called podocytes

Thus neither the capillary endothelium nor the lining cells of Bowman's capsule constitute an effective barrier to the diffusion of large molecules, though the formed elements of the blood are retained within the vessels by the endothelium.

4 - Large molecules

1 - Neither the capillary endothelium nor the lining cells of the Bowman's capsule constitute an effective barrier to the diffusion of large molecules

2 - Basement membrane

3 - The formed elements of the blood are retained within the vessels by the endothelium

The true barrier to diffusion is the rather amorphous layer of **basement membrane** between the endothelial cells and the podocytes. This layer acts as if it had holes of diameter 7–10 nm, and allows all the crystalloids dissolved in the blood to pass into the filtrate, but excludes the colloids like albumin and globulin.

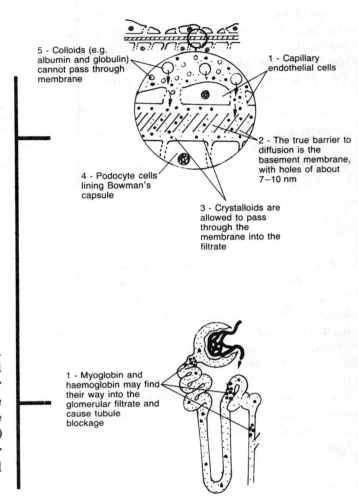

5 - Colloids (e.g. albumin and globulin) cannot pass through membrane

1 - Capillary endothelial cells

2 - The true barrier to diffusion is the basement membrane, with holes of about 7–10 nm

4 - Podocyte cells lining Bowman's capsule

3 - Crystalloids are allowed to pass through the membrane into the filtrate

Smaller proteins like myoglobin (which can be present in the blood following severe trauma to muscle) or even haemoglobin (if it is free in the plasma, having been released from the red cells during haemolytic processes) may find their way into the glomerular filtrate and cause blockage of the renal tubules.

1 - Myoglobin and haemoglobin may find their way into the glomerular filtrate and cause tubule blockage

PRINCIPLES OF RENAL FUNCTION MEASUREMENT

The concept of **clearance** is fundamental to much of renal physiology. If a substance is excreted in the urine, then the amount appearing in the urine depends on both the concentration in the plasma and the rate of secretion or absorption by the kidney tubules. If a substance is present in the plasma in small concentrations and yet appears in large quantities in the urine, it is obviously being treated differently from a substance which is present in high concentrations in both plasma and urine.

It is not very useful simply to describe the concentration of a substance in the urine; the water content of urine is controlled independently of most other components, so the simple concentrations of these other constituents may not reflect the rate of excretion.

The absolute amount appearing in the urine (i.e. the concentration multiplied by the volume of urine) may give a better indication, though it says nothing about the gradient between plasma concentration and the amount in the urine. One of the best indicators, which takes into account plasma levels and the amount in the urine, is the **clearance**.

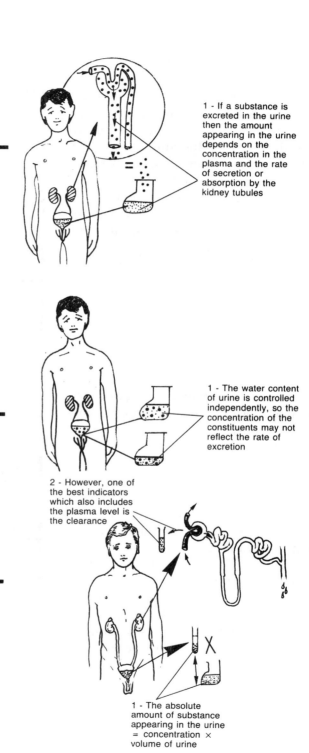

1 - If a substance is excreted in the urine then the amount appearing in the urine depends on the concentration in the plasma and the rate of secretion or absorption by the kidney tubules

1 - The water content of urine is controlled independently, so the concentration of the constituents may not reflect the rate of excretion

2 - However, one of the best indicators which also includes the plasma level is the clearance

1 - The absolute amount of substance appearing in the urine = concentration × volume of urine

Rather than trying to say that 25% of the substance present in plasma is excreted in the urine, it has become usual to talk of the volume of plasma that would be **completely** cleared of that substance. This is, of course, a purely artificial notion, as very few substances are completely eliminated from the plasma, but it is a useful concept for understanding how the kidney handles various types of substance.

Suppose the blood flow through a kidney were 1 litre per minute; suppose the concentration of a substance in the blood were 100 g per litre, and 25 g of this substance were excreted in the urine each minute. One way of expressing this would be to say that the plasma had one-quarter of the substance removed by the kidney; another way would be to say that one-quarter of the blood flowing through the kidney was completely cleared of the substance, or the clearance was 0.25 litres per minute. (These values are merely examples for illustration, and do not necessarily correspond to any values normally found in the real kidney.)

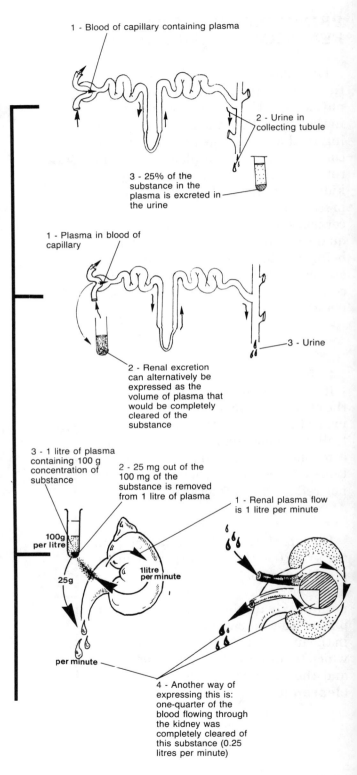

1 - Blood of capillary containing plasma

2 - Urine in collecting tubule

3 - 25% of the substance in the plasma is excreted in the urine

1 - Plasma in blood of capillary

3 - Urine

2 - Renal excretion can alternatively be expressed as the volume of plasma that would be completely cleared of the substance

3 - 1 litre of plasma containing 100 g concentration of substance

2 - 25 mg out of the 100 mg of the substance is removed from 1 litre of plasma

1 - Renal plasma flow is 1 litre per minute

100g per litre

25g

1 litre per minute

per minute

4 - Another way of expressing this is: one-quarter of the blood flowing through the kidney was completely cleared of this substance (0.25 litres per minute)

Clearance is always expressed in units of volume flow per minute (or hour). It is calculated as

$$\frac{U \times V}{P}$$

where U is the concentration in the urine, V is the volume flow of urine, and P is the concentration in plasma.

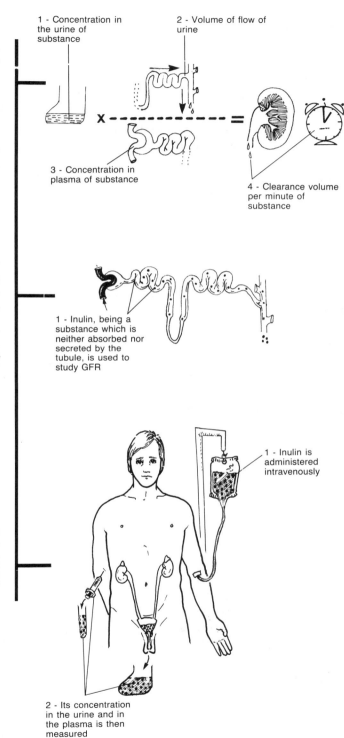

1 - Concentration in the urine of substance

2 - Volume of flow of urine

3 - Concentration in plasma of substance

4 - Clearance volume per minute of substance

The **glomerular filtration rate (GFR)** is exactly equal to the clearance of any substance which is filtered by the kidney, but is neither secreted nor reabsorbed by the tubules. One such substance is inulin (previously encountered as an impermeant marker of extracellular space).

1 - Inulin, being a substance which is neither absorbed nor secreted by the tubule, is used to study GFR

In order to measure clearance inulin is infused intravenously until a steady plasma concentration is reached, and then its concentrations in plasma and urine are measured.

1 - Inulin is administered intravenously

2 - Its concentration in the urine and in the plasma is then measured

Another substance which is widely used for estimating glomerular filtration rate, though it does not strictly meet these criteria, is creatinine. It is both secreted and absorbed by the tubules, but the rates of secretion and absorption are almost exactly equal, so it behaves as if it were a purely filtered substance. The advantage of using creatinine is that it is a completely natural endogenous substance, requiring no infusion or injection.

1 - The rates of secretion and absorption of creatinine are almost equal, so it behaves as a completely filtered substance and may be used instead of inulin

Creatinine clearance is best calculated by collecting the urine for 24 hours and measuring the total volume and the concentration of creatinine; a representative blood sample is taken at some time during the day, and then U, V and P are all known and can be inserted into the clearance equation, referred to earlier.

1 - Creatinine clearance is best calculated by collecting the volume of urine for 24 hours

2 - A representative blood sample is taken during the day

If the clearance measured for a particular substance (which is filtered) is less than the GFR, this means that the substance is actively reabsorbed; if clearance is greater than GFR then the substance is being actively secreted.

1 - When the clearance is less than the GFR the substance is actively reabsorbed

2 - When clearance is greater than GFR the substance is being actively secreted

Renal blood flow can be measured using the Fick principle. It could be calculated from measurements on *any* substance which appears in the urine, by dividing the rate of appearance of that substance in the urine by the arteriovenous difference.

However, to avoid having to make separate measurements of arterial and venous concentrations, which would involve cannulating the renal artery and vein, it is convenient to use a substance which is totally excreted by the kidney, so that none of it appears in the renal venous blood (the venous concentration is zero).

Then the arteriovenous difference is equal to the concentration in the arteries, or in fact in any sample of peripheral blood, even from a capillary or vein.

Para-aminohippuric acid (PAH) is such a substance, excreted totally by the kidney (provided the plasma concentration is not too high), and having the advantages of being inert and non-toxic. The renal clearance of PAH is exactly equal to the renal plasma flow, and represents the maximum value that clearance could possibly take.

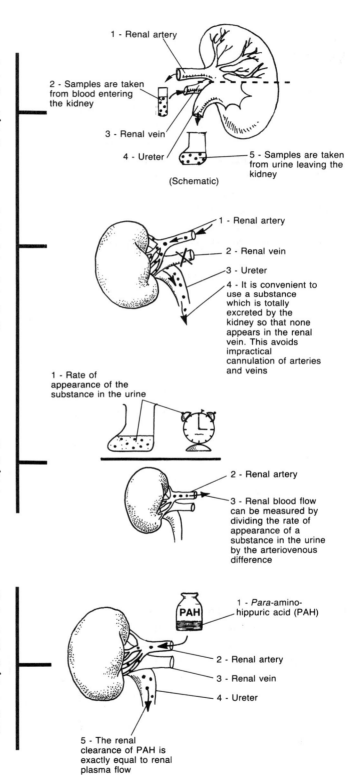

1 - Renal artery

2 - Samples are taken from blood entering the kidney

3 - Renal vein

4 - Ureter

5 - Samples are taken from urine leaving the kidney

(Schematic)

1 - Renal artery

2 - Renal vein

3 - Ureter

4 - It is convenient to use a substance which is totally excreted by the kidney so that none appears in the renal vein. This avoids impractical cannulation of arteries and veins

1 - Rate of appearance of the substance in the urine

2 - Renal artery

3 - Renal blood flow can be measured by dividing the rate of appearance of a substance in the urine by the arteriovenous difference

1 - *Para*-amino-hippuric acid (PAH)

2 - Renal artery

3 - Renal vein

4 - Ureter

5 - The renal clearance of PAH is exactly equal to renal plasma flow

TUBULAR SECRETION AND ABSORPTION

Many of the substances handled by the proximal and distal convoluted tubules are actively transported. There are two main classes of active transport: in the first, all of the substrate presented to the mechanism is transported, until a maximum amount is reached and the mechanism is saturated; in the second, the rate of transport is adaptive, depending on the concentration gradient present and the time available for transport.

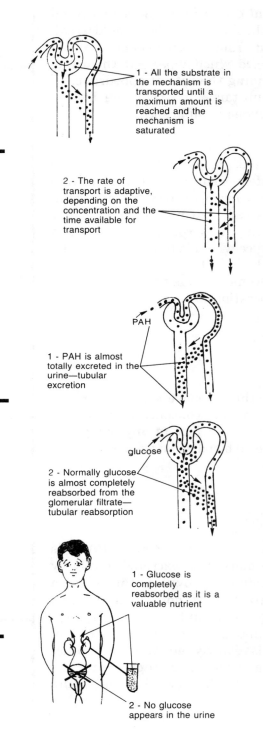

1 - All the substrate in the mechanism is transported until a maximum amount is reached and the mechanism is saturated

2 - The rate of transport is adaptive, depending on the concentration and the time available for transport

The first type of transport is called **transport maximum (T_m) limited** (sometimes tubular maximum, sometimes transfer maximum), and is the method by which PAH is secreted into the urine; it is also the way in which glucose is reabsorbed from the glomerular filtrate.

PAH

1 - PAH is almost totally excreted in the urine—tubular excretion

glucose

2 - Normally glucose is almost completely reabsorbed from the glomerular filtrate—tubular reabsorption

Glucose is a valuable nutrient, well worth conserving in the body, and normally all of the glucose present in the glomerular filtrate is reabsorbed during the passage along the proximal convoluted tubule; none appears in the urine, and the clearance of glucose is zero. As well as glucose, other sugars like galactose and xylose are reabsorbed by a common carrier.

1 - Glucose is completely reabsorbed as it is a valuable nutrient

2 - No glucose appears in the urine

If glucose is present in the plasma in excessive amounts, and hence appears in higher than normal amounts in the filtrate, then a certain fixed amount gets reabsorbed, and the rest appears in the urine. The amount appearing in the urine is less than the plasma concentration, but is proportional to the amount by which the concentration exceeds the 'renal threshold'.

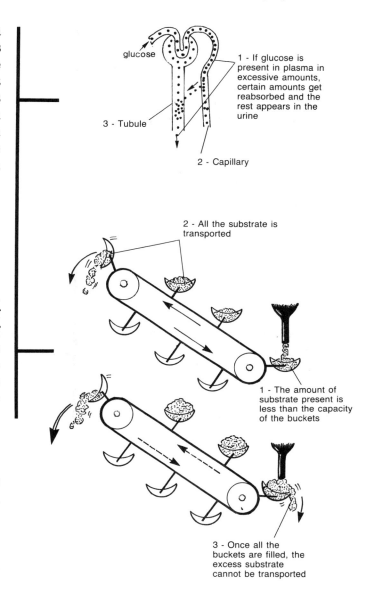

glucose

1 - If glucose is present in plasma in excessive amounts, certain amounts get reabsorbed and the rest appears in the urine

3 - Tubule

2 - Capillary

2 - All the substrate is transported

1 - The amount of substrate present is less than the capacity of the buckets

3 - Once all the buckets are filled, the excess substrate cannot be transported

We can draw an analogy with a conveyor belt having a fixed number of buckets; so long as the amount of substrate presented is less than the capacity of the buckets, all of the substrate is transported. Once all of the buckets are filled, the excess substrate cannot be transported.

Glucose in the urine (**glycosuria**) occurs in diabetic patients who have a high plasma concentration of glucose, and hence a high concentration in the glomerular filtrate, saturating the transport system. It can also occur in normal women during pregnancy when the renal threshold becomes lowered for reasons which are not understood.

The amino acids are also absorbed by T_m-limited carriers; there are at least three different carriers for different classes of amino acids. Other substances reabsorbed by T_m-limited mechanisms include sulphate, phosphate and various organic anions such as citrate and lactate. The way in which phosphate reabsorption is regulated is described in the chapter on the endocrine system.

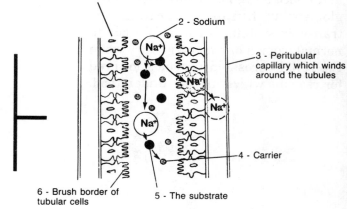

1 - Amino acids
Sulphate
Phosphate
Lactate
Citrate
} Organic anions

It is likely that the carriers for glucose and amino acids in the kidney are similar to or identical to the carriers for these molecules present in the small intestine, and are described in the chapter on the digestive system.

2 - The carriers for glucose in the kidney are perhaps identical to those found in the small intestine

1 - Glucose molecule

3 - Small intestine

These mechanisms involve the formation of a ternary complex between the carrier, the substrate and the sodium ion, and it is the concentration gradient for sodium which provides the driving force to move the complex across the cell membrane.

1 - Proximal tubule
2 - Sodium
3 - Peritubular capillary which winds around the tubules
4 - Carrier
5 - The substrate
6 - Brush border of tubular cells

T_m-limited carriers are also responsible for the active **secretion** of a number of important substances, including many organic acids and bases, and the various glucuronides produced by the liver in the process of detoxication. The type of substance most likely to be actively excreted is the lipid-soluble non-ionized molecule which easily crosses cell membranes.

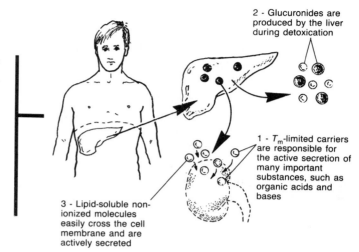

2 - Glucuronides are produced by the liver during detoxication

1 - T_m-limited carriers are responsible for the active secretion of many important substances, such as organic acids and bases

3 - Lipid-soluble non-ionized molecules easily cross the cell membrane and are actively secreted

Another important substance which is actively secreted is the antibiotic penicillin, and its excretion by the kidney is so successful that it is difficult to maintain high therapeutic concentrations in the plasma.

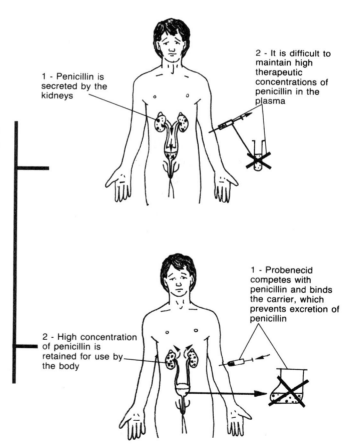

1 - Penicillin is secreted by the kidneys

2 - It is difficult to maintain high therapeutic concentrations of penicillin in the plasma

It is thus often found necessary to administer another drug such as probenecid, which binds strongly to the same carrier and competitively prevents the excretion of penicillin.

1 - Probenecid competes with penicillin and binds the carrier, which prevents excretion of penicillin

2 - High concentration of penicillin is retained for use by the body

The second adaptive transport mechanism is referred to as **gradient-time limited** transport, and the best example of this is the transport of sodium, though it also applies to calcium, magnesium and other cations. The rate of sodium transport depends upon the amount of the ion presented to the tubular cells, and the higher the concentration the more the transport mechanism is stimulated.

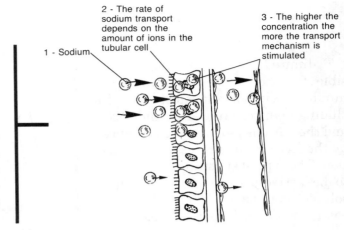

1 - Sodium

2 - The rate of sodium transport depends on the amount of ions in the tubular cell

3 - The higher the concentration the more the transport mechanism is stimulated

The rate also depends on the length of time for which the substrate is in contact with the tubular membrane, so if there is a high rate of urine flow due to a high glomerular filtration rate then there is less time available for sodium to be transported.

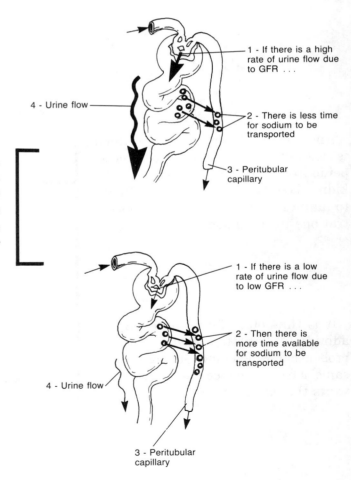

1 - If there is a high rate of urine flow due to GFR . . .

4 - Urine flow

2 - There is less time for sodium to be transported

3 - Peritubular capillary

1 - If there is a low rate of urine flow due to low GFR . . .

2 - Then there is more time available for sodium to be transported

4 - Urine flow

3 - Peritubular capillary

With this type of transport, an almost constant **proportion** of the substrate is transported no matter what the concentration in the filtrate. The proximal convoluted tubule reabsorbs about 75% of the filtered sodium, whatever the concentration. The fine adjustment of sodium levels occurs in the distal tubule where the transport mechanism is different, and the fraction of the remainder which gets reabsorbed is determined by the concentrations of various hormones in the blood.

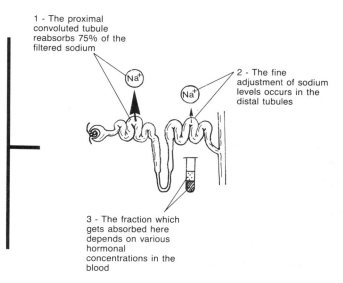

1 - The proximal convoluted tubule reabsorbs 75% of the filtered sodium

2 - The fine adjustment of sodium levels occurs in the distal tubules

3 - The fraction which gets absorbed here depends on various hormonal concentrations in the blood

There are three distinct mechanisms of sodium transport available in the kidney tubule. The first is the Na–K pump previously described in the chapter on the nervous system and present on the membranes of almost all cells, including the red blood cells; it is also present in the kidney tubule, but operates at the surface of the cell furthest from the lumen, closest to the renal capillary. Sodium is transported out of the cell into the blood, in exchange for potassium ions which are imported into the cell from the blood. This mechanism is not quantitatively the most important but is useful for establishing the normal trans-membrane ionic gradients.

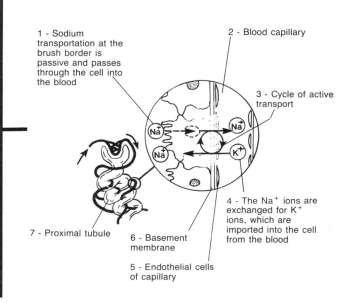

1 - Sodium transportation at the brush border is passive and passes through the cell into the blood

2 - Blood capillary

3 - Cycle of active transport

4 - The Na^+ ions are exchanged for K^+ ions, which are imported into the cell from the blood

5 - Endothelial cells of capillary

6 - Basement membrane

7 - Proximal tubule

The second mechanism, the most important in quantitative terms, is the active transport of sodium out of the tubular cell into the intercellular cleft at the lateral surface of the cells. As sodium ions are pumped out, they are followed by an equal number of chloride ions (to balance the positive charges) and an osmotically appropriate quantity of water. This encourages the passive entry of sodium, chloride and water into the cell from the fluid in the tubular lumen, down a concentration gradient. The accumulation of fluid in the intercellular clefts increases the hydrostatic pressure, and water, sodium and chloride move into the peritubular fluid and thence into the capillaries.

2 - They are followed by an osmotically appropriate quantity of water and chloride ions

1 - As sodium ions are pumped out of the tubular cell into the intercellular cleft

Na^+ + H_2O +

3 - The accumulation of fluid in the intercellular cleft increases the hydrostatic pressure

5 - This encourages the passive entry of sodium, chloride and water into the cell

4 - Sodium and chloride then move into the peritubular fluid and then into the capillaries

The third mechanism for sodium and potassium transport is the one found predominantly in the distal tubule. It is a linked sodium–potassium exchange, but more sodium than potassium is transported.

1 - More sodium than potassium is transported

5 - Lumen of tubule

Na^+
Na^+
Na^+
K^+

2 - Peritubular capillary

3 - Sodium and potassium transport is found predominantly in the distal tubule

4 - Distal tubule of the kidney

The rate of sodium reabsorption by this mechanism is controlled (increased) by the hormone **aldosterone**, secreted by the adrenal cortex; the hormone also promotes the excretion of potassium.

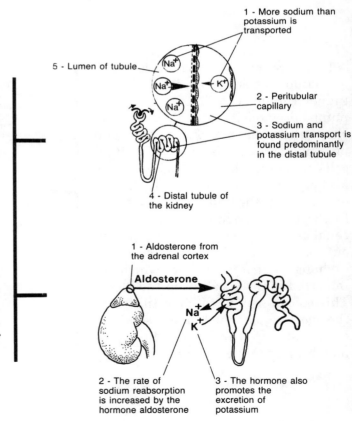

1 - Aldosterone from the adrenal cortex

Aldosterone

Na^+
K^+

2 - The rate of sodium reabsorption is increased by the hormone aldosterone

3 - The hormone also promotes the excretion of potassium

Aldosterone, a steroid, works by entering the renal tubular cell, combining with an intracellular receptor and then entering the nucleus, where it stimulates the nucleic acid mechanisms to synthesize new membrane carrier proteins for transporting the ions. There is a delay of some 45 minutes between the release of aldosterone and the recognition of its effect on sodium excretion; this is accounted for by the time taken to make the new proteins.

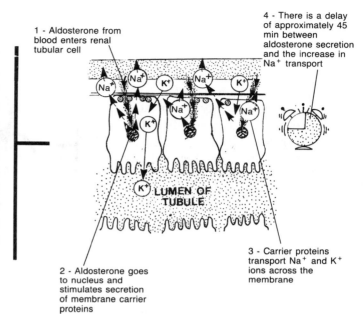

1 - Aldosterone from blood enters renal tubular cell

4 - There is a delay of approximately 45 min between aldosterone secretion and the increase in Na^+ transport

2 - Aldosterone goes to nucleus and stimulates secretion of membrane carrier proteins

3 - Carrier proteins transport Na^+ and K^+ ions across the membrane

Another substance which is important in regulating sodium transport is **atrial natriuretic hormone** (or peptide, or factor), a small peptide (released from the atrium of the heart) which inhibits sodium reabsorption and thus acts in the opposite direction to aldosterone. It has a relaxant effect on smooth muscle (producing arterial hypotension) yet increases glomerular filtration rate, presumably by relaxing the afferent arterioles; this increases sodium excretion.

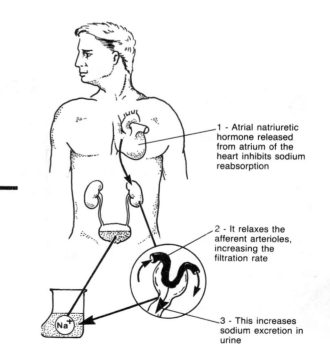

1 - Atrial natriuretic hormone released from atrium of the heart inhibits sodium reabsorption

2 - It relaxes the afferent arterioles, increasing the filtration rate

3 - This increases sodium excretion in urine

It also diminishes active sodium reabsorption, possibly by an effect on both proximal and distal tubules, and may also affect sodium permeability of tubular or collecting duct cells in the medulla. Its net effect is to increase the urinary output of sodium.

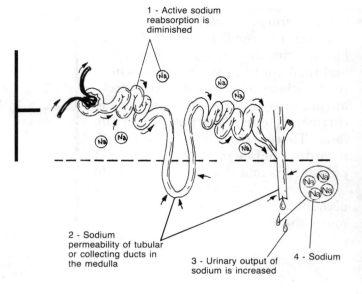

1 - Active sodium reabsorption is diminished

2 - Sodium permeability of tubular or collecting ducts in the medulla

3 - Urinary output of sodium is increased

4 - Sodium

Potassium ions are almost completely reabsorbed from the glomerular filtrate by active transport in the proximal tubule; the K$^+$ found in the urine has been secreted by the distal tubule. Some of the secretion is passive along concentration or electrical gradients, and some occurs under the control of the aldosterone-sensitive Na−K exchange mechanism. There may be other mechanisms available for the active excretion of potassium. The final concentration of potassium in the plasma is probably regulated mainly by the aldosterone mechanism.

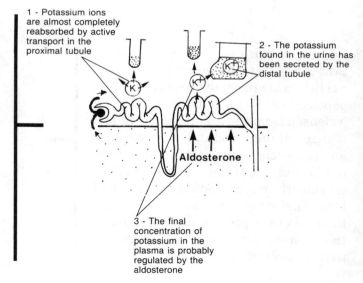

1 - Potassium ions are almost completely reabsorbed by active transport in the proximal tubule

2 - The potassium found in the urine has been secreted by the distal tubule

Aldosterone

3 - The final concentration of potassium in the plasma is probably regulated by the aldosterone

THE LOOP OF HENLE

The tubular fluid leaving the proximal convoluted tubule enters the descending limb of the loop of Henle. The loop runs from the cortex deep into the medulla and then up again into the cortex, returning to a point close to where it left.

The descending limb of the loop is fairly permeable to water and most ions; the ascending limb has thicker cells in its wall which are relatively impermeable to water but contain an active transport mechanism for chloride ions.

As fluid flows along the loop, it is subjected to a process of **counter-current multiplication**. The cells of the ascending limb pump chloride ions into the interstitial fluid; sodium ions follow to maintain electroneutrality, but water molecules cannot follow, despite the resultant osmotic gradient.

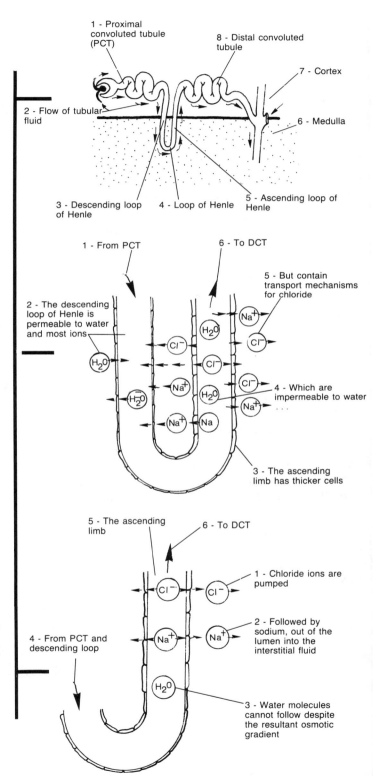

1 - Proximal convoluted tubule (PCT)

8 - Distal convoluted tubule

7 - Cortex

2 - Flow of tubular fluid

6 - Medulla

3 - Descending loop of Henle

4 - Loop of Henle

5 - Ascending loop of Henle

1 - From PCT

6 - To DCT

5 - But contain transport mechanisms for chloride

2 - The descending loop of Henle is permeable to water and most ions

4 - Which are impermeable to water . . .

3 - The ascending limb has thicker cells

5 - The ascending limb

6 - To DCT

1 - Chloride ions are pumped

2 - Followed by sodium, out of the lumen into the interstitial fluid

4 - From PCT and descending loop

3 - Water molecules cannot follow despite the resultant osmotic gradient

The parts of the tubule at the very bottom of the loop lose ions to the interstitium; some of the excess ions enter the descending limb, so that the tubular fluid becomes progressively more concentrated as it passes deeper into the medulla, then becomes more and more dilute as it passes upward out of the medulla.

The fluid entering the descending limb of Henle's loop is virtually isosmotic with plasma, and the fluid leaving the loop to enter the distal convoluted tubule is again virtually isosmotic with plasma. What happens in between, the progressive increase and then decrease in osmolality and in the strength of the interstitial fluid, is vital to the regulation of water excretion and the ability of the kidney to excrete a concentrated urine.

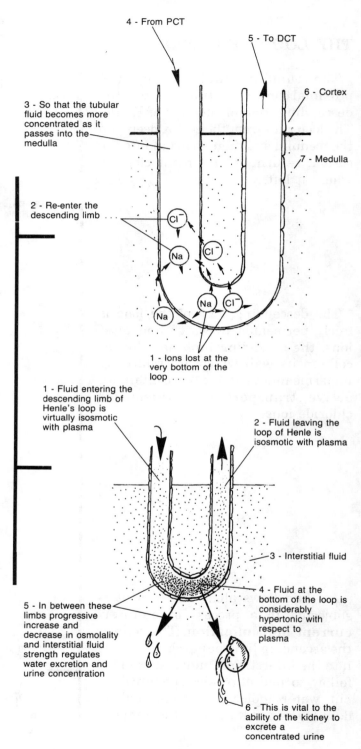

4 - From PCT

5 - To DCT

6 - Cortex

7 - Medulla

3 - So that the tubular fluid becomes more concentrated as it passes into the medulla

2 - Re-enter the descending limb

1 - Ions lost at the very bottom of the loop . . .

1 - Fluid entering the descending limb of Henle's loop is virtually isosmotic with plasma

2 - Fluid leaving the loop of Henle is isosmotic with plasma

3 - Interstitial fluid

4 - Fluid at the bottom of the loop is considerably hypertonic with respect to plasma

5 - In between these limbs progressive increase and decrease in osmolality and interstitial fluid strength regulates water excretion and urine concentration

6 - This is vital to the ability of the kidney to excrete a concentrated urine

Following its passage through the distal tubule (where the fine adjustment of excretion of many substances occurs) the fluid passes into the collecting ducts, which run through the renal medulla and empty into the pelvis of the kidney.

The walls of the collecting ducts are ordinarily impermeable to water, but the **antidiuretic hormone** of the posterior lobe of the pituitary gland can render the walls of the collecting duct permeable to water.

As the duct passes through regions of the medulla with progressively more and more concentrated interstitial fluid, the water is drawn out of the collecting ducts and into the interstitium, with a resultant increase in the concentration of solutes in the urine.

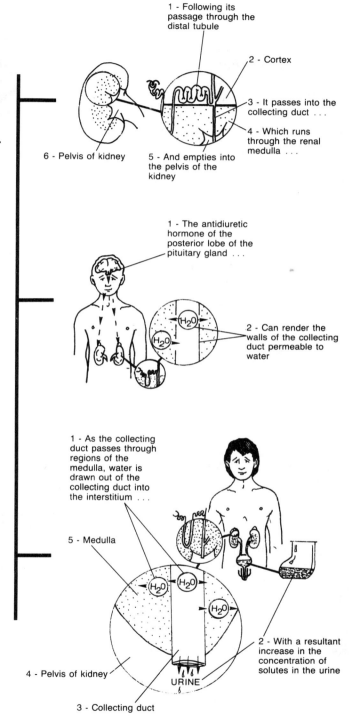

1 - Following its passage through the distal tubule

2 - Cortex

3 - It passes into the collecting duct . . .

4 - Which runs through the renal medulla . . .

5 - And empties into the pelvis of the kidney

6 - Pelvis of kidney

1 - The antidiuretic hormone of the posterior lobe of the pituitary gland . . .

2 - Can render the walls of the collecting duct permeable to water

1 - As the collecting duct passes through regions of the medulla, water is drawn out of the collecting duct into the interstitium . . .

5 - Medulla

4 - Pelvis of kidney

3 - Collecting duct

2 - With a resultant increase in the concentration of solutes in the urine

URINE

This elaborate procedure for creating a concentration gradient through the renal medulla would rapidly become negated if the blood vessels through the medulla were to carry blood straight through at high flow rates; areas of high osmolality would rapidly become diluted by passage of fluid out of the plasma, and areas of low osmolality would rapidly transfer water to the blood.

However, the vessels to the medulla, the **vasa recta**, are looped just like the renal tubules, and run in parallel with them. Furthermore the blood flow through them is rather sluggish, just enough to maintain the metabolism of the tubular cells.

The result is that blood in the descending limb is allowed to come into equilibrium with the interstitial fluid in the medulla, becoming more and more concentrated; as blood flows in the ascending limb back towards the cortex it becomes less concentrated again, and the end result is that the blood returning to the cortex has had its composition altered very little, and the concentration gradients in the medulla have not been disturbed.

All that has happened is that some of the excess water, extracted from the collecting ducts, is carried away by the blood leaving the vasa recta.

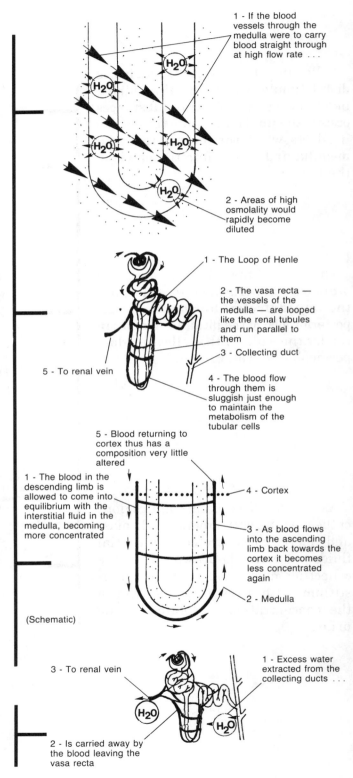

1 - If the blood vessels through the medulla were to carry blood straight through at high flow rate . . .

2 - Areas of high osmolality would rapidly become diluted

1 - The Loop of Henle

2 - The vasa recta — the vessels of the medulla — are looped like the renal tubules and run parallel to them

3 - Collecting duct

4 - The blood flow through them is sluggish just enough to maintain the metabolism of the tubular cells

5 - To renal vein

5 - Blood returning to cortex thus has a composition very little altered

1 - The blood in the descending limb is allowed to come into equilibrium with the interstitial fluid in the medulla, becoming more concentrated

4 - Cortex

3 - As blood flows into the ascending limb back towards the cortex it becomes less concentrated again

2 - Medulla

(Schematic)

1 - Excess water extracted from the collecting ducts . . .

3 - To renal vein

2 - Is carried away by the blood leaving the vasa recta

EXCRETION OF UREA AND OTHER WASTE PRODUCTS OF METABOLISM

Many substances like urea have no specific carrier for their secretion or absorption; they are freely filterd, and then passively reabsorbed. The clearance of urea is normally around 85 ml/min, or rather less than the GFR, but this clearance depends on the rate of urine flow.

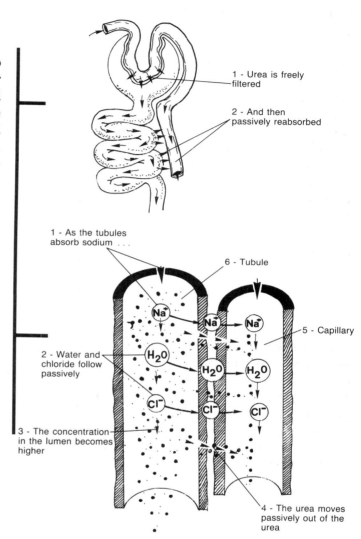

1 - Urea is freely filtered

2 - And then passively reabsorbed

1 - As the tubules absorb sodium . . .

6 - Tubule

5 - Capillary

2 - Water and chloride follow passively

3 - The concentration in the lumen becomes higher

4 - The urea moves passively out of the urea

As the tubules absorb sodium and the water and chloride follow passively, the concentration of urea left in the lumen becomes higher and urea moves passively out of the tubule. The more concentrated the urine becomes, the bigger is the gradient for urea and the more is absorbed; at high urine flows with a dilute urine less urea is absorbed and more is excreted.

Urea does not remain at a constant concentration in the tubular water because it is less permeant that water, and becomes partly 'trapped' in the tubule. Usually only 50–60% of the filtered urea is reabsorbed, and the rest is excreted.

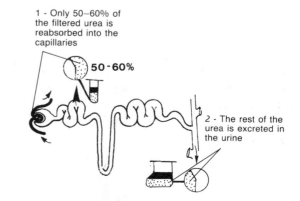

1 - Only 50–60% of the filtered urea is reabsorbed into the capillaries

50-60%

2 - The rest of the urea is excreted in the urine

CONTROL OF RENAL BLOOD FLOW AND GFR

The kidney is capable of maintaining its blood flow and the glomerular filtration rate remarkably constant over a very wide range of systemic blood pressures: the kidney performs **autoregulation**. Although sympathetic nerves can have profound effects on renal blood flow, they are not necessary for this regulation, as the denervated or even the transplanted kidney can autoregulate blood flow. Several mechanisms have been advanced to explain this.

In one, an increase in systemic pressure would increase renal perfusion pressure and hence cause the exudation of more fluid from capillaries; this would increase interstitial pressure, and since the kidney has a fibrous capsule the increased intracapsular pressure would oppose any further rise in blood flow.

Another explanation relies on the property of smooth muscle, once stretched, to develop active tension; distension of afferent arterioles by high pressure would cause them to constrict, reducing blood flow.

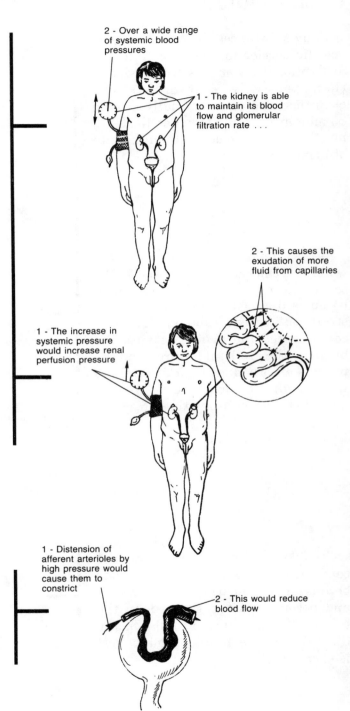

2 - Over a wide range of systemic blood pressures

1 - The kidney is able to maintain its blood flow and glomerular filtration rate . . .

2 - This causes the exudation of more fluid from capillaries

1 - The increase in systemic pressure would increase renal perfusion pressure

1 - Distension of afferent arterioles by high pressure would cause them to constrict

2 - This would reduce blood flow

The explanation which receives most support is one involving local chemical reflexes. If pressure falls in the renal blood vessels, this is sensed by the **juxtaglomerular apparatus**, consisting of a specialized part of the afferent arteriole linked to the **macula densa** in the distal tubule.

The juxtaglomerular cells in the media of the afferent arterioles do not look like smooth muscle; instead they have granules which are released in response to low arterial pressure, and may also be released when the cells of the macula densa detect low concentrations of sodium in the distal tubular fluid; this would happen if GFR fell as a consequence of decreased renal blood flow. The precise way in which the macula densa communicates with the arteriolar cells is still a mystery.

The granules released from juxtaglomerular cells contain **renin**, a proteolytic enzyme which acts on a specific alpha$_2$-globulin in the plasma (and presumably in the renal interstitial fluid), producing the decapeptide **angiotensin I**. This is further modified in the renal tissue fluid or during the passage of blood through the lungs by **angiotensin-converting enzyme** (**ACE**) to form the octopeptide **angiotensin II**.

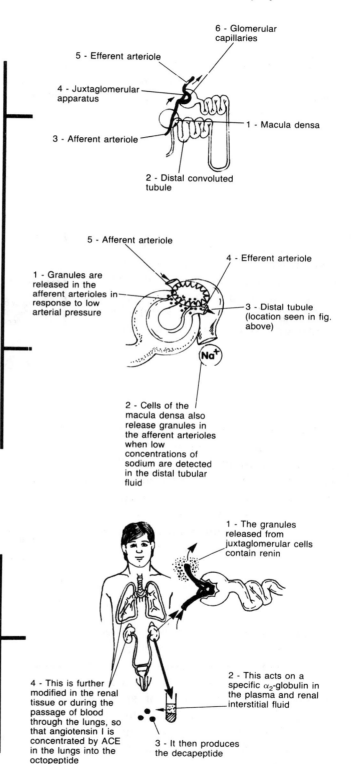

6 - Glomerular capillaries

5 - Efferent arteriole

4 - Juxtaglomerular apparatus

3 - Afferent arteriole

1 - Macula densa

2 - Distal convoluted tubule

5 - Afferent arteriole

4 - Efferent arteriole

1 - Granules are released in the afferent arterioles in response to low arterial pressure

3 - Distal tubule (location seen in fig. above)

2 - Cells of the macula densa also release granules in the afferent arterioles when low concentrations of sodium are detected in the distal tubular fluid

Na$^+$

1 - The granules released from juxtaglomerular cells contain renin

2 - This acts on a specific α_2-globulin in the plasma and renal interstitial fluid

3 - It then produces the decapeptide

4 - This is further modified in the renal tissue or during the passage of blood through the lungs, so that angiotensin I is concentrated by ACE in the lungs into the octopeptide angiotensin II

The role of the local renal fraction of angiotensin is to constrict the efferent arteriole, raising the glomerular pressure and increasing GFR.

If renal blood flow rises, the control mechanism acts in the reverse way: the release of renin is decreased, and the production of angiotensin is reduced, allowing the efferent arterioles to dilate and restore blood flow to normal.

The systemically circulating angiotensin is an extremely potent vasoconstrictor, about 40 times as effective as noradrenaline, and causes a rapid rise in blood pressure; consequently renal perfusion pressure increases by this systemic mechanism as well as by the local intrarenal pathway.

As well as its effects on blood vessels, angiotensin has a very important effect on the secretion of aldosterone by the adrenal cortex. This steroid hormone promotes the resorption of salt and water by the distal tubule, thus expanding the extracellular fluid volume and plasma volume and raising cardiac output.

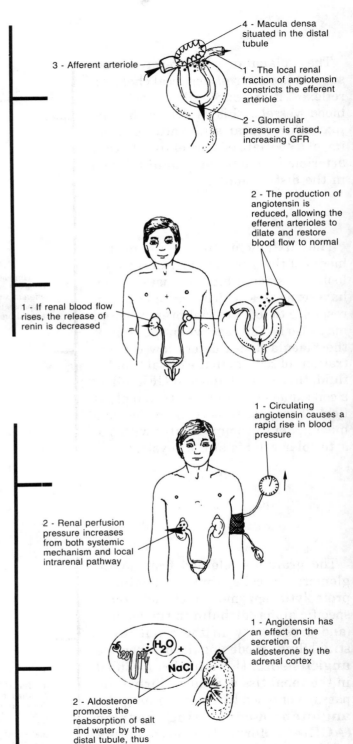

4 - Macula densa situated in the distal tubule

3 - Afferent arteriole

1 - The local renal fraction of angiotensin constricts the efferent arteriole

2 - Glomerular pressure is raised, increasing GFR

2 - The production of angiotensin is reduced, allowing the efferent arterioles to dilate and restore blood flow to normal

1 - If renal blood flow rises, the release of renin is decreased

1 - Circulating angiotensin causes a rapid rise in blood pressure

2 - Renal perfusion pressure increases from both systemic mechanism and local intrarenal pathway

1 - Angiotensin has an effect on the secretion of aldosterone by the adrenal cortex

2 - Aldosterone promotes the reabsorption of salt and water by the distal tubule, thus increasing plasma volume and cardiac output

There is also a small negative feedback effect; angiotensin in the plasma inhibits the further secretion of renin by the juxtaglomerular apparatus.

Angiotensin is eventually broken down in the kidney by the enzyme angiotensinase.

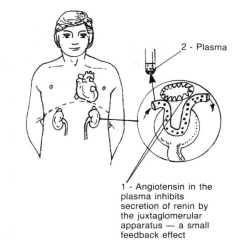

2 - Plasma

1 - Angiotensin in the plasma inhibits secretion of renin by the juxtaglomerular apparatus — a small feedback effect

RENAL REGULATION OF PLASMA COMPOSITION

Control of plasma osmolality

The osmolality of the blood is normally kept within close limits. If the osmolality is increased, for example by ingestion of excess salt or the loss of water in sweat, then this is detected by **osmoreceptors** in the **supraoptic** nucleus of the hypothalamus.

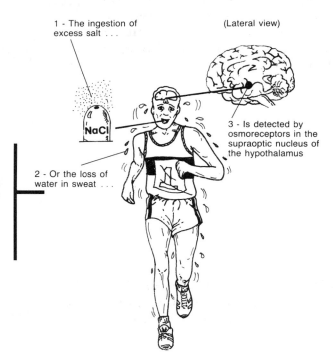

1 - The ingestion of excess salt . . .

(Lateral view)

3 - Is detected by osmoreceptors in the supraoptic nucleus of the hypothalamus

2 - Or the loss of water in sweat . . .

Some cells in the nearby **lateral preoptic** nucleus are also sensitive to the osmolality of tissue fluid, and stimulate the **thirst** mechanism, initiating drinking of water.

1 - Cells in the lateral preoptic nucleus are sensitive to the osmolality of tissue fluid

2 - These cells stimulate the thirst mechanism, initiating drinking of water

The cells of the supraoptic nucleus give rise to axons which pass along the pituitary stalk into the posterior lobe of the pituitary. Osmotic stimulation causes action potentials to pass along these axons, triggering the **neuro-secretion** of **antidiuretic hormone** (**ADH**) into the blood.

1 - The cells of the supraoptic nucleus give rise to axons which pass along the pituitary stalk

2 - The cells then pass into the posterior lobe of the pituitary . . .

ADH

3 - Triggering the neurosecretion of ADH into the blood

The hormone acts on the cells lining the collecting ducts of the kidney, increasing their permeability to water.

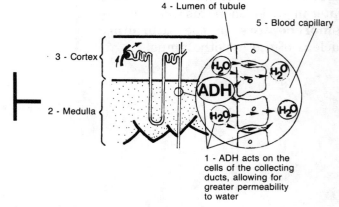

4 - Lumen of tubule

5 - Blood capillary

3 - Cortex

2 - Medulla

ADH

H_2O

1 - ADH acts on the cells of the collecting ducts, allowing for greater permeability to water

In the absence of **ADH** the ducts are relatively impermeable to water, very little of which leaves the luminal fluid, even though the ducts pass through the cortex of the kidney where the osmotic strength of the interstitial fluid is considerably hypertonic to plasma.

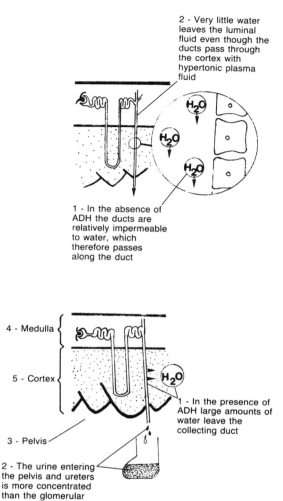

2 - Very little water leaves the luminal fluid even though the ducts pass through the cortex with hypertonic plasma fluid

1 - In the absence of ADH the ducts are relatively impermeable to water, which therefore passes along the duct

In the presence of **ADH**, when water permeability is increased, large amounts of water leave the collecting duct in response to the large osmotic gradient, and the urine entering the pelvis and ureters is much more concentrated than the original glomerular filtrate.

4 - Medulla

5 - Cortex

1 - In the presence of ADH large amounts of water leave the collecting duct

3 - Pelvis

2 - The urine entering the pelvis and ureters is more concentrated than the glomerular filtrate

If the plasma osmolality is reduced, for example by drinking a large volume of water, this is detected by the osmoreceptors and the secretion of **ADH** is reduced, so that water is not reabsorbed from the collecting duct but passes instead into the ureters for excretion.

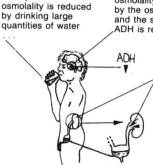

1 - If plasma osmolality is reduced by drinking large quantities of water

2 - This change in osmolality is detected by the osmoreceptors and the secretion of ADH is reduced

ADH

3 - As a result there is reduced ADH secretion; water is not reabsorbed from the collecting duct but passes out of the kidneys for excretion

The regulation of plasma osmolality is a good example of a homeostatic mechanism. The detectors are the osmoreceptors in the hypothalamus, the controlling centre is the supraoptic nucleus, the signal is carried as a hormone by the blood, and the effector is the collecting duct of the kidney. The system also contains a means for increasing water intake — the thirst mechanism.

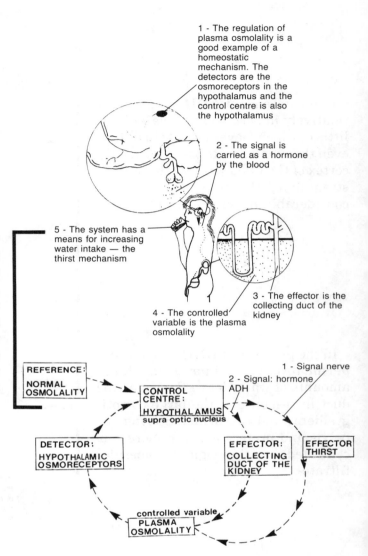

1 - The regulation of plasma osmolality is a good example of a homeostatic mechanism. The detectors are the osmoreceptors in the hypothalamus and the control centre is also the hypothalamus

2 - The signal is carried as a hormone by the blood

5 - The system has a means for increasing water intake — the thirst mechanism

3 - The effector is the collecting duct of the kidney

4 - The controlled variable is the plasma osmolality

Several other factors influence the production of **ADH** and hence the excretion of water by the kidney. Distension of the gut by ingested fluid, even if it is isotonic (for instance 0.9% saline), can reflexly inhibit secretion of **ADH**; ethanol and several other drugs inhibit ADH secretion and cause a diuresis (increase in urine output). Large blood losses, for example haemorrhage by more than 10% of normal blood volume, stimulate the production of **ADH** as well as exciting the thirst mechanism.

A diuresis can be caused by factors other than absence of **ADH**. For instance, if substances appear in the glomerular filtrate which cannot subsequently be reabsorbed but remain in the tubular fluid, they exert an osmotic force opposing the reabsorption of water (even though the collecting ducts may be permeable) and causing an **osmotic diuresis**. Ethanol has this effect in addition to its inhibitory effect on the pituitary; excessive glucose in the urine of diabetics also has this effect and is responsible for the severe dehydration which is experienced.

Infusions of **mannitol** are sometimes given to promote osmotic diuresis in cases of poisoning when it is desired to eliminate the toxin in the urine.

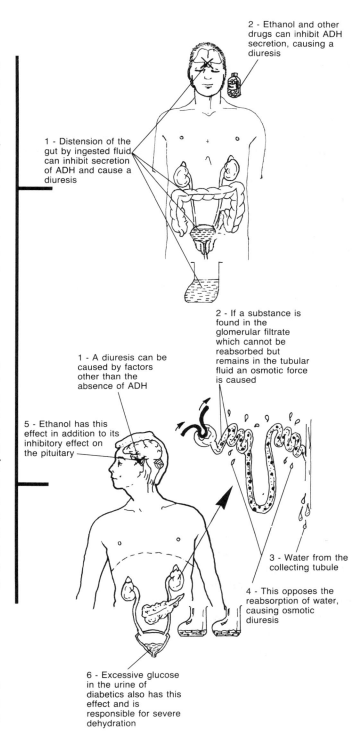

2 - Ethanol and other drugs can inhibit ADH secretion, causing a diuresis

1 - Distension of the gut by ingested fluid can inhibit secretion of ADH and cause a diuresis

2 - If a substance is found in the glomerular filtrate which cannot be reabsorbed but remains in the tubular fluid an osmotic force is caused

1 - A diuresis can be caused by factors other than the absence of ADH

5 - Ethanol has this effect in addition to its inhibitory effect on the pituitary

3 - Water from the collecting tubule

4 - This opposes the reabsorption of water, causing osmotic diuresis

6 - Excessive glucose in the urine of diabetics also has this effect and is responsible for severe dehydration

Control of blood volume

The ADH system can readily cope with changes in the water intake or output, but cannot cope so easily with changes in salt content. For example, drinking a litre of pure water promotes a rapid diuresis, but drinking or infusing a litre of isotonic (0.9%) saline has almost no stimulant effect on the osmoreceptors, and there is often no diuresis for a number of hours. The excess salt and water must be eliminated at some stage, and the mechanisms for achieving this are rather more complex.

The main effect of isotonic infusion or ingestion is to increase the plasma volume and the interstitial fluid volume. An increased plasma volume increases the venous return to the heart, and could theoretically increase stroke volume, cardiac output and blood pressure.

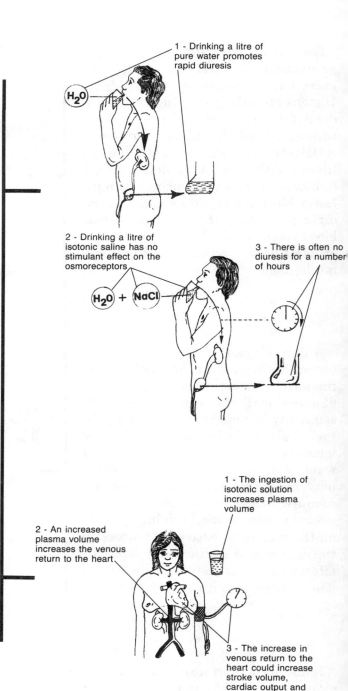

1 - Drinking a litre of pure water promotes rapid diuresis

2 - Drinking a litre of isotonic saline has no stimulant effect on the osmoreceptors

3 - There is often no diuresis for a number of hours

1 - The ingestion of isotonic solution increases plasma volume

2 - An increased plasma volume increases the venous return to the heart

3 - The increase in venous return to the heart could increase stroke volume, cardiac output and blood pressure

The raised systemic arterial pressure could increase GFR, and could also stimulate arterial baroreceptors, causing reflex alterations in the secretion of hormones active on the kidney. In practice it seems that this mechanism is not very important, but rather it is the effect on the volume of blood in the great veins and right atrium which acts as a stimulant for the excretion of salt and water.

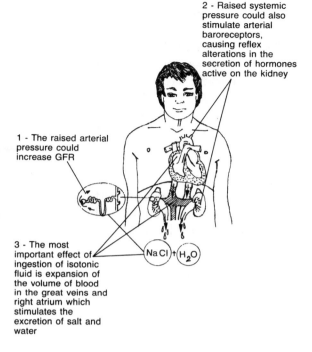

2 - Raised systemic pressure could also stimulate arterial baroreceptors, causing reflex alterations in the secretion of hormones active on the kidney

1 - The raised arterial pressure could increase GFR

3 - The most important effect of ingestion of isotonic fluid is expansion of the volume of blood in the great veins and right atrium which stimulates the excretion of salt and water

There are volume receptors in the great veins of the thorax and in the atria. Distension of the venous system stimulates these receptors, which have a number of effects. They cause the sympathetic nervous system to produce peripheral vasodilatation, lowering the blood pressure; the sympathetic nerves constricting the afferent arterioles in the kidney are inhibited, improving blood flow and increasing GFR.

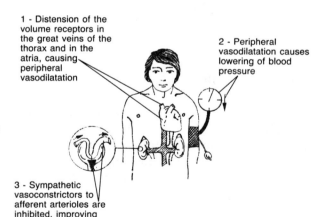

1 - Distension of the volume receptors in the great veins of the thorax and in the atria, causing peripheral vasodilatation

2 - Peripheral vasodilatation causes lowering of blood pressure

3 - Sympathetic vasoconstrictors to afferent arterioles are inhibited, improving glomerular filtration

There is also a reflex decrease in the secretion of aldosterone from the adrenal cortex, caused partly by suppression of ACTH release from the anterior pituitary, but partly by reduction in renin release from the kidney.

Above all the distension of the right atrium releases **atrial natriuretic hormone**, which promotes the excretion of sodium and hence water, eliminating the excess which was infused or ingested.

A decrease in plasma volume causes the reverse changes: there is increased absorption of salt and water due to stimulation of aldosterone and inhibition of atrial natriuretic hormone with retention of fluid by the kidney.

Control of plasma pH

The carbon dioxide/carbonic acid/ bicarbonate buffer system offers the kidney a means for influencing the pH of plasma. Although it may not be the most powerful buffer system present in the blood (since the proteins are quantitatively more important and the phosphates, too, have a large buffering power), it is the only system whose components can be increased or decreased readily and rapidly in response to the body's needs. We have already considered how the lung can modify pH by increasing or decreasing the excretion of carbon dioxide in the expired air.

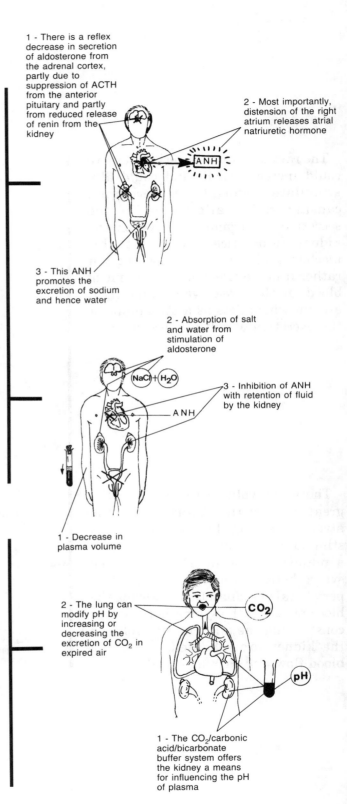

1 - There is a reflex decrease in secretion of aldosterone from the adrenal cortex, partly due to suppression of ACTH from the anterior pituitary and partly from reduced release of renin from the kidney

2 - Most importantly, distension of the right atrium releases atrial natriuretic hormone

3 - This ANH promotes the excretion of sodium and hence water

2 - Absorption of salt and water from stimulation of aldosterone

3 - Inhibition of ANH with retention of fluid by the kidney

1 - Decrease in plasma volume

2 - The lung can modify pH by increasing or decreasing the excretion of CO_2 in expired air

1 - The CO_2/carbonic acid/bicarbonate buffer system offers the kidney a means for influencing the pH of plasma

2 - The kidney can also manufacture new bicarbonate ions for addition to the plasma

HCO_3^-

H^+

1 - The kidney can increase or decrease the excretion of H^+ ions in the urine

The kidney can modify the other end of the equilibrium by increasing or decreasing the excretion of hydrogen ions in the urine and by manufacturing new bicarbonate ions for addition to the plasma.

1 - The PCT reabsorbs all bicarbonate in the filtrate

HCO_3^-

The proximal tubule usually reabsorbs all of the bicarbonate in the glomerular filtrate, but the nephron can make new bicarbonate ions in addition to the ones which are reabsorbed.

2 - The nephron can make new bicarbonate ions

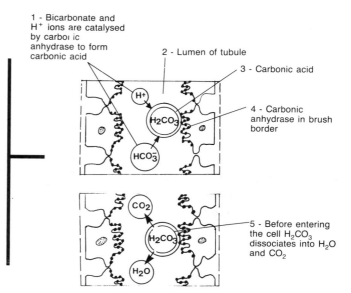

1 - Bicarbonate and H^+ ions are catalysed by carbonic anhydrase to form carbonic acid

2 - Lumen of tubule

3 - Carbonic acid

4 - Carbonic anhydrase in brush border

5 - Before entering the cell H_2CO_3 dissociates into H_2O and CO_2

Bicarbonate ions are not absorbed directly, as the tubular epithelium is impermeable to this ion and there is no active transport mechanism. However, the tubular cells have the enzyme **carbonic anhydrase** on their brush border membranes, and this enzyme catalyses the combination of bicarbonate with hydrogen ions to form carbonic acid, which in turn dissociates into carbon dioxide and water:

$$H^+ + HCO_3^- \rightleftharpoons H_2CO_3 \rightleftharpoons H_2O + CO_2$$

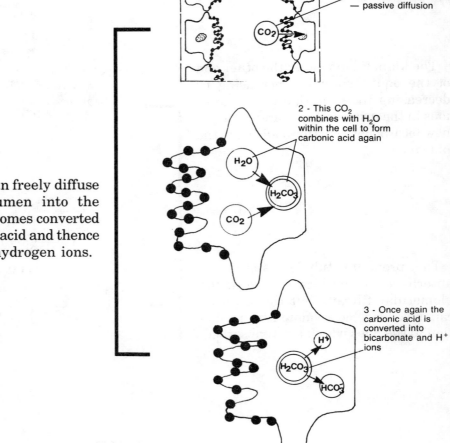

1 - The CO_2 freely enters the tubular cell — passive diffusion

2 - This CO_2 combines with H_2O within the cell to form carbonic acid again

3 - Once again the carbonic acid is converted into bicarbonate and H^+ ions

The carbon dioxide can freely diffuse out of the tubular lumen into the tubular cell; there it becomes converted once more into carbonic acid and thence into bicarbonate and hydrogen ions.

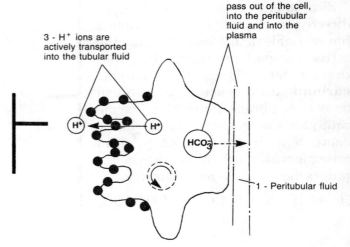

2 - Bicarbonate ions pass out of the cell, into the peritubular fluid and into the plasma

3 - H^+ ions are actively transported into the tubular fluid

1 - Peritubular fluid

The bicarbonate ions pass out of the cell into the peritubular fluid and the plasma, while the hydrogen ions are actively transported back into the tubular fluid.

Their place in the cell is taken by sodium ions entering passively from the lumen; these are subsequently actively transported across the membrane into the peritubular fluid and the plasma. The net result is the reabsorption of a bicarbonate ion and the uptake of a sodium ion. This may seem to be a round-about way of absorbing bicarbonate ions, but it is necessary because of the impermeability of the luminal membrane to bicarbonate ions.

5 - Na^+ ions enter passively from the lumen into the cell and later into the peritubular fluid and the plasma. Net results are reabsorption of bicarbonate ions (see fig. above) and uptake of Na^+ ions

4 - Since the luminal membrane is impermeable to bicarbonate ions, they have to be absorbed in an apparently round-about way

As well as reabsorbing filtered bicarbonate from the proximal tubular fluid, the kidney can manufacture new bicarbonate from its cellular metabolism; this occurs in the distal tubule.

1 - The cellular metabolism in the distal tubule can manufacture new bicarbonate

Carbon dioxide produced within the cell can be converted to carbonic acid and thence to bicarbonate and hydrogen ions; the bicarbonate ions are available to add to the plasma if the hydrogen ion concentration becomes too high, while the accompanying hydrogen ions are passed into the tubular fluid, resulting in the net elimination of acid from the body.

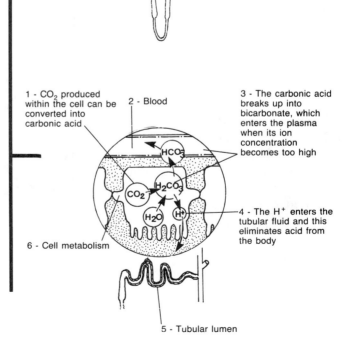

1 - CO_2 produced within the cell can be converted into carbonic acid

2 - Blood

3 - The carbonic acid breaks up into bicarbonate, which enters the plasma when its ion concentration becomes too high

4 - The H^+ enters the tubular fluid and this eliminates acid from the body

6 - Cell metabolism

5 - Tubular lumen

It was once thought that potassium and hydrogen ions competed for the same secretory carrier in the distal tubule, as acidosis results in increased excretion of hydrogen ions and decreased secretion of potassium; however, it now seems more likely that intracellular acidosis partly paralyses the pump mechanisms responsible for potassium secretion, and there is no real competition between hydrogen and potassium ions.

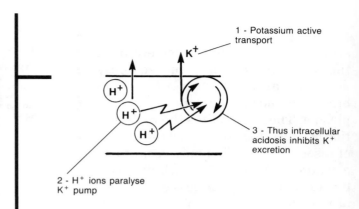

1 - Potassium active transport

3 - Thus intracellular acidosis inhibits K⁺ excretion

2 - H⁺ ions paralyse K⁺ pump

If hydrogen ions accumulate in the tubular fluid they inhibit the further excretion of acid and hence the production of bicarbonate; thus it is necessary to buffer the urine in some way.

2 - Further excretion of acid becomes inhibited. Thus it is desirable to buffer urine

1 - If H⁺ ions accumulate in the tubular fluid . . .

There are several mechanisms available for this; the divalent monohydrogen phosphate ion in the tubular lumen can accept hydrogen ions and become the monovalent dihydrogen phosphate ion, thus:

$$H^+ + HPO_4^{2-} \rightleftharpoons H_2PO_4^-$$

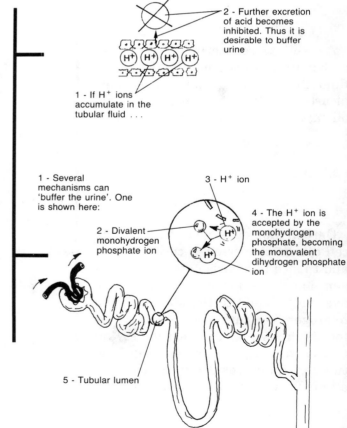

1 - Several mechanisms can 'buffer the urine'. One is shown here:

2 - Divalent monohydrogen phosphate ion

3 - H⁺ ion

4 - The H⁺ ion is accepted by the monohydrogen phosphate, becoming the monovalent dihydrogen phosphate ion

5 - Tubular lumen

Glutamine produced in the cell can be broken down to ammonia, which appears in the tubular fluid; this can accept hydrogen ions to become the ammonium ion, thus:

$$H^+ + NH_3 \rightleftharpoons NH_4^+$$

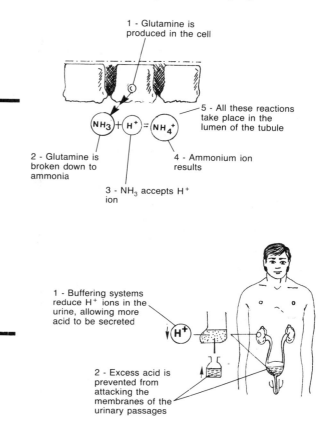

1 - Glutamine is produced in the cell

5 - All these reactions take place in the lumen of the tubule

2 - Glutamine is broken down to ammonia

3 - NH_3 accepts H^+ ion

4 - Ammonium ion results

These buffering systems reduce the concentration of free hydrogen ions in the urine and hence allow more acid to be excreted; they also prevent excessive acid from attacking the membranes of the urinary passages.

1 - Buffering systems reduce H^+ ions in the urine, allowing more acid to be secreted

2 - Excess acid is prevented from attacking the membranes of the urinary passages

THE URETERS, BLADDER AND URETHRA

Urine collected in the pelvis of each kidney passes without further modification along the ureters into the bladder for storage; at intervals the bladder is emptied through the urethra. These functions are under the control of autonomic nerves, and are also amenable to a certain degree of voluntary control.

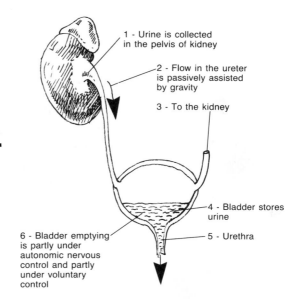

1 - Urine is collected in the pelvis of kidney

2 - Flow in the ureter is passively assisted by gravity

3 - To the kidney

4 - Bladder stores urine

5 - Urethra

6 - Bladder emptying is partly under autonomic nervous control and partly under voluntary control

The flow of urine along the ureters is probably largely passive: as urine is formed by the kidney the pressure in the pelvis rises and forces flow along the ureter, and this flow is often assisted by gravity. However, the ureter is lined with smooth muscle cells which undergo regular spontaneous peristaltic contractions which could help to propel urine. At its lower end the ureter passes through the thick muscular wall of the bladder, and this usually keeps the lumen of the ureter closed. When the bladder contracts the pinching action of the muscle prevents the reflux of urine up the ureter; the bladder needs to be relaxed for flow to occur from ureter to bladder.

The bladder is an organ of storage for urine, receiving the urine in small quantities as it is formed, and then expelling a large accumulated volume at convenient intervals.

1 - The ureter is lined with smooth muscle cells, which contract to propel the urine along the ureter

3 - When the bladder contracts the muscle prevents the reflux of urine up the ureter

2 - At its lower end the ureter passes through the thick bladder wall

It has no role in modifying the composition of urine in man, although in amphibians the bladder epithelium has some important absorptive functions. The bladder is composed of several layers of smooth muscle, lined by a **transitional** epithelium, whose structure allows for large changes in the surface area being covered as the bladder becomes distended or contracted.

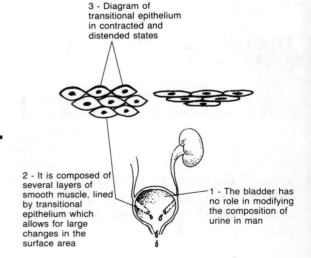

3 - Diagram of transitional epithelium in contracted and distended states

2 - It is composed of several layers of smooth muscle, lined by transitional epithelium which allows for large changes in the surface area

1 - The bladder has no role in modifying the composition of urine in man

As urine flows into the bladder the volume increases and the pressure rises. When the pressure in the bladder exceeds a certain level, stretch receptors in the bladder wall are excited and sensory impulses pass along the **pelvic visceral nerves** to the sacral segments of the spinal cord. There they synaptically excite parasympathetic preganglionic neurones whose axons run in the **nervi erigentes** to the bladder; the postganglionic neurones in the bladder wall have short axons which release acetylcholine to make the bladder muscle contract, expelling urine. At the same time the urethral sphincter relaxes. This is known as the **micturition** reflex.

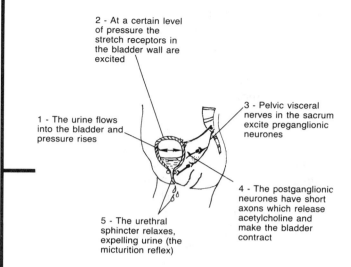

2 - At a certain level of pressure the stretch receptors in the bladder wall are excited

3 - Pelvic visceral nerves in the sacrum excite preganglionic neurones

1 - The urine flows into the bladder and pressure rises

4 - The postganglionic neurones have short axons which release acetylcholine and make the bladder contract

5 - The urethral sphincter relaxes, expelling urine (the micturition reflex)

The contraction of the smooth muscle in the bladder can be augmented by contraction of voluntary muscles of the abdominal wall, and the relaxation of the urethral sphincter is accompanied by relaxation of voluntary muscles of the pelvic floor.

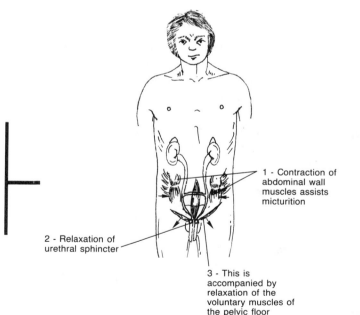

1 - Contraction of abdominal wall muscles assists micturition

2 - Relaxation of urethral sphincter

3 - This is accompanied by relaxation of the voluntary muscles of the pelvic floor

The micturition reflex can be modified by impulses from higher centres. If it is socially inconvenient for urine to be voided, voluntary inhibition is applied. Not only are the parasympathetic neurones inhibited to prevent bladder contraction; the sympathetic nerves supplying the bladder are excited and cause relaxation of the smooth muscle. The pressure in the bladder consequently falls, the urge to micturate becomes less, and a further increment can occur in the volume of the bladder before it is again stretched enough to initiate the micturition reflex. The sympathetic nerves also cause constriction of the urethral sphincter, and the striated muscles of the pelvic floor can be contracted voluntarily to augment the sphincter effect.

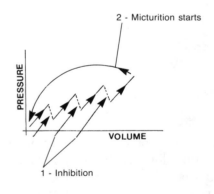

1 - Parasympathetic neurones are inhibited to prevent bladder contraction

2 - Sympathetic nerves supplying the bladder are excited and cause smooth muscle relaxation

Sacrum

← pressure

3 - Sympathetic nerves also cause constriction of the urethral sphincter

4 - The muscles of the pelvic floor can be contracted voluntarily to augment the sphincter effect

(Schematic)

The bladder may undergo several cycles of filling, pressure rise, stimulation of the urge to micturate, voluntary inhibition and further filling; eventually the walls become so stretched that no further inhibition is possible and the urge to micturate is uncontrollable.

2 - Micturition starts

PRESSURE

VOLUME

1 - Inhibition

One usually arranges to visit a suitable convenience before this stage is reached; here micturition can be initiated voluntarily by contracting the abdominal muscles to raise the pressure in the bladder, and relaxing the muscles of the pelvic floor.

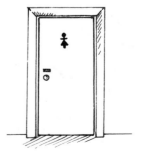

Once the micturition reflex is initiated, the bladder muscle contracts very vigorously, raising the pressure within the bladder and producing forceful expulsion of the urine; the bladder is normally left with very little residual urine at the end of micturition.

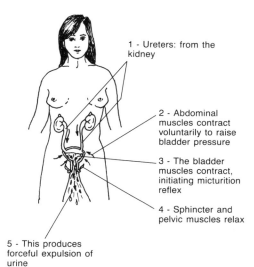

1 - Ureters: from the kidney

2 - Abdominal muscles contract voluntarily to raise bladder pressure

3 - The bladder muscles contract, initiating micturition reflex

4 - Sphincter and pelvic muscles relax

5 - This produces forceful expulsion of urine

The Endocrine System

The endocrine glands (meaning 'glands of internal secretion') form one of the most important regulatory systems in the body, complementing the nervous system in controlling bodily functions. Whilst nervous control, using discrete permanent cable-like pathways, is usually rapid, bringing about change within a few milliseconds or at most a few minutes, endocrine control, using circulating chemical messengers, occurs more slowly and has a longer duration; many endocrine effects take minutes, hours or even days or years. There are also some endocrine effects which are very rapid, and there are several places where the nervous and endocrine systems interact, allowing for very complex regulatory processes.

The endocrine glands produce hormones, i.e. secretions which are delivered internally into the blood rather than into ducts; in fact, they are often referred to as the ductless glands. Many of the glands have a very similar microscopic structure: they are extremely cellular, with small clumps of cells surrounded by a dense network of capillaries, so that the products of cellular activity can be delivered to the circulation.

Most glands in the body are derived from epithelial structures, but whereas the exocrine glands retain their connection with the epithelial surfaces via ducts, the endocrine glands lose their ducts and secrete directly into the blood vessels.

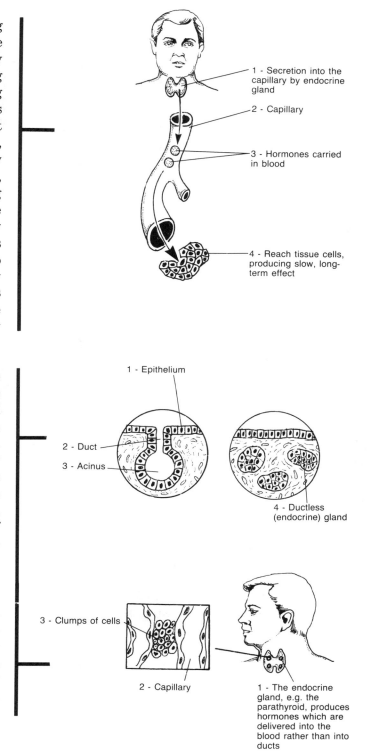

1 - Secretion into the capillary by endocrine gland

2 - Capillary

3 - Hormones carried in blood

4 - Reach tissue cells, producing slow, long-term effect

1 - Epithelium

2 - Duct

3 - Acinus

4 - Ductless (endocrine) gland

3 - Clumps of cells

2 - Capillary

1 - The endocrine gland, e.g. the parathyroid, produces hormones which are delivered into the blood rather than into ducts

The endocrine system is arranged in a hierarchical manner, with several levels of control. At the lowest level are the glands producing the final hormones which affect the end organs; examples are the thyroid gland producing thyroxine, which stimulates cellular metabolism generally, the adrenal cortex which produces several hormones regulating cellular metabolism and renal function, and the reproductive glands (testis and ovary) which produce hormones affecting the secondary sexual characteristics.

At the next level is the pituitary gland secreting **trophic** hormones, which stimulate the function of other endocrine glands. Examples are thyroid-stimulating hormone or thyrotrophin, which regulates thyroid function, adrenocortical trophic hormone which regulates the adrenal gland, and the gonadotrophins which modify the activity of the sexual glands.

In the case of each of these hormones, the pituitary gland is sensitive to the plasma concentrations of the end-organ hormones and produces more or less trophic hormone in response to falls or rises in the activity of the glands at the lower level. For example, a fall in the concentration of thyroxine (T_4) causes the pituitary to secrete more thyrotrophin so that the thyroid gland is stimulated to produce more thyroxine; an increase in plasma thyroxine has an inhibitory effect on the pituitary.

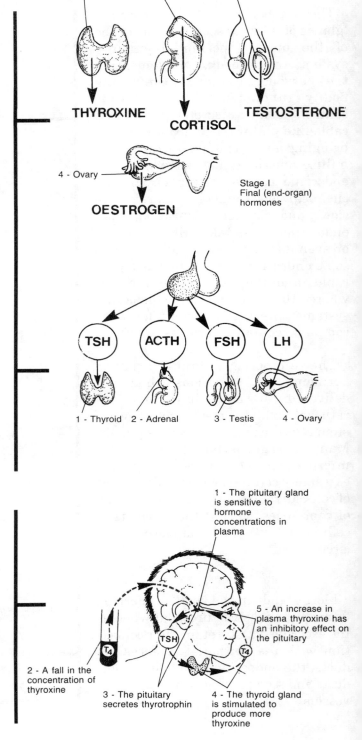

3 - Thyroid   2 - Adrenal   1 - Testis

THYROXINE   TESTOSTERONE
          CORTISOL

4 - Ovary

OESTROGEN

Stage I
Final (end-organ)
hormones

TSH   ACTH   FSH   LH

1 - Thyroid   2 - Adrenal   3 - Testis   4 - Ovary

1 - The pituitary gland is sensitive to hormone concentrations in plasma

5 - An increase in plasma thyroxine has an inhibitory effect on the pituitary

2 - A fall in the concentration of thyroxine

3 - The pituitary secretes thyrotrophin

4 - The thyroid gland is stimulated to produce more thyroxine

There is a still higher level of control: the pituitary in its turn is controlled by cells in the hypothalamus which secrete releasing factors, and there is a releasing factor for each type of trophic hormone. For example, thyrotrophin-releasing factor stimulates the release of thyrotrophin which in turn stimulates the thyroid gland to secrete thyroxine; the hypothalamus is sensitive to the concentrations of both thyrotrophin and thyroxine in the circulation, and modifies its secretion of releasing factor in response to changes in either hormone. The hypothalamus also provides a pathway for the central nervous system to influence the function of the endocrine system directly, though the extent to which this happens varies greatly from hormone to hormone.

1 - The pituitary is controlled by the cells of the hypothalamus

2 - Thyrotrophin releasing factor stimulates the release of thyrotrophin

4 - The hypothalamus also provides a pathway for the CNS to influence the function of the endocrine system

3 - This in turn stimulates the thyroid gland to produce thyroxine

This multi-level organization of the endocrine system allows for **amplification** of effect; a tiny amount of a releasing factor produced in the hypothalamus and liberated into the portal system causes the release of a much larger amount of the trophic hormone by the pituitary gland, which in turn causes the target gland to produce a very much larger amount of the final end-organ stimulating hormone.

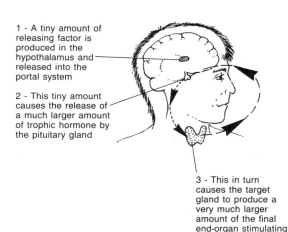

1 - A tiny amount of releasing factor is produced in the hypothalamus and released into the portal system

2 - This tiny amount causes the release of a much larger amount of trophic hormone by the pituitary gland

3 - This in turn causes the target gland to produce a very much larger amount of the final end-organ stimulating hormone

Not all of the endocrine glands are controlled in this hierarchical way. The parathyroid glands (regulating plasma calcium), the pancreas (producing insulin), the adrenal medulla (producing adrenaline) and the various parts of the gut (producing hormones to regulate motility and secretion) are outside the control of the pituitary gland, and some of the hormones of the pituitary gland itself are end-organ hormones rather than trophic hormones.

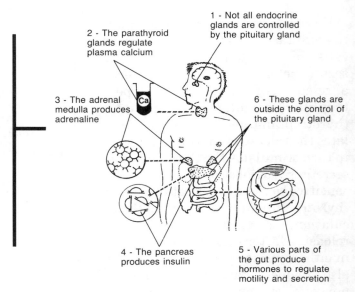

1 - Not all endocrine glands are controlled by the pituitary gland

2 - The parathyroid glands regulate plasma calcium

3 - The adrenal medulla produces adrenaline

6 - These glands are outside the control of the pituitary gland

4 - The pancreas produces insulin

5 - Various parts of the gut produce hormones to regulate motility and secretion

THE NATURE OF HORMONES

Most of the hormones belong to one of three classes: simple amines, peptides or steroids. The first group consists of relatively small molecules, usually related to amino acids, and including adrenaline and thyroxine (both derived from tyrosine).

The second group consists of small polypeptide molecules like insulin, the hypothalamic releasing factors and the hormones of the posterior pituitary, or larger peptides, almost proteins, like the anterior pituitary trophic hormones.

The third group consists of the steroids, lipid analogues of cholesterol, and includes the hormones from the adrenal cortex and the sex glands.

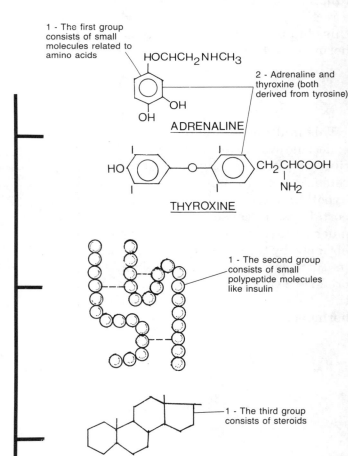

1 - The first group consists of small molecules related to amino acids

2 - Adrenaline and thyroxine (both derived from tyrosine)

ADRENALINE

THYROXINE

1 - The second group consists of small polypeptide molecules like insulin

1 - The third group consists of steroids

Many of the hormones, having a very complex molecular structure, take a long time to synthesize, so the cells produce them almost continuously and they are pre-packaged in vesicles which are stored in the cytoplasm (or in the case of the thyroid gland, in large follicles between cells). The action of the stimulant hormones or other trigger factors is thus to promote release of the pre-formed hormone.

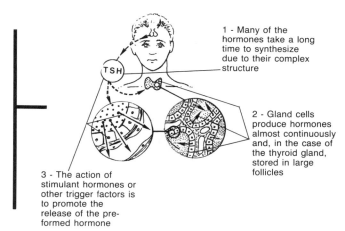

1 - Many of the hormones take a long time to synthesize due to their complex structure

2 - Gland cells produce hormones almost continuously and, in the case of the thyroid gland, stored in large follicles

3 - The action of stimulant hormones or other trigger factors is to promote the release of the pre-formed hormone

The exception to this is the steroid hormones, which are not stored but are synthesized right away as soon as the cells receive their signal from the trophic hormone or other trigger factor.

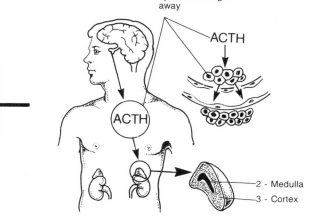

1 - Steroid hormones are not stored but are synthesized right away

2 - Medulla

3 - Cortex

4 - Hormones are synthesized as soon as the cells receive a signal from the trophic hormones

The modes of operation of the three classes of hormone are quite different. The simple amino acid derivatives often produce permeability changes at the cell membrane, causing ion movements and the resultant contraction of smooth muscle or secretion from exocrine glands. They work rather like neurotransmitters, and are often chemically related to them (for example, adrenaline is very like noradrenaline).

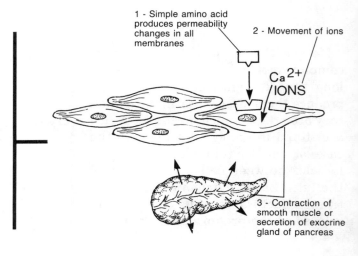

1 - Simple amino acid produces permeability changes in all membranes

2 - Movement of ions

Ca^{2+} / IONS

3 - Contraction of smooth muscle or secretion of exocrine gland of pancreas

Schematic diagram

The **peptides** act mainly by binding to specific receptors on the cell membrane, and stimulating the enzyme **adenyl cyclase**. This catalyses the conversion of adenosine triphosphate (ATP) to cyclic 3′,5′-adenosine monophosphate (cAMP), which acts as an intracellular second messenger (the first messenger is the hormone itself). Cyclic AMP triggers various intracellular events such as the transport of calcium, the activation of various metabolic pathways, or the release of other hormones. (Some of the simple amino acid type hormones also work in this way.)

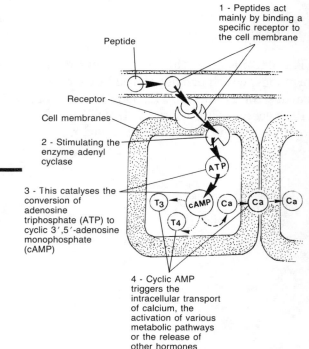

1 - Peptides act mainly by binding a specific receptor to the cell membrane

Peptide

Receptor

Cell membranes

2 - Stimulating the enzyme adenyl cyclase

3 - This catalyses the conversion of adenosine triphosphate (ATP) to cyclic 3′,5′-adenosine monophosphate (cAMP)

ATP

T_3 cAMP   Ca   Ca   Ca

T_4

4 - Cyclic AMP triggers the intracellular transport of calcium, the activation of various metabolic pathways or the release of other hormones

The steroids do not have receptors on the cell membrane; being lipids, they can diffuse across the membrane and into the cells, where they interact with their receptors which are located in or near the nucleus. They stimulate the nucleic acid systems, activating ribosomes to produce more proteins which perform various cellular regulatory functions. For example, extra enzymes can be made to promote glucose breakdown, or membrane transport protein can be made in order to increase ionic pumping.

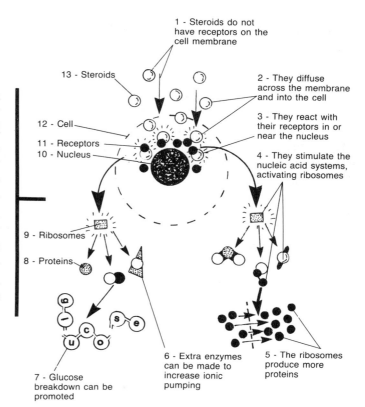

1 - Steroids do not have receptors on the cell membrane

2 - They diffuse across the membrane and into the cell

3 - They react with their receptors in or near the nucleus

4 - They stimulate the nucleic acid systems, activating ribosomes

5 - The ribosomes produce more proteins

6 - Extra enzymes can be made to increase ionic pumping

7 - Glucose breakdown can be promoted

8 - Proteins

9 - Ribosomes

10 - Nucleus

11 - Receptors

12 - Cell

13 - Steroids

The individual endocrine glands will now be described; discussion of the endocrine functions of the reproductive system will be found in the relevant chapter.

THE PITUITARY GLAND

The pituitary (meaning 'hanging down') is actually two separate glands with very different functions. The anterior lobe develops from an upward growth of the fetal pharynx and is called the **adenohypophysis**, while the posterior lobe is derived from a downward growth of the fetal brain and is called the **neurohypophysis**.

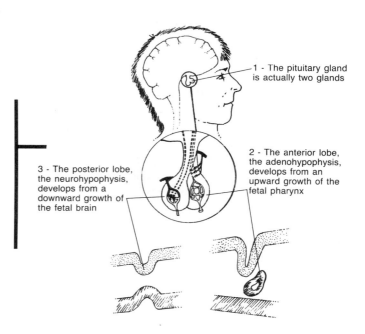

1 - The pituitary gland is actually two glands

2 - The anterior lobe, the adenohypophysis, develops from an upward growth of the fetal pharynx

3 - The posterior lobe, the neurohypophysis, develops from a downward growth of the fetal brain

The structures are quite different, the mechanisms of secretion are quite different, and the types of hormone and their functions are quite different. The two parts of the gland come together almost as an accident of development, and the posterior lobe remains attached to the brain by the pituitary stalk; this stalk is important in the function of both lobes, because it contains the axons of neurones which take part directly in the function of the posterior lobe, but it also contains capillaries which act as a portal system carrying releasing factors from the hypothalamus to the anterior lobe.

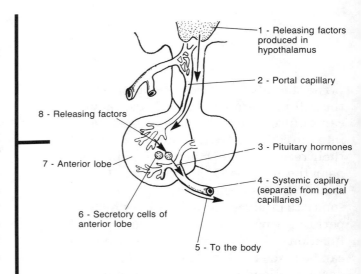

1 - Releasing factors produced in hypothalamus

2 - Portal capillary

8 - Releasing factors

3 - Pituitary hormones

7 - Anterior lobe

4 - Systemic capillary (separate from portal capillaries)

6 - Secretory cells of anterior lobe

5 - To the body

Posterior pituitary

The structure of the posterior lobe of the pituitary gland is unlike that of any other endocrine gland; instead of the highly cellular appearance typical of most endocrines, the neurohypophysis consists simply of neurones which originate in the supraoptic and paraventricular nuclei of the hypothalamus. The hypothalamic neurones synthesize the hormones which are then transported down microtubules in the axons of the pituitary stalk to lie in vesicles in the nerve terminals of the posterior lobe; this process can take several weeks.

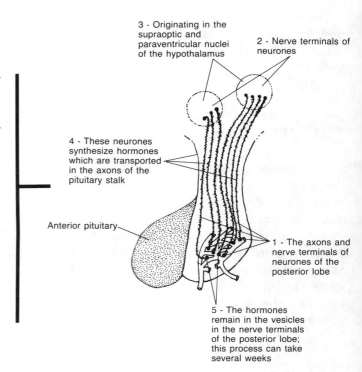

3 - Originating in the supraoptic and paraventricular nuclei of the hypothalamus

2 - Nerve terminals of neurones

4 - These neurones synthesize hormones which are transported in the axons of the pituitary stalk

Anterior pituitary

1 - The axons and nerve terminals of neurones of the posterior lobe

5 - The hormones remain in the vesicles in the nerve terminals of the posterior lobe; this process can take several weeks

Stimulation of the hypothalamic neurones by various influences causes action potentials to pass down the axons and release the hormones into the blood. The hormones are really neurotransmitters carried by the blood, and the process of their liberation is **neurosecretion**.

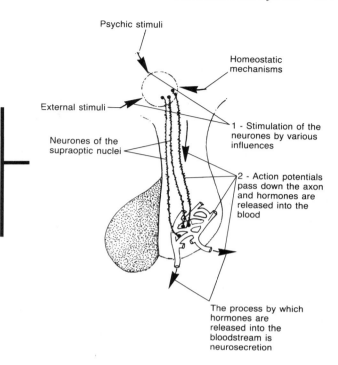

Psychic stimuli

Homeostatic mechanisms

External stimuli

Neurones of the supraoptic nuclei

1 - Stimulation of the neurones by various influences

2 - Action potentials pass down the axon and hormones are released into the blood

The process by which hormones are released into the bloodstream is neurosecretion

The hormones of the posterior pituitary are **oxytocin** and **vasopressin** (or antidiuretic hormone ADH). The function of antidiuretic hormone in regulating plasma osmolality is considered in the chapter on the kidney; the functions of oxytocin in regulating uterine motility and milk secretion are considered in the chapter on reproduction.

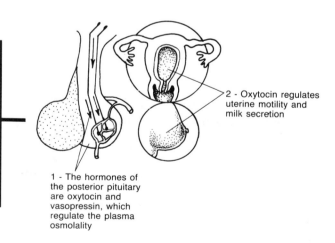

2 - Oxytocin regulates uterine motility and milk secretion

1 - The hormones of the posterior pituitary are oxytocin and vasopressin, which regulate the plasma osmolality

Both oxytocin and ADH are short-chain peptides consisting of eight amino acid residues; they function by promoting the formation of AMP in the target cells. In the kidney this alters the permeability of collecting ducts to water; in uterine muscle or the myo-epithelial cells of the mammary gland it enhances contractility. Since the two hormones are structurally very similar, it is not surprising that there is some overlap in their functions. ADH has an effect on smooth muscle, and its ability to constrict blood vessels is responsible for its other name, vasopressin. In fact it needs much higher concentrations of vasopressin than those normally found in plasma to cause much vasoconstriction.

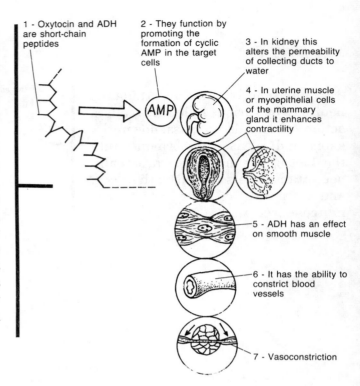

1 - Oxytocin and ADH are short-chain peptides

2 - They function by promoting the formation of cyclic AMP in the target cells

3 - In kidney this alters the permeability of collecting ducts to water

4 - In uterine muscle or myoepithelial cells of the mammary gland it enhances contractility

5 - ADH has an effect on smooth muscle

6 - It has the ability to constrict blood vessels

7 - Vasoconstriction

Deficient production of ADH results in **diabetes insipidus**, a condition in which there is excretion of copious watery urine and the inability to produce concentrated urine. In order to cope with an increased volume output of urine, there is permanent thirst, with the drinking of large volumes of fluid.

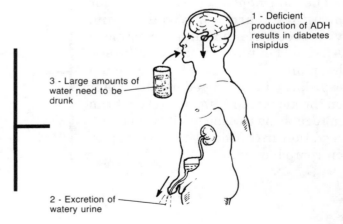

1 - Deficient production of ADH results in diabetes insipidus

3 - Large amounts of water need to be drunk

2 - Excretion of watery urine

Anterior pituitary

This gland produces a large number of hormones. Some of these are trophic hormones regulating other endocrine glands, and some are end-organ hormones producing their own specific effects on their target tissues.

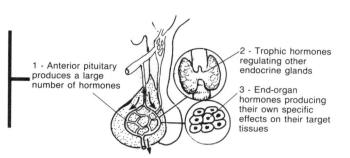

1 - Anterior pituitary produces a large number of hormones

2 - Trophic hormones regulating other endocrine glands

3 - End-organ hormones producing their own specific effects on their target tissues

The adenohypophysis has a structure typical of endocrine glands: the cells are arranged in clumps which are richly supplied with blood vessels. Three distinct cell types can be distinguished by normal histological techniques, although if specific histochemical methods are used it is possible to identify a separate cell type producing each hormone. The **acidophils** produce growth hormone and prolactin; the **basophils** produce luteinizing hormone, follicle-stimulating hormone and thyroid-stimulating hormone; the **chromophobes** (taking up neither acidic nor basic stains) produce adrenocortical-stimulating hormone.

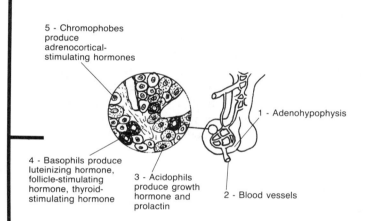

5 - Chromophobes produce adrenocortical-stimulating hormones

4 - Basophils produce luteinizing hormone, follicle-stimulating hormone, thyroid-stimulating hormone

3 - Acidophils produce growth hormone and prolactin

1 - Adenohypophysis

2 - Blood vessels

The hormones of the anterior pituitary are:

End-organ hormones — growth hormone (**GH**) melanocyte-stimulating hormone (**MSH**), prolactin;

Trophic hormones — thyroid-stimulating hormone (**TSH**), adrenocortical trophic hormone (**ACTH**), follicle-stimulating hormone (**FSH**) and luteinizing hormone (**LH**).

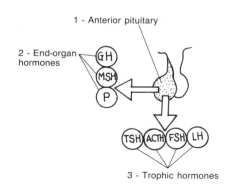

1 - Anterior pituitary

2 - End-organ hormones

3 - Trophic hormones

Growth hormone (somatotrophin) is a small peptide (188 amino acids) which stimulates growth in almost all tissues of the body. It stimulates both increase in cell size and cell division.

1 - Growth hormone is a small peptide

2 - It stimulates growth in all tissues

3 - Increase in cell size

4 - Cell division

In young individuals it promotes bone growth and increases stature, but once the epiphyses of the long bones have fused no further increase in height is possible; however, the width and thickness of bones can still increase, and growth of other tissues such as muscle is still possible.

1 - In young individuals it promotes bone growth and increases stature, but once the epiphyses of the long bones have fused no further increase in height is possible but the width and thickness of bones can still increase

2 - Growth of muscle is still possible

Growth hormone works by stimulating protein synthesis (enhancing amino acid transport into cells, increasing ribosomal activity and decreasing protein catabolism), reducing utilization of carbohydrate (so that the blood glucose concentration can rise, producing a form of diabetes) and mobilizing fats. It produces its effects on bone and cartilage indirectly by stimulating liver cells to produce **somatomedin**; in this respect the hormone is acting like a trophic hormone, although in most other respects it is an end-organ hormone.

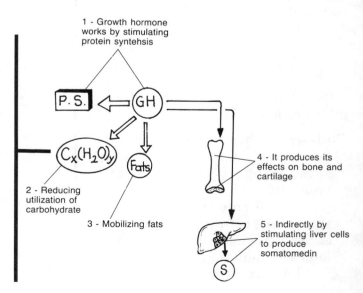

1 - Growth hormone works by stimulating protein syntehsis

P. S.

$C_x(H_2O)_y$

Fats

GH

2 - Reducing utilization of carbohydrate

3 - Mobilizing fats

4 - It produces its effects on bone and cartilage

5 - Indirectly by stimulating liver cells to produce somatomedin

S

Excess of growth hormone in a young person produces **gigantism**; some individuals have grown over seven feet tall. If the excessive secretion occurs after fusion of epiphyses has taken place then it produces **acromegaly**, with thickening of the jaw and skull bones and lengthening of the fingers and toes. Lack of growth hormone causes **dwarfism**.

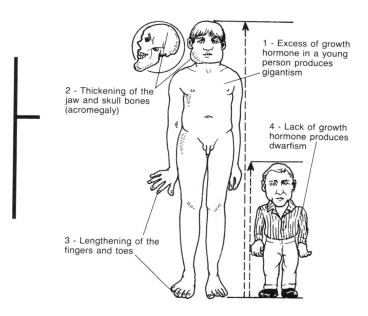

1 - Excess of growth hormone in a young person produces gigantism

2 - Thickening of the jaw and skull bones (acromegaly)

4 - Lack of growth hormone produces dwarfism

3 - Lengthening of the fingers and toes

The production of growth hormone is regulated by the hypothalamus; **growth hormone-releasing factor** is secreted into the portal capillaries by cells of the lateral ventromedial nucleus, and there is also a **growth hormone release inhibitory hormone** which counteracts the stimulant hormone. It is the balance between the action of these two factors which determines the secretion of growth hormone by the anterior pituitary.

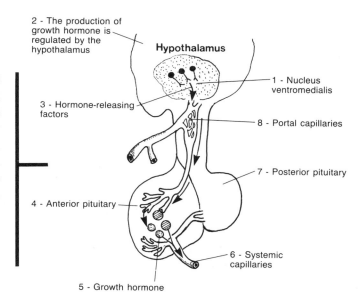

2 - The production of growth hormone is regulated by the hypothalamus

Hypothalamus

3 - Hormone-releasing factors

1 - Nucleus ventromedialis

8 - Portal capillaries

7 - Posterior pituitary

4 - Anterior pituitary

6 - Systemic capillaries

5 - Growth hormone

Melanocyte-stimulating hormone (**MSH**) has two forms, alpha and beta, which are short polypeptide chains of 13 and 22 amino acids respectively. It causes darkening of the skin by stimulating the melanin-producing cells between the epidermis and dermis. Its release is regulated by two hypothalamic hormones, MSH-releasing hormone (MRH) and MSH release inhibitory hormone (MRIH) which act in a reciprocal manner. The function and significance of the MSH system in man is not fully understood.

Prolactin is a protein (198 amino acids) whose release is regulated by prolactin inhibitory factor (PIF) from the hypothalamus. It promotes growth and development of the breasts in the female, and its concentration rises during pregnancy and during the period of infant feeding. Its functions will be discussed more fully in connection with the reproductive system.

Thyroid-stimulating hormone (**TSH**, thyrotrophin) is a glycoprotein with a molecular weight of 30 000. It stimulates the cells of the thyroid gland to produce thyroxine and triiodothyronine. Its release is regulated by **thyrotrophin-releasing factor** (or hormone, **TRH**) from cells in the paraventricular area of the hypothalamus, and by a feedback control mechanism in response to circulating levels of thyroid hormones.

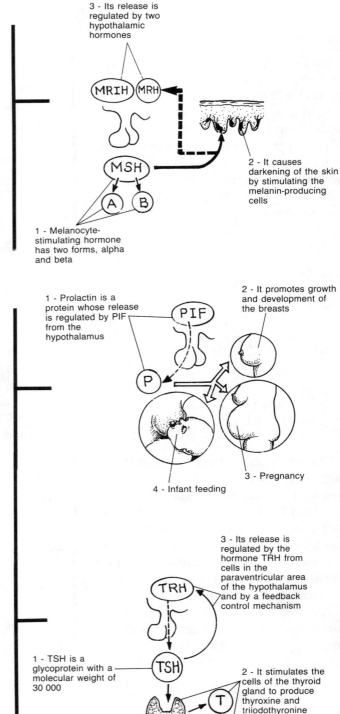

3 - Its release is regulated by two hypothalamic hormones

2 - It causes darkening of the skin by stimulating the melanin-producing cells

1 - Melanocyte-stimulating hormone has two forms, alpha and beta

1 - Prolactin is a protein whose release is regulated by PIF from the hypothalamus

2 - It promotes growth and development of the breasts

3 - Pregnancy

4 - Infant feeding

3 - Its release is regulated by the hormone TRH from cells in the paraventricular area of the hypothalamus and by a feedback control mechanism

1 - TSH is a glycoprotein with a molecular weight of 30 000

2 - It stimulates the cells of the thyroid gland to produce thyroxine and triiodothyronine

The nervous system has a link with the endocrine system in the production of TRH, and in many animals a decrease in the temperature of the body's core or of the environment can trigger the release of TRH, TSH and thyroxine to stimulate metabolic heat production.

Adrenocortical trophic hormone (ACTH, corticotrophin) is a short polypeptide (39 amino acids) which stimulates secretion of steroids by the cells of the adrenal cortex. Its release is controlled by **corticotrophin-releasing factor (CRF)** from the posterior part of the hypothalamus, and is also subject to feedback control based on the levels of circulating corticosteroids.

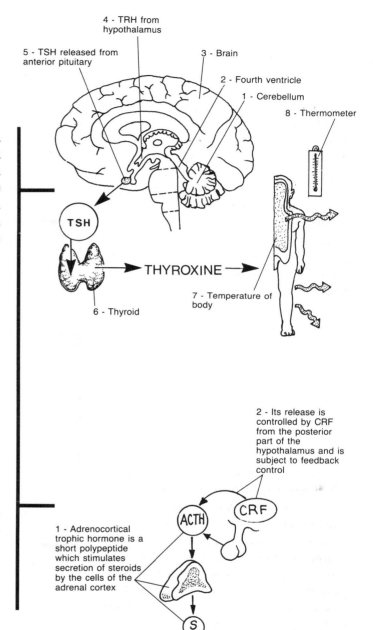

4 - TRH from hypothalamus

5 - TSH released from anterior pituitary

3 - Brain

2 - Fourth ventricle

1 - Cerebellum

8 - Thermometer

TSH

THYROXINE

7 - Temperature of body

6 - Thyroid

2 - Its release is controlled by CRF from the posterior part of the hypothalamus and is subject to feedback control

1 - Adrenocortical trophic hormone is a short polypeptide which stimulates secretion of steroids by the cells of the adrenal cortex

ACTH

CRF

S

There is a considerable circadian variation in blood concentrations of ACTH and consequently of cortisol; the rhythm is presumably dictated by the hypothalamus, which is in turn influenced by a number of environmental triggering factors such as day and night, or cycles of rest and activity. The occurrence of stress such as illness, trauma or surgery is also communicated to the hypothalamus with consequent increase in the activity of the pituitary—andrenocortical axis.

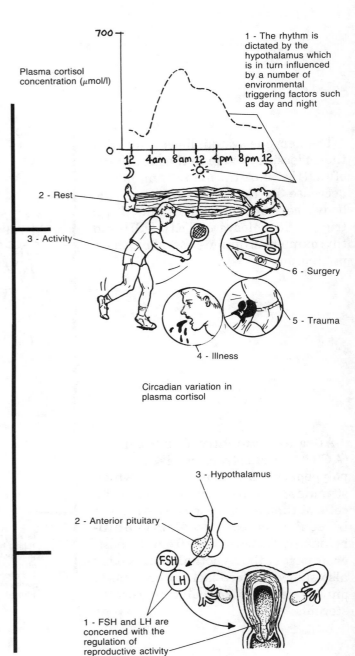

Plasma cortisol concentration (μmol/l)

700

12   4am   8am   12   4pm   8pm   12

1 - The rhythm is dictated by the hypothalamus which is in turn influenced by a number of environmental triggering factors such as day and night

2 - Rest

3 - Activity

6 - Surgery

5 - Trauma

4 - Illness

Circadian variation in plasma cortisol

Follicle-stimulating hormone (FSH) and **luteinizing hormone (LH)** are concerned with the regulation of reproductive activity, and are discussed in more detail in the chapter on the reproductive system. Like most of the other hormones of the anterior pituitary, they are small proteins whose release is regulated by hypothalamic releasing or inhibitory factors.

3 - Hypothalamus

2 - Anterior pituitary

FSH

LH

1 - FSH and LH are concerned with the regulation of reproductive activity

THE THYROID GLAND

The metabolic rate of most of the tissues in the body is regulated by the hormones of the thyroid gland. This is a centrally placed organ, located in the neck just below the larynx and in front of the trachea. It has a rather granular texture and a very high blood flow. Its histological structure is unlike that of other endocrine glands: it consists of clumps of cuboidal epithelial cells surrounding **follicles** containing a specialized protein, **thyroglobulin**. The cells secrete the protein into the follicles, and the thyroid hormones are made in the follicles, attached to the protein; when the body needs more thyroid hormones they are recovered by the epithelial cells from their storage site in the follicles and liberated into the circulation.

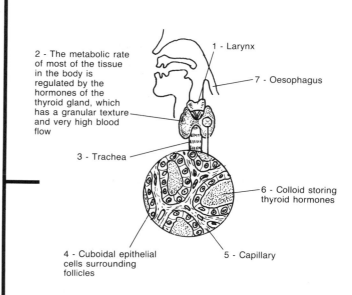

1 - Larynx

2 - The metabolic rate of most of the tissue in the body is regulated by the hormones of the thyroid gland, which has a granular texture and very high blood flow

7 - Oesophagus

3 - Trachea

6 - Colloid storing thyroid hormones

4 - Cuboidal epithelial cells surrounding follicles

5 - Capillary

The hormones of the thyroid gland are a series of iodinated amino acids, principally **triiodothyronine** (T_3) and **thyroxine** (tetraiodothyronine, T_4). These substances have a strong stimulant effect on the metabolic rate of almost all cells in the body; T_3 has a stronger stimulant effect and a more rapid onset of action than T_4, but it is present at lower concentrations in the blood and has a shorter-lasting effect, and therefore thyroxine or T_4 is the predominant thyroid hormone in the blood.

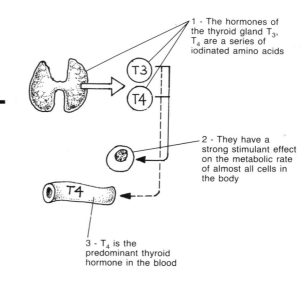

1 - The hormones of the thyroid gland T_3, T_4 are a series of iodinated amino acids

2 - They have a strong stimulant effect on the metabolic rate of almost all cells in the body

3 - T_4 is the predominant thyroid hormone in the blood

There are several important stages in the synthesis of thyroid hormones. The first of these is the **trapping** of iodine. Dietary iodine is almost always in the form of iodide ions, and these are absorbed in the gut. A large proportion (66%) of the ingested iodide is lost in the urine, but almost all of the iodide that remains within the body is trapped in the thyroid. The cells take up the iodide ions, concentrating them about 25 times (or, at peak activity, up to 350 times) and converting them to un-ionized iodine. This requires the enzyme **peroxidase**.

1 - There are several important stages in the synthesis of thyroid hormones. The first of these is the trapping of iodine

SYNTHESIS T.H.

I

2 - Iodide ions are absorbed in the gut

3 - 66% of the ingested iodide is lost in the urine

4 - The remaining iodine within the body is trapped in the thyroid

+ P

U.I.

5 - The cells convert them to un-ionized iodine; this requires the enzyme peroxidase

The second stage is the synthesis of thyroglobulin; this is a secretory product of the thyroid cells, which deposits large quantities of the protein within the follicles. The next stage is the secretion of iodine into the follicles, where it becomes mixed with the thyroglobulin. There now follows the enzymatic iodination of specific amino acids (thyrosine) actually incorporated within the thyroglobulin protein.

2 - Capillary

3 - Cuboidal cells secrete both protein (as amino acids) and iodine

PROTEIN
IODINE
IODINATION OF AMINO ACIDS

1 - Follicle or large area between cuboidal cells

4 - The iodination of amino acids results in the formation of thyroglobulin

The stages are:

conversion of tyrosine to monoiodotyrosine (T_1) and diiodotyrosine (T_2); combination of one molecule of T_2 with either T_1 or T_2 to form T_3 or T_4.

The T_3 or T_4 remain locked in the thyroglobulin molecule as amino acid residues, joined to other amino acids, until required by the body.

When extra thyroid hormones are required the thyroid cells perform pinocytosis — pinching off vesicles containing thyroglobulin from the follicular surface; to these are added proteolytic enzymes (from lysosomal vesicles) which break off the iodinated amino acids from the main protein. The active thyroid hormones are discharged into the capillaries to be carried to the rest of the body. Once they reach the plasma the hormones rapidly become bound to carrier proteins such as albumin; the concentration of free thyroid hormones in the plasma and tissue fluid is rather low, and the protein-bound thyroid hormones remain in the plasma for a long time.

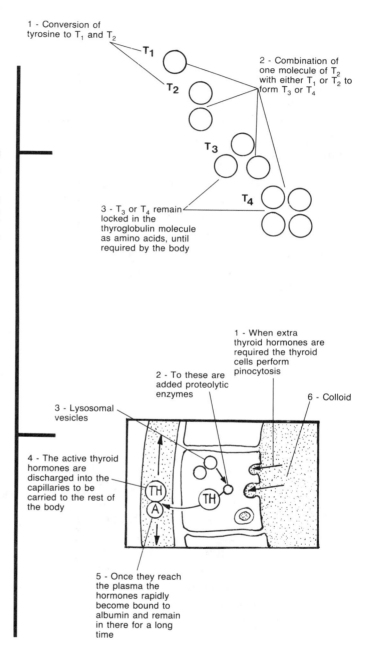

1 - Conversion of tyrosine to T_1 and T_2

2 - Combination of one molecule of T_2 with either T_1 or T_2 to form T_3 or T_4

3 - T_3 or T_4 remain locked in the thyroglobulin molecule as amino acids, until required by the body

1 - When extra thyroid hormones are required the thyroid cells perform pinocytosis

2 - To these are added proteolytic enzymes

6 - Colloid

3 - Lysosomal vesicles

4 - The active thyroid hormones are discharged into the capillaries to be carried to the rest of the body

5 - Once they reach the plasma the hormones rapidly become bound to albumin and remain in there for a long time

Actions of thyroid hormones

The thyroid hormones have a general stimulant effect upon metabolism. The **basal metabolic rate** (**BMR**) can be measured by recording the rate of oxygen consumption of the fasting resting subject lying quietly in a thermoneutral room; thyroxine or T_3 can stimulate the BMR to increase 60–100% above the normal value. The measurement of BMR was often used as a diagnostic test for hyper- or hypothyroidism before sensitive chemical tests for the hormones became available, but the BMR is so variable from subject to subject, and is susceptible to so many sources of error, that it is not often used as a clinical test nowadays.

The mechanism whereby the hormones stimulate cellular metabolism are still not fully known, but in many cells they stimulate adenyl cyclase producing intracellular cAMP. Many cells undergo increased protein synthesis; many cellular enzymes increase in concentration, particularly those involved in energy release (for example, those contributing to degradation of carbohydrate); the mitochondria of many cells increase in size and number; there is a stimulant effect on bone growth (though the epiphyses can be provoked to fuse at an earlier age than normal, so that long-term stature may be decreased).

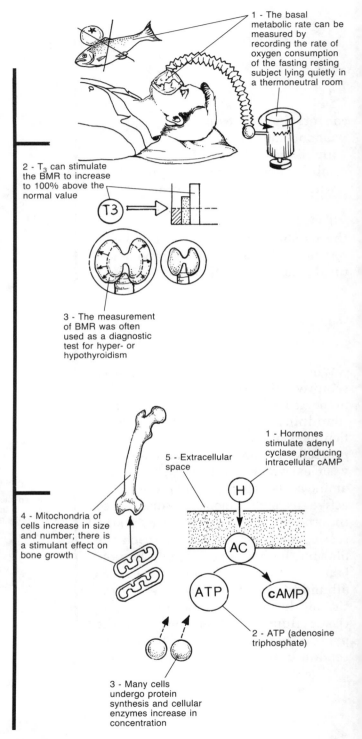

1 - The basal metabolic rate can be measured by recording the rate of oxygen consumption of the fasting resting subject lying quietly in a thermoneutral room

2 - T_3 can stimulate the BMR to increase to 100% above the normal value

3 - The measurement of BMR was often used as a diagnostic test for hyper- or hypothyroidism

1 - Hormones stimulate adenyl cyclase producing intracellular cAMP

5 - Extracellular space

4 - Mitochondria of cells increase in size and number; there is a stimulant effect on bone growth

2 - ATP (adenosine triphosphate)

3 - Many cells undergo protein synthesis and cellular enzymes increase in concentration

The increased rate of metabolism in tissues stimulated by the thyroid causes increased peripheral blood flow and therefore greater demands upon the heart; there is a reflex stimulant effect on cardiac output. There is probably also a direct stimulant effect of the hormones on the heart, causing increased force and rate of beating.

1 - Increased rate of metabolism in tissues stimulated by the thyroid causes increased blood flow and great demands upon the heart

2 - Cardiac output

3 - Increased force and rate of heart beat

Patients with deficiency of thyroid hormones, caused either by an inadequate dietary intake of iodine or by primary thyroid disease, have a depressed metabolism. Hypothyroid children have stunted growth and development, and congenitally hypothyroid infants become mentally retarded; they are called **cretins**.

All hypothyroid individuals are sluggish; they tend to feel the cold because they do not generate enough internal metabolic heat; they have a slow heart rate and a low cardiac output. They tend to become overweight despite a poor appetite.

1 - Patients with thyroid deficiency have a depressed metabolism

5 - Depressed appetite

4 - Cretin with stunted growth and poor mental development

2 - They feel the cold

3 - Overweight and sluggish

There is a feature of the clinical syndrome that is not so easy to explain in metabolic terms; this is **myxoedema**, the deposition of glycoprotein in many of the tissues. There is a coarsening of the features, with a thickening of the skin and a non-pitting oedema of the subcutaneous tissue.

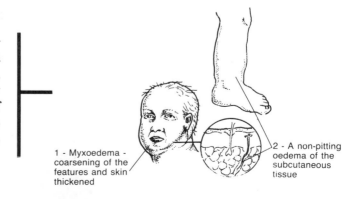

1 - Myxoedema - coarsening of the features and skin thickened

2 - A non-pitting oedema of the subcutaneous tissue

Overactivity of the thyroid gland, or **thyrotoxicosis**, can be caused by benign or malignant tumours of the thyroid gland. It can also be caused by an autoimmune inflammatory disease of the gland, which first stimulates activity, and then, as the gland becomes progressively damaged, produces the hypothyroid state. Thyrotoxicosis is characterized by hyperactivity and excitability, with a raised metabolic rate and therefore overproduction of heat. The patient feels hot and sweaty, and there is a tendency to weight loss despite a voracious appetite. The circulation is hyperdynamic, with dilated peripheries, a bounding rapid pulse and high cardiac output, and there is a rapid tremor of the muscles.

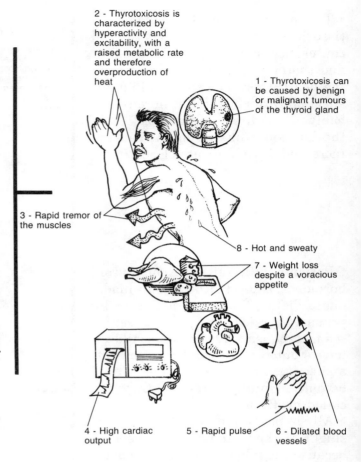

2 - Thyrotoxicosis is characterized by hyperactivity and excitability, with a raised metabolic rate and therefore overproduction of heat

1 - Thyrotoxicosis can be caused by benign or malignant tumours of the thyroid gland

3 - Rapid tremor of the muscles

8 - Hot and sweaty

7 - Weight loss despite a voracious appetite

4 - High cardiac output

5 - Rapid pulse

6 - Dilated blood vessels

A feature which is difficult to explain in terms of increased metabolic rate is **exophthalmos**, the protrusion of the eyeballs due to the deposition of mucopolysaccharides at the back of the orbit. In severe cases the protrusion is so great that the eyelids cannot close and corneal ulceration can result.

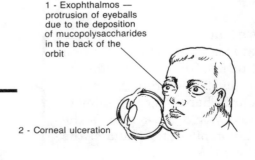

1 - Exophthalmos — protrusion of eyeballs due to the deposition of mucopolysaccharides in the back of the orbit

2 - Corneal ulceration

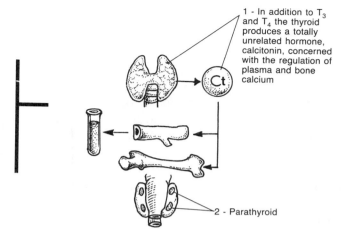

1 - In addition to T_3 and T_4 the thyroid produces a totally unrelated hormone, calcitonin, concerned with the regulation of plasma and bone calcium

2 - Parathyroid

In addition to T_3 and T_4, the thyroid produces a totally unrelated hormone, **calcitonin** concerned with the regulation of plasma and bone calcium. Its function will be considered in conjunction with that of the parathyroid glands a little later.

Control of thyroid secretion

The function of the thyroid gland is under the control of thyroid-stimulating hormone (**TSH**; thyrotrophin) released by the anterior pituitary gland. **TSH** stimulates a number of stages in the production of thyroxine and T_3: it increases iodine trapping by the thyroid cells, it increases the deposition of thyroglobulin in the follicles, it stimulates the enzymes for iodination of tyramine in the follicles, and it stimulates the pinocytotic uptake of thyroglobulin by the thyroid cells for extraction of the active amino acids and release of the hormones into the capillaries.

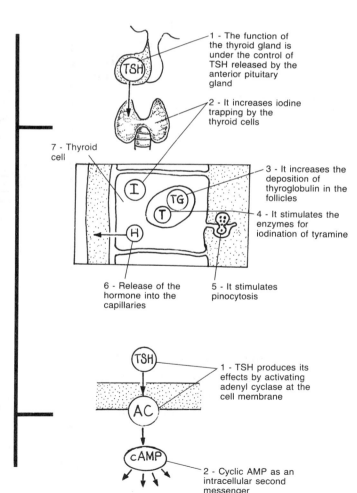

1 - The function of the thyroid gland is under the control of TSH released by the anterior pituitary gland

2 - It increases iodine trapping by the thyroid cells

7 - Thyroid cell

3 - It increases the deposition of thyroglobulin in the follicles

4 - It stimulates the enzymes for iodination of tyramine

6 - Release of the hormone into the capillaries

5 - It stimulates pinocytosis

TSH produces its effects by activating adenyl cyclase at the cell membrane; this causes the production of **AMP** as an intracellular second messenger which triggers the various biochemical events described above.

1 - TSH produces its effects by activating adenyl cyclase at the cell membrane

2 - Cyclic AMP as an intracellular second messenger

The rate of production of **TSH** is subject to feedback regulation by the level of circulating thyroxine and T_3; as the level of hormones rises, the production of **TSH** decreases, and as the level of thyroxine or T_3 falls, the secretion of TSH rises to stimulate the thyroid gland to produce more hormone.

The concentrations of T_3 and T_4 in the plasma also affect the secretion of thyrotrophin-releasing factor (**TRF**) from the hypothalamus: this is called 'long-loop' feedback control, where an organ two levels lower in the hierarchy is controlling a higher-order organ.

'Short-loop' feedback is where an organ just one level lower is controlling the higher organ, such as the control of **TSH** release from the pituitary by the concentration of thyroxine from the thyroid.

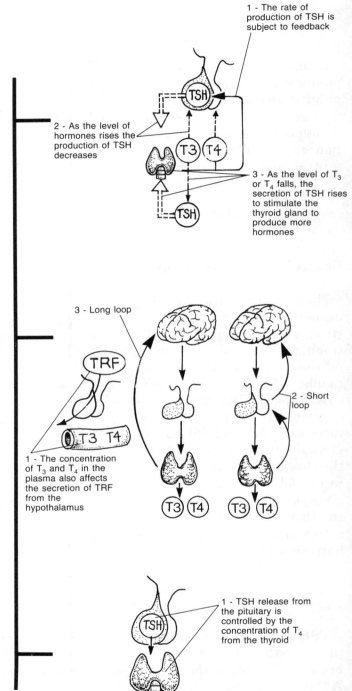

1 - The rate of production of TSH is subject to feedback

2 - As the level of hormones rises the production of TSH decreases

3 - As the level of T_3 or T_4 falls, the secretion of TSH rises to stimulate the thyroid gland to produce more hormones

3 - Long loop

2 - Short loop

1 - The concentration of T_3 and T_4 in the plasma also affects the secretion of TRF from the hypothalamus

1 - TSH release from the pituitary is controlled by the concentration of T_4 from the thyroid

If the thyroid malfunctions and is unable to produce enough hormones, the pituitary is provoked into producing extra TSH in an attempt to stimulate the thyroid gland. For instance if the diet is deficient in iodine, the thyroid cannot iodinate tyrosine and insufficient hormone is produced. The low level of circulating thyroid hormones provokes the pituitary to produce large amounts of **TSH**, stimulating the thyroid cells to secrete large amounts of thyroglobulin. This accumulates in enormously distended follicles, resulting in a hugely swollen gland, a **goitre**. The gland is extremely active, producing vast quantities of totally useless thyroglobulin. The patients are clinically hypothyroid; the condition is readily reversed by oral administration of iodine, and this is most conveniently achieved by adding small quantities of sodium iodide to the cooking salt.

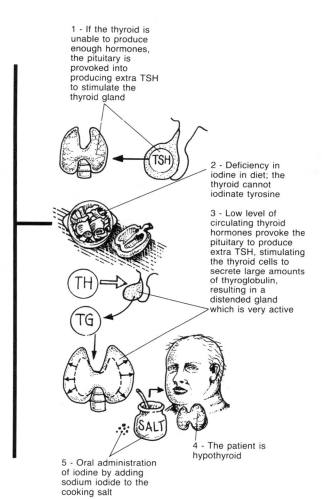

1 - If the thyroid is unable to produce enough hormones, the pituitary is provoked into producing extra TSH to stimulate the thyroid gland

2 - Deficiency in iodine in diet; the thyroid cannot iodinate tyrosine

3 - Low level of circulating thyroid hormones provoke the pituitary to produce extra TSH, stimulating the thyroid cells to secrete large amounts of thyroglobulin, resulting in a distended gland which is very active

4 - The patient is hypothyroid

5 - Oral administration of iodine by adding sodium iodide to the cooking salt

THE ADRENAL GLANDS

There are two adrenal (suprarenal) glands, one situated at the superior pole of each kidney. Each gland consists of two parts, a cortex and medulla, which are functionally quite separate and arise from quite different embryonic structures. The cortex develops from the coelomic epithelium of the primitive mesoderm, while the medulla is derived from the neural tube and is structurally and functionally related to the ganglia of the sympathetic chain.

Adrenal medulla

The functions of the medulla have largely been described in connection with the autonomic nervous system. The hormones of the medulla are the **catecholamines** noradrenaline and adrenaline, made from phenylalanine and tyrosine; the gland produces four times as much adrenaline as nor-adrenaline (in the USA these hormones are called epinephrine and norepin-ephrine).

The hormones are pre-formed and stored in granules in the ganglion cells, and are secreted directly into the adrenal vessels during the release of acetylcholine (nicotinic effect) following excitation of the sympathetic pre-ganglionic fibres.

The catecholamines are eventually broken down by the enzymes **monoamine oxidase (MAO)** and **catechol O-methyl transferase (COMT)**, found both in the tissues and in the blood.

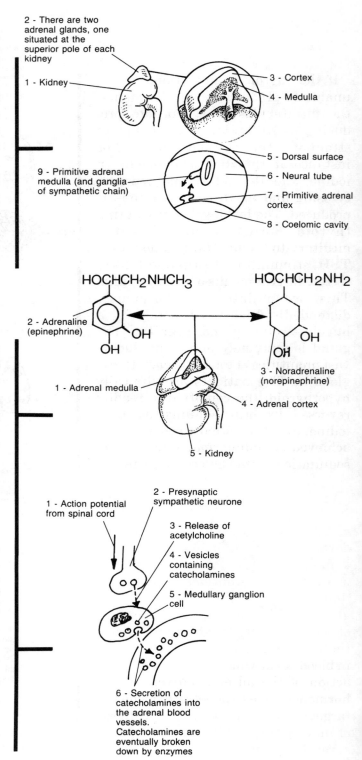

2 - There are two adrenal glands, one situated at the superior pole of each kidney

1 - Kidney

3 - Cortex

4 - Medulla

9 - Primitive adrenal medulla (and ganglia of sympathetic chain)

5 - Dorsal surface

6 - Neural tube

7 - Primitive adrenal cortex

8 - Coelomic cavity

$HOCHCH_2NHCH_3$

$HOCHCH_2NH_2$

2 - Adrenaline (epinephrine)

3 - Noradrenaline (norepinephrine)

1 - Adrenal medulla

4 - Adrenal cortex

5 - Kidney

1 - Action potential from spinal cord

2 - Presynaptic sympathetic neurone

3 - Release of acetylcholine

4 - Vesicles containing catecholamines

5 - Medullary ganglion cell

6 - Secretion of catecholamines into the adrenal blood vessels. Catecholamines are eventually broken down by enzymes

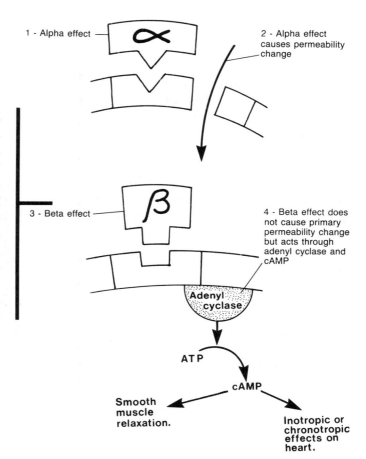

1 - Alpha effect

2 - Alpha effect causes permeability change

3 - Beta effect

4 - Beta effect does not cause primary permeability change but acts through adenyl cyclase and cAMP

Adenyl cyclase

ATP

cAMP

Smooth muscle relaxation.

Inotropic or chronotropic effects on heart.

The distinction has already been made between the alpha and beta effects of catecholamines; most alpha effects are manifest as permeability changes at cell membranes, while most beta effects are mediated by activating adenyl cyclase to produce **AMP**. This regulates the translocation of calcium ions across the membrane of smooth muscle cells, causing relaxation, has positive inotropic and chronotropic effects on the myocardium, and has other important metabolic effects.

In the liver it promotes the breakdown of glycogen to glucose, and thus it makes metabolic substrate rapidly available for situations of 'fight or flight'. This rapid mobilization of glucose, which can happen in a matter of seconds, should be contrasted with the slower but more sustained increase in blood sugar which is produced by the action of the adrenal **cortex**, whose hormones have to penetrate inside the target cells and stimulate the synthesis of new protein, all of which takes several minutes or hours.

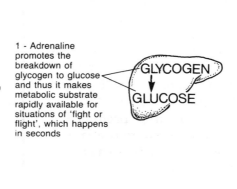

1 - Adrenaline promotes the breakdown of glycogen to glucose and thus it makes metabolic substrate rapidly available for situations of 'fight or flight', which happens in seconds

GLYCOGEN

GLUCOSE

Adrenal cortex

The cortex consists of three structurally separate zones, each of which produces a different group of hormones. The outermost layer, the **zona glomerulosa**, has its cells arranged in small clumps like glomeruli, with a dense supply of capillaries running between the clumps. This structure is very similar to the 'typical' endocrine gland described earlier. The next layer, the **zona fasciculata**, consists of long thin columns or fascicles of cells, with capillaries running in between the columns. The third layer, the **zona reticularis**, has its cells arranged in shorter interlocking cords, forming a network (or reticulum). All of the layers are richly supplied with capillaries to carry away their hormones.

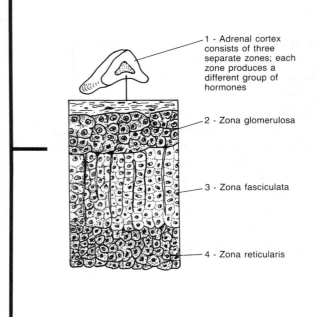

1 - Adrenal cortex consists of three separate zones; each zone produces a different group of hormones

2 - Zona glomerulosa

3 - Zona fasciculata

4 - Zona reticularis

The hormones produced by the adrenal cortex are all **steroids**, derived from the cholesterol molecule. Some forty different steroids have been isolated from human adrenal cortex. They differ from one another in minor detail, having slightly different side-chains and radicals at various places on the molecule, but these small changes can result in enormous changes in the hormones' biological properties and activity. The two hormones which are produced in greatest quantity are **aldosterone** and **cortisol**, and these are functionally the most important.

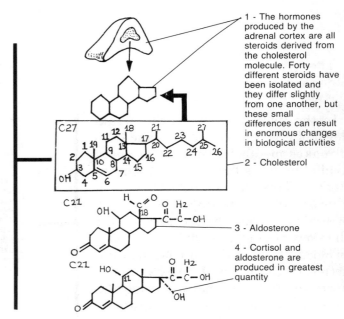

1 - The hormones produced by the adrenal cortex are all steroids derived from the cholesterol molecule. Forty different steroids have been isolated and they differ slightly from one another, but these small differences can result in enormous changes in biological activities

2 - Cholesterol

3 - Aldosterone

4 - Cortisol and aldosterone are produced in greatest quantity

The hormones of the zona glomerulosa are **mineralocorticoids**; they control the metabolism of minerals or inorganic materials. The chief hormone is **aldosterone**, whose actions in regulating transport of sodium and potassium by the kidney tubules are described elsewhere. Briefly, aldosterone promotes the reabsorption of sodium by the distal convoluted tubule, with the excretion of potassium.

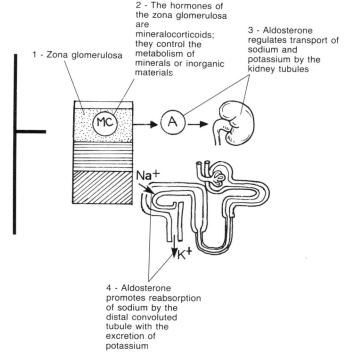

1 - Zona glomerulosa

2 - The hormones of the zona glomerulosa are mineralocorticoids; they control the metabolism of minerals or inorganic materials

3 - Aldosterone regulates transport of sodium and potassium by the kidney tubules

4 - Aldosterone promotes reabsorption of sodium by the distal convoluted tubule with the excretion of potassium

The synthesis and release of aldosterone is controlled by a number of factors: a rise in the plasma concentration of potassium stimulates aldosterone production, resulting in enhanced secretion of K^+ by the distal renal tubule; angiotensin produced as a result of renin release from the kidney stimulates production of aldosterone with consequent retention of sodium and water and excretion of potassium.

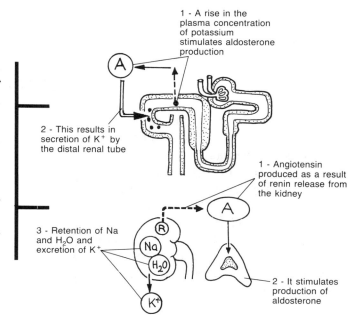

1 - A rise in the plasma concentration of potassium stimulates aldosterone production

2 - This results in secretion of K^+ by the distal renal tube

1 - Angiotensin produced as a result of renin release from the kidney

3 - Retention of Na and H_2O and excretion of K^+

2 - It stimulates production of aldosterone

ACTH from the anterior pituitary gland has a small stimulant effect on the release of aldosterone, but the trophic hormone is by no means essential for the control of this system.

1 - ACTH from the pituitary gland has a small stimulant effect on the release of aldosterone

The hormones of the zona fasciculata are the **glucocorticoids**; they regulate the metabolism of glucose and other organic materials. The most important hormone of this group is **cortisol**, or hydrocortisone. The main function of these hormones is to promote glucose production, largely by **gluconeogenesis** or the synthesis of glucose from new sources such as amino acids. They also promote the breakdown of fats and the dephosphorylation of glucose 6-phosphate, so that the blood sugar concentration becomes increased; glucocorticoids are said to have an anti-insulin function.

Glucocorticoids seem to be important in mediating the body's metabolic responses to stress (such as trauma or surgery), presumably by making glucose available from many sources. They also reduce the intensity of inflammatory and allergic responses by stabilizing cell and lysosomal membranes so that mast cells and other inflammatory cells are less easily degranulated.

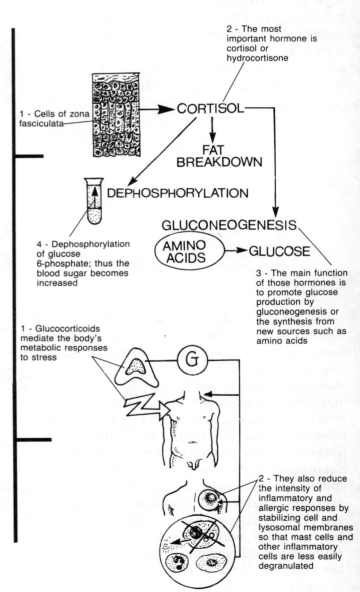

1 - Cells of zona fasciculata

2 - The most important hormone is cortisol or hydrocortisone

CORTISOL

FAT BREAKDOWN

DEPHOSPHORYLATION

GLUCONEOGENESIS

AMINO ACIDS → GLUCOSE

3 - The main function of those hormones is to promote glucose production by gluconeogenesis or the synthesis from new sources such as amino acids

4 - Dephosphorylation of glucose 6-phosphate; thus the blood sugar becomes increased

1 - Glucocorticoids mediate the body's metabolic responses to stress

2 - They also reduce the intensity of inflammatory and allergic responses by stabilizing cell and lysosomal membranes so that mast cells and other inflammatory cells are less easily degranulated

Hormones of this group rarely have a pure glucocorticoid activity, but usually have some effect on mineral metabolism as well; as a consequence, if the hormones are being administered therapeutically for some desired metabolic or anti-inflammatory effect, they often produce unwanted side-effects like salt and water retention.

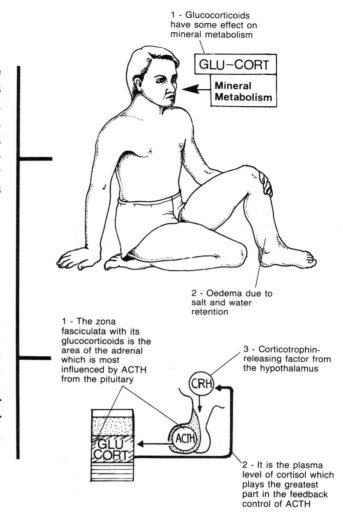

1 - Glucocorticoids have some effect on mineral metabolism

GLU-CORT
Mineral Metabolism

2 - Oedema due to salt and water retention

The zona fasciculata, with its glucocorticoids, is the area of the adrenal which is most influenced by **ACTH** from the pituitary; it is the plasma level of cortisol which plays the greatest part in the feedback control of ACTH release and the production of corticotrophin-releasing factor from the hypothalamus.

1 - The zona fasciculata with its glucocorticoids is the area of the adrenal which is most influenced by ACTH from the pituitary

3 - Corticotrophin-releasing factor from the hypothalamus

CRH

ACTH

GLU CORT

2 - It is the plasma level of cortisol which plays the greatest part in the feedback control of ACTH

Many of the other endocrine glands have prominent granules in their cells, and store their hormone in pre-packaged form for subsequent release. The cells of the adrenal cortex have no such storage granules; the hormones have to be synthesized as and when they are needed, and the function of **ACTH** is to activate adenyl cyclase to produce AMP, which acts as an intracellular second messenger, promoting the various cellular reactions involved in steroid synthesis.

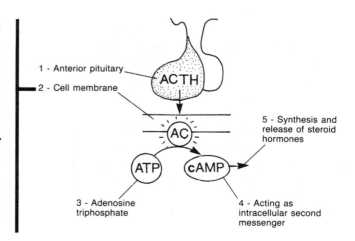

1 - Anterior pituitary
2 - Cell membrane

ACTH

AC

ATP

cAMP

5 - Synthesis and release of steroid hormones

3 - Adenosine triphosphate

4 - Acting as intracellular second messenger

The output of steroids from the cortex occurs several minutes after ACTH is first applied.

The hormones of the zona reticularis are the **sex hormones**, predominantly the **androgens** or male sex hormones. These are present in both sexes, and produce male secondary sexual characteristics such as facial hair growth, increased muscle bulk and aggressive behavioural tendencies.

In the female their activity is largely counteracted by the female hormones produced by the ovaries, though the adrenal remains the only source of some essential androgens.

In the male they augment the sex hormones produced by the testes. The androgens as a group have metabolic effects which are opposite to those of the glucocorticoids; they are **anabolic** or body-building steroids whereas the glucocorticoids are **catabolic** or breaking-down steroids.

There is very little effect of **ACTH** on the rate of production or release of androgens from the zona reticularis. Androgens have little influence on the rate of release of ACTH or of corticitrophin-releasing factor.

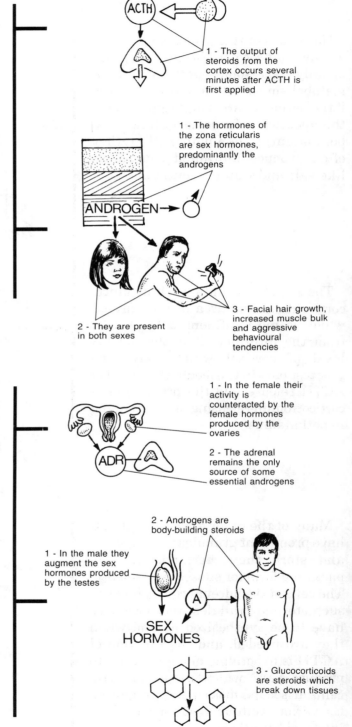

1 - The output of steroids from the cortex occurs several minutes after ACTH is first applied

1 - The hormones of the zona reticularis are sex hormones, predominantly the androgens

ANDROGEN →

2 - They are present in both sexes

3 - Facial hair growth, increased muscle bulk and aggressive behavioural tendencies

1 - In the female their activity is counteracted by the female hormones produced by the ovaries

ADR

2 - The adrenal remains the only source of some essential androgens

2 - Androgens are body-building steroids

1 - In the male they augment the sex hormones produced by the testes

A

SEX HORMONES

3 - Glucocorticoids are steroids which break down tissues

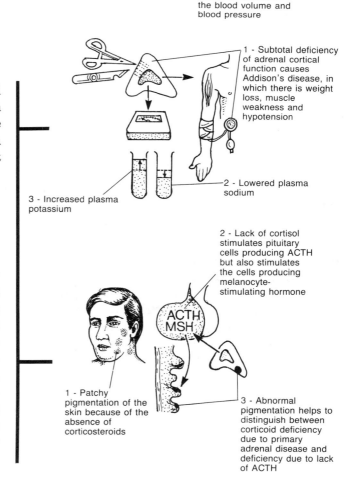

1 - If the adrenal cortex is diseased and its production of hormones is deficient

2 - Total removal of the cortex results in death

3 - In the absence of aldosterone the body loses sodium and is unable to maintain the blood volume and blood pressure

If the adrenal cortex is diseased and its production of hormones is deficient, certain well-recognized clinical effects occur. Total removal of the cortex results in death within a few days, the most important deficiency being that of aldosterone. In its absence, the body loses sodium and is unable to maintain the blood volume and blood pressure.

1 - Subtotal deficiency of adrenal cortical function causes Addison's disease, in which there is weight loss, muscle weakness and hypotension

2 - Lowered plasma sodium

3 - Increased plasma potassium

Subtotal deficiency of adrenal cortical function causes **Addison's** disease, in which there is weight loss, muscle weakness and hypotension, with a lowered plasma sodium and a slight increase in plasma potassium.

2 - Lack of cortisol stimulates pituitary cells producing ACTH but also stimulates the cells producing melanocyte-stimulating hormone

ACTH MSH

1 - Patchy pigmentation of the skin because of the absence of corticosteroids

3 - Abnormal pigmentation helps to distinguish between corticoid deficiency due to primary adrenal disease and deficiency due to lack of ACTH

There is also a characteristic patchy pigmentation of the skin; this is because the absence of corticosteroids not only stimulates the pituitary cells producing **ACTH**, but also non-specifically stimulates the cells producing melanocyte-stimulating hormone. The presence of abnormal pigmentation thus helps to distinguish between corticoid deficiency due to primary adrenal disease and deficiency due to lack of **ACTH**.

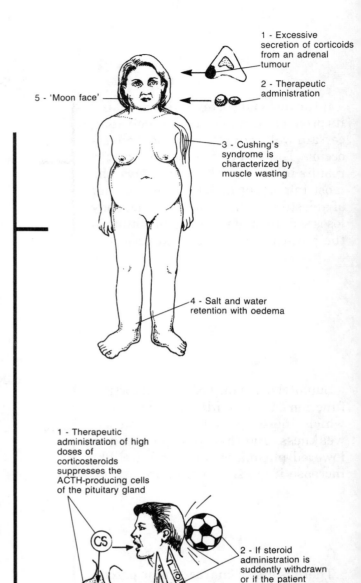

1 - Excessive secretion of corticoids from an adrenal tumour

2 - Therapeutic administration

5 - 'Moon face'

3 - Cushing's syndrome is characterized by muscle wasting

4 - Salt and water retention with oedema

1 - Therapeutic administration of high doses of corticosteroids suppresses the ACTH-producing cells of the pituitary gland

2 - If steroid administration is suddenly withdrawn or if the patient experiences trauma or surgery, the pituitary is unable to stimulate higher production of cortisol to meet the crisis

An increase in circulating corticoids, due either to excessive secretion from an adrenal tumour or to therapeutic administration, causes a condition called **Cushing's** syndrome. This is characterized by muscle wasting due to the breakdown of amino acids for gluco-neogenesis, together with salt and water retention with oedema (due to mineralocorticoid actions), and a swollen 'moon face'.

The therapeutic administration of high doses of corticosteroids suppresses the **ACTH**-producing cells of the pituitary gland. This can be dangerous if steroid administration is suddenly withdrawn or if the patient experiences trauma or surgery; the pituitary is unable to stimulate the production of the higher levels of cortisol which are required to meet the crisis.

If the cells of the zona reticularis are overactive the effect is scarcely noticeable in adult males; in young boys it can cause precocious puberty, with early development of external genitalia, and in females it can produce unfortunate results such as excessive facial hair growth and the loss of the feminine body shape (virilization). In female babies it can produce abnormal growth of the external genitalia, and may make it difficult to determine a baby's sex at birth.

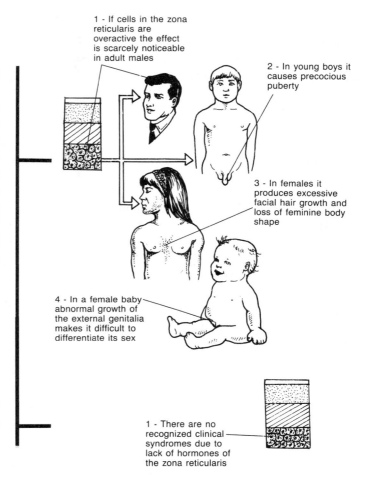

1 - If cells in the zona reticularis are overactive the effect is scarcely noticeable in adult males

2 - In young boys it causes precocious puberty

3 - In females it produces excessive facial hair growth and loss of feminine body shape

4 - In a female baby abnormal growth of the external genitalia makes it difficult to differentiate its sex

There are no recognized clinical syndromes due to lack of the hormones of the zona reticularis.

1 - There are no recognized clinical syndromes due to lack of hormones of the zona reticularis

THE PARATHYROID GLANDS

The level of calcium in the blood and the state of mineralization of the bones, is regulated by the parathyroid glands — four small glands about the size of peas, attached to the top and bottom poles of the thyroid gland on its posterior surface (they are thus particularly vulnerable to damage during thyroid surgery).

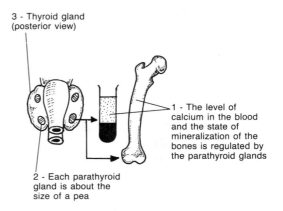

3 - Thyroid gland (posterior view)

1 - The level of calcium in the blood and the state of mineralization of the bones is regulated by the parathyroid glands

2 - Each parathyroid gland is about the size of a pea

The structure of the parathyroid glands is typical of endocrine glands; there are small clumps of cells with a very extensive capillary blood supply. The cells are of two types: **chief cells** and **oxyntic cells**. The parathyroid hormone is secreted by chief cells; the function of the oxyntic cells is quite unknown.

Parathyroid hormone (parathormone, PTH) is a protein (84 amino acids) with a molecular weight of 8500. Its release from the gland is regulated by the plasma calcium concentration; a fall in calcium causes a rise in **PTH** and **vice versa**. Its secretion is not under nervous control or control by any other hormone or releasing factor.

The function of parathormone is to raise the plasma concentration of calcium ions. It does this by reabsorbing calcium from bone, by promoting intestinal absorption of calcium from dietary sources, and by reducing renal reabsorption of phosphate.

Despite its hard appearance, bone is a dynamic tissue which is subject to continuous remodelling. **Osteoblasts** are continually depositing new bone — both the protein matrix and the calcium phosphate crystals. At the same time **osteoclasts** are continuously reabsorbing calcium and breaking down the bone at other sites.

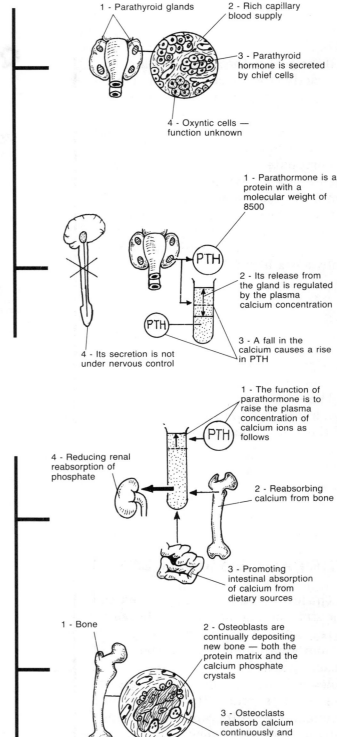

1 - Parathyroid glands

2 - Rich capillary blood supply

3 - Parathyroid hormone is secreted by chief cells

4 - Oxyntic cells — function unknown

1 - Parathormone is a protein with a molecular weight of 8500

2 - Its release from the gland is regulated by the plasma calcium concentration

3 - A fall in the calcium causes a rise in PTH

4 - Its secretion is not under nervous control

1 - The function of parathormone is to raise the plasma concentration of calcium ions as follows

4 - Reducing renal reabsorption of phosphate

2 - Reabsorbing calcium from bone

3 - Promoting intestinal absorption of calcium from dietary sources

1 - Bone

2 - Osteoblasts are continually depositing new bone — both the protein matrix and the calcium phosphate crystals

3 - Osteoclasts reabsorb calcium continuously and break down the bone at other sites

Parathormone acts principally to stimulate osteoclast activity, with increased bone reabsorption; it also inhibits osteoblasts and reduces deposition of new bone. If a fragment of parathyroid gland is implanted on the surface of a piece of bone in a Petri dish, it will cause a hollow of reabsorption to form within a couple of days.

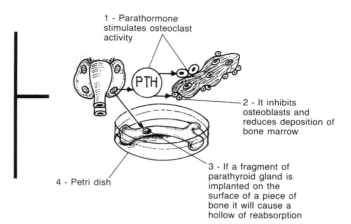

1 - Parathormone stimulates osteoclast activity

2 - It inhibits osteoblasts and reduces deposition of bone marrow

3 - If a fragment of parathyroid gland is implanted on the surface of a piece of bone it will cause a hollow of reabsorption

4 - Petri dish

The action of PTH on intestinal absorption of calcium is probably indirect: the hormone modifies the activity of vitamin D.

Cholecalciferol (vitamin D_3), ingested in the diet or made in the skin by the action of ultraviolet light rays, requires to be converted by the liver to 25-hydroxycholecalciferol (25-HC), and then is further converted by the kidney to 1,25-dihydroxycholecalciferol (1,25-DHC). It is this latter step that is activated by parathormone, and the resulting substance, a steroid, acts very like a hormone; it enters the intestinal epithelial cells and stimulates the manufacture of **calcium-binding protein**, which is essential for the active uptake of calcium by the intestine.

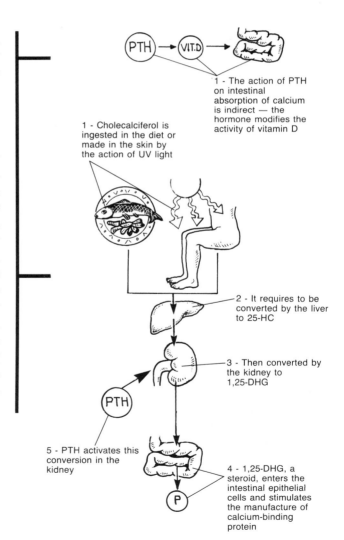

1 - The action of PTH on intestinal absorption of calcium is indirect — the hormone modifies the activity of vitamin D

1 - Cholecalciferol is ingested in the diet or made in the skin by the action of UV light

2 - It requires to be converted by the liver to 25-HC

3 - Then converted by the kidney to 1,25-DHG

5 - PTH activates this conversion in the kidney

4 - 1,25-DHG, a steroid, enters the intestinal epithelial cells and stimulates the manufacture of calcium-binding protein

The plasma concentration of calcium is also affected by **calcitonin**, a hormone produced in the thyroid gland. This is a large polypeptide (32 amino acids; molecular weight 3000) which stimulates osteoblasts, inhibits osteoclasts and thus reduces plasma calcium concentration.

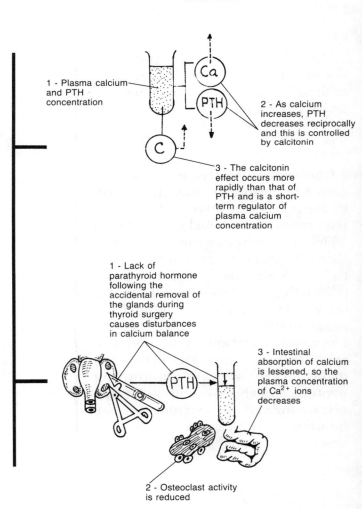

1 - Calcitonin, a hormone produced by the thyroid gland — molecular weight 3000

2 - It stimulates osteoblasts

3 - It inhibits osteoclasts

4 - It thus reduces plasma calcium concentration

Its rate of production is regulated by the plasma calcium concentration and proceeds in a reciprocal manner to the regulation of PTH: as calcium increases, PTH decreases and calcitonin increases. The calcitonin effects occur much more rapidly than those due to PTH, and last for a shorter time; thus calcitonin functions as a short-term regulator of calcium while PTH is a long-term regulator.

1 - Plasma calcium and PTH concentration

2 - As calcium increases, PTH decreases reciprocally and this is controlled by calcitonin

3 - The calcitonin effect occurs more rapidly than that of PTH and is a short-term regulator of plasma calcium concentration

1 - Lack of parathyroid hormone following the accidental removal of the glands during thyroid surgery causes disturbances in calcium balance

3 - Intestinal absorption of calcium is lessened, so the plasma concentration of Ca^{2+} ions decreases

A lack of parathyroid hormone, which might follow the accidental removal of the glands during thyroid surgery, causes disturbances in calcium balance. Osteoclast activity is reduced and intestinal absorption of calcium is lessened, so the plasma concentration of calcium ions decreases.

2 - Osteoclast activity is reduced

The main effect of this is to render cell membranes hyperexcitable; calcium ions in the extracellular fluid control the membrane permeability to sodium ions, and if calcium ions are deficient then the nerve and muscle cell membranes are more likely to discharge spontaneous action potentials due to sodium entering the cell.

The clinical manifestation of this decreased calcium concentration is **tetany** (not to be confused with the disease **tetanus**). There is a tendency for muscles to go into spasm because of spontaneous activity in the motor nerves: this is commonly seen in the muscles controlling the hands and feet, producing **carpopedal spasm**.

In cases where overt spasm has not yet occurred it is possible to provoke it by inflating a venous-occluding cuff around a limb (Trousseau's sign); it is also possible to elicit abnormally active reflexes, such as a jerk of the jaw when the chin is tapped (Chvostek's sign).

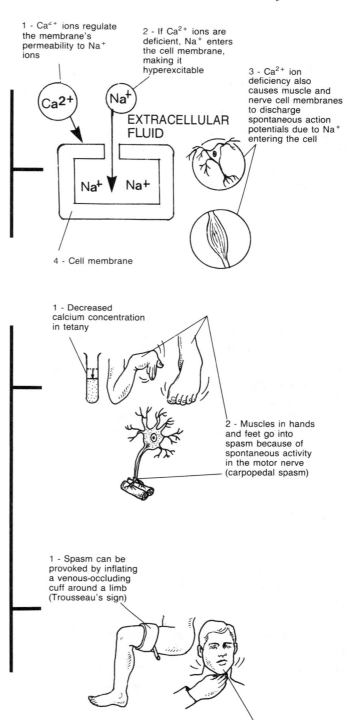

1 - Ca²⁺ ions regulate the membrane's permeability to Na⁺ ions

2 - If Ca²⁺ ions are deficient, Na⁺ enters the cell membrane, making it hyperexcitable

3 - Ca²⁺ ion deficiency also causes muscle and nerve cell membranes to discharge spontaneous action potentials due to Na⁺ entering the cell

4 - Cell membrane

1 - Decreased calcium concentration in tetany

2 - Muscles in hands and feet go into spasm because of spontaneous activity in the motor nerve (carpopedal spasm)

1 - Spasm can be provoked by inflating a venous-occluding cuff around a limb (Trousseau's sign)

2 - A jerk of the jaw when the chin is tapped (Chvostek's sign)

Calcium ions are, of course, important for blood clotting. However, in order to demonstrate a defect in clotting one would have to reduce plasma calcium to levels which would be lethal due to neuromuscular hyperactivity and in particular to cardiac hyperactivity (probably ventricular fibrillation).

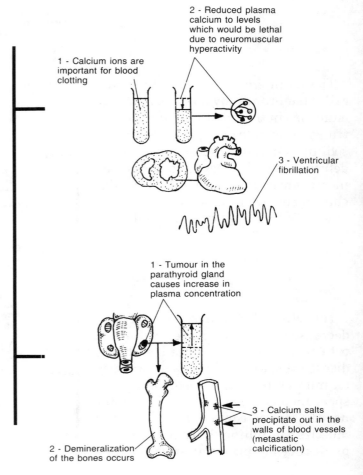

1 - Calcium ions are important for blood clotting

2 - Reduced plasma calcium to levels which would be lethal due to neuromuscular hyperactivity

3 - Ventricular fibrillation

Overactivity of the parathyroid glands, due usually to a tumour, causes an increase in plasma calcium, with demineralization of the bones. The plasma calcium concentration is often so high that calcium salts precipitate out, commonly in the walls of blood vessels (**metastatic calcification**).

1 - Tumour in the parathyroid gland causes increase in plasma concentration

2 - Demineralization of the bones occurs

3 - Calcium salts precipitate out in the walls of blood vessels (metastatic calcification)

THE PANCREAS

As well as its important role in manufacturing digestive enzymes, the pancreas has a major role as an endocrine organ. In between the exocrine acini are found small clumps of cells called the **islets of Langerhans**, and these constitute the endocrine part of this organ. The cells can be distinguished, on the basis of their histological staining reaction, into alpha and beta cells. The alpha cells produce **insulin**; the beta cells produce **glucagon**.

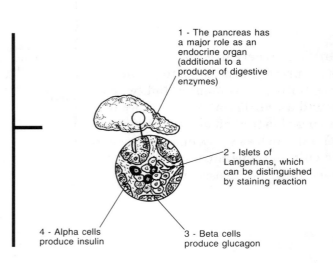

1 - The pancreas has a major role as an endocrine organ (additional to a producer of digestive enzymes)

2 - Islets of Langerhans, which can be distinguished by staining reaction

3 - Beta cells produce glucagon

4 - Alpha cells produce insulin

Insulin is a small protein consisting of two interconnecting chains and having a molecular weight of 6000; it has 51 amino acid residues. It is stored in granules in the islet cells of the pancreas; if the concentration of glucose exceeds the normal range of values (about 2.5−5 mmol/l) the islet cells discharge action potentials and the granules are released into the blood.

Glucagon is also a small peptide (29 amino acids; molecular weight 3482) and its secretion is stimulated when blood glucose levels fall too low.

Insulin's main action is to reduce the plasma concentration of glucose, and glucagon's action is to increase it. Other hormones such as cortisol, growth hormone and adrenaline also increase blood glucose; insulin is about the only one which reduces it, and is thus very important in the control of the supply of glucose to the tissues.

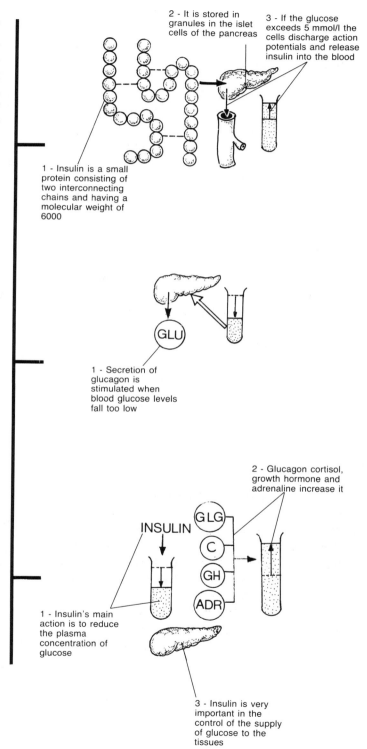

2 - It is stored in granules in the islet cells of the pancreas

3 - If the glucose exceeds 5 mmol/l the cells discharge action potentials and release insulin into the blood

1 - Insulin is a small protein consisting of two interconnecting chains and having a molecular weight of 6000

GLU

1 - Secretion of glucagon is stimulated when blood glucose levels fall too low

2 - Glucagon cortisol, growth hormone and adrenaline increase it

INSULIN

GLG
C
GH
ADR

1 - Insulin's main action is to reduce the plasma concentration of glucose

3 - Insulin is very important in the control of the supply of glucose to the tissues

Insulin works by promoting the uptake of glucose into cells across the cell membrane. The maximal rate of insulin-stimulated transport is about twenty times the minimum rate in the absence of insulin. This uptake of glucose is not an active transport mechanism and does not require energy expenditure, but is a carrier-mediated facilitated diffusion. The movement of glucose is not against a concentration gradient, as the glucose becomes phosphorylated by intracellular enzyme systems as soon as it enters the cell. Insulin presumably acts by combining with the glucose carrier in the cell membrane, making it bind more effectively to the glucose molecule and thus facilitating the transport. The increase in glucose uptake occurs within seconds or minutes of the addition of insulin, indicating that the receptor site is on the cell membrane.

The tissues in which insulin is most effective are the muscles (skeletal, cardiac and smooth) and adipose tissue. It has very little effect on the brain (which is absolutely dependent upon an adequate level of blood glucose for its nutrition), or on red cells; it has no effect upon the T_m (transport maximum) limited glucose transport of the renal tubule or the intestinal epithelium.

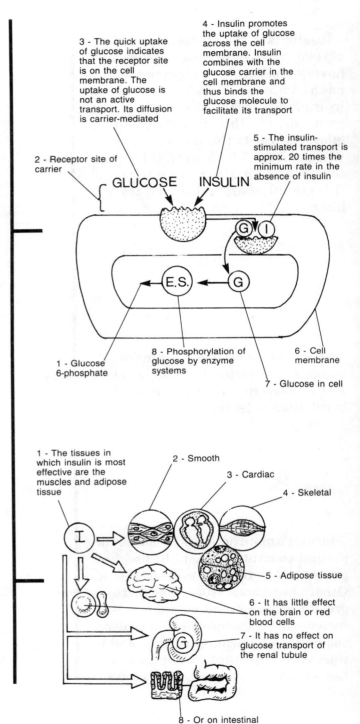

3 - The quick uptake of glucose indicates that the receptor site is on the cell membrane. The uptake of glucose is not an active transport. Its diffusion is carrier-mediated

4 - Insulin promotes the uptake of glucose across the cell membrane. Insulin combines with the glucose carrier in the cell membrane and thus binds the glucose molecule to facilitate its transport

2 - Receptor site of carrier

5 - The insulin-stimulated transport is approx. 20 times the minimum rate in the absence of insulin

GLUCOSE   INSULIN

1 - Glucose 6-phosphate

8 - Phosphorylation of glucose by enzyme systems

6 - Cell membrane

7 - Glucose in cell

1 - The tissues in which insulin is most effective are the muscles and adipose tissue

2 - Smooth

3 - Cardiac

4 - Skeletal

5 - Adipose tissue

6 - It has little effect on the brain or red blood cells

7 - It has no effect on glucose transport of the renal tubule

8 - Or on intestinal epithelium

Insulin has a special effect on liver cells, whose membrane is freely permeable to glucose in both directions; insulin does not influence transport of glucose across the membrane, but it does affect the fate of glucose once it enters the hepatic cell. By promoting the synthesis of glycogen, insulin increases the storage of carbohydrate in the liver; insulin also promotes the conversion of glucose by the liver into fat. Both of these mechanisms reduce the intracellular concentration of glucose and hence stimulate the further uptake of free glucose from the plasma.

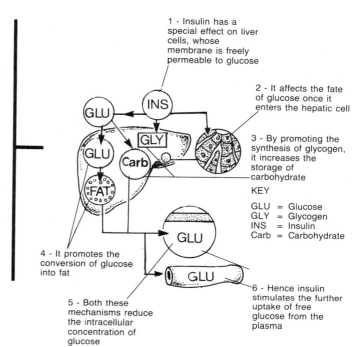

1 - Insulin has a special effect on liver cells, whose membrane is freely permeable to glucose

2 - It affects the fate of glucose once it enters the hepatic cell

3 - By promoting the synthesis of glycogen, it increases the storage of carbohydrate

KEY

GLU = Glucose
GLY = Glycogen
INS = Insulin
Carb = Carbohydrate

4 - It promotes the conversion of glucose into fat

5 - Both these mechanisms reduce the intracellular concentration of glucose

6 - Hence insulin stimulates the further uptake of free glucose from the plasma

CONTROL OF BLOOD GLUCOSE

If a meal of carbohydrate is ingested, there is a rapid uptake of glucose from the intestine, and a rise of glucose concentration in the portal venous blood. The pancreatic islet cells sense the rise in blood sugar and stimulate the release of insulin, which facilitates the uptake of glucose by the liver and other cells throughout the body.

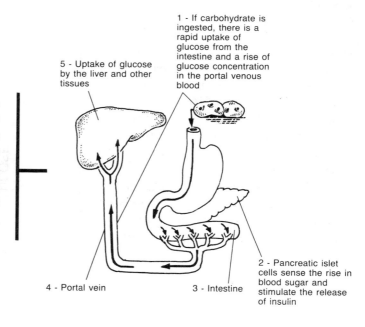

1 - If carbohydrate is ingested, there is a rapid uptake of glucose from the intestine and a rise of glucose concentration in the portal venous blood

5 - Uptake of glucose by the liver and other tissues

2 - Pancreatic islet cells sense the rise in blood sugar and stimulate the release of insulin

4 - Portal vein

3 - Intestine

Later, after the meal has been fully absorbed, if glucose levels start to drop, the secretion of insulin ceases and other hormones such as glucagon or cortisol (or in an emergency, adrenaline) cause the release of glucose into the blood. This glucose comes from the breakdown of liver glycogen, or from an enhanced rate of gluconeogenesis, and these mechanisms serve to ensure that there is an adequate supply of glucose for the cells even though several hours may have elapsed since the last meal.

The function of the pancreas (and the other glucose-regulating endocrine glands) can be tested by performing a **glucose tolerance test**. A standard oral or intravenous dose of glucose is given to the fasting subject, and blood samples are taken at regular intervals (15 or 30 minutes) for measurement of glucose levels (and, if facilities are available, for assay of insulin, cortisol and glucagon). In normal subjects the blood glucose level rises to about 1.5 times the fasting level, but returns to normal within one or two hours; this is a reflection of an almost parallel rise in insulin secretion. In the absence of insulin, the glucose tolerance curve is much higher and more prolonged.

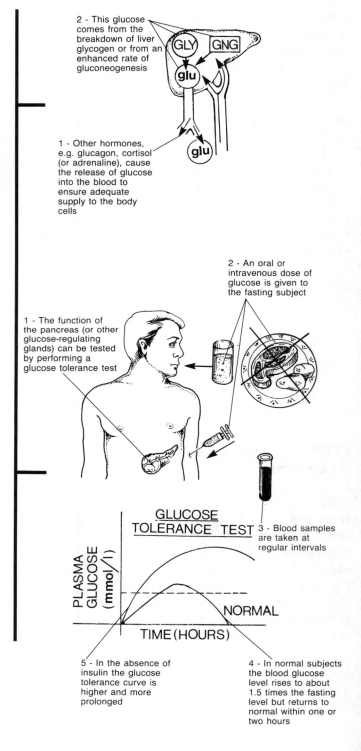

2 - This glucose comes from the breakdown of liver glycogen or from an enhanced rate of gluconeogenesis

GLY GNG

glu

1 - Other hormones, e.g. glucagon, cortisol (or adrenaline), cause the release of glucose into the blood to ensure adequate supply to the body cells

glu

2 - An oral or intravenous dose of glucose is given to the fasting subject

1 - The function of the pancreas (or other glucose-regulating glands) can be tested by performing a glucose tolerance test

GLUCOSE TOLERANCE TEST

3 - Blood samples are taken at regular intervals

PLASMA GLUCOSE (mmol/l)

NORMAL

TIME (HOURS)

5 - In the absence of insulin the glucose tolerance curve is higher and more prolonged

4 - In normal subjects the blood glucose level rises to about 1.5 times the fasting level but returns to normal within one or two hours

A lack of insulin secretion causes **diabetes mellitus**, a condition in which blood glucose is excessively raised. Urinary glucose excretion is increased as the tubular maximum for reabsorption is exceeded, and the presence of glucose in the tubular fluid causes an osmotic diuresis. Patients typically suffer from polyuria (large amount of urine), and the urine is sweet (hence the name of the disease). They also suffer from polydipsia (excessive drinking due to the dehydration caused by osmotic diuresis).

Although the blood glucose is increased, the cells cannot utilize it, as glucose is not transported across cell membranes; the cells have to obtain their energy for metabolism from other sources. The breakdown of fats is greatly increased in diabetics, and as fat metabolism never proceeds as fully as carbohydrate metabolism, the body is left with a lot of incomplete products of breakdown, the **keto acids**. The diabetic patient often suffers from metabolic acidosis.

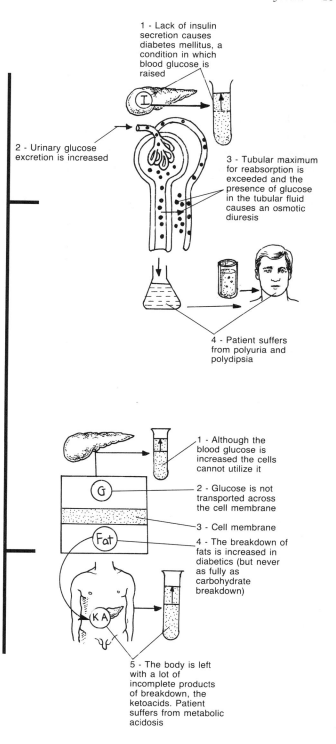

1 - Lack of insulin secretion causes diabetes mellitus, a condition in which blood glucose is raised

2 - Urinary glucose excretion is increased

3 - Tubular maximum for reabsorption is exceeded and the presence of glucose in the tubular fluid causes an osmotic diuresis

4 - Patient suffers from polyuria and polydipsia

1 - Although the blood glucose is increased the cells cannot utilize it

2 - Glucose is not transported across the cell membrane

3 - Cell membrane

4 - The breakdown of fats is increased in diabetics (but never as fully as carbohydrate breakdown)

5 - The body is left with a lot of incomplete products of breakdown, the ketoacids. Patient suffers from metabolic acidosis

The very real problems of diabetes mellitus are treated with insulin; as it is a protein it cannot be taken orally (it would be digested by gastric or duodenal enzymes), so it has to be injected subcutaneously every day (often several times a day). If a diabetic takes too much insulin, or fails to eat the prescribed level of food while being treated with insulin, he is liable to develop **hypoglycaemia** with possible faintness and dizziness, proceeding sometimes to coma.

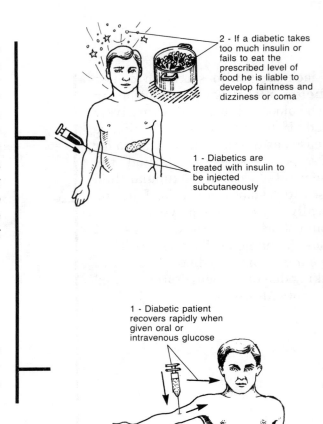

2 - If a diabetic takes too much insulin or fails to eat the prescribed level of food he is liable to develop faintness and dizziness or coma

1 - Diabetics are treated with insulin to be injected subcutaneously

It is often spectacular to watch the rapid recovery from coma of a hypoglycaemic diabetic patient when given oral or intravenous glucose.

1 - Diabetic patient recovers rapidly when given oral or intravenous glucose

The Reproductive System

Reproduction consists of the fusion of two cells, one from the male and one from the female, to form a new individual who is nurtured within the female's body until able to lead an independent existence.

The human adult has 46 chromosomes or 23 pairs (diploid state), but the reproductive cells (**gametes**) contain half of this number (haploid state); the new diploid individual formed by the fusion of two haploid gametes derives half the complement of genetic material from each of the parents.

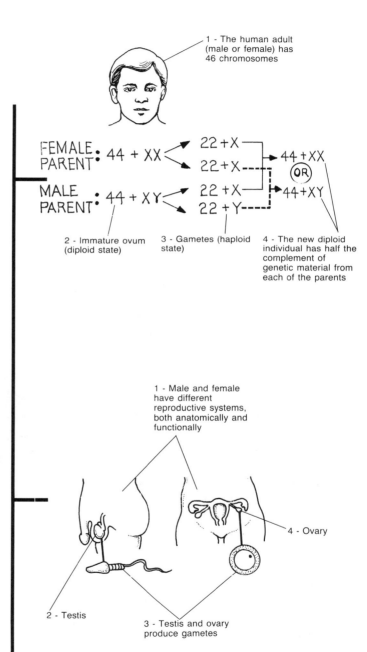

1 - The human adult (male or female) has 46 chromosomes

2 - Immature ovum (diploid state)

3 - Gametes (haploid state)

4 - The new diploid individual has half the complement of genetic material from each of the parents

The two sexes, male and female, have very different reproductive systems, both anatomically and functionally. In each sex there are primary reproductive organs producing the cells which will fuse to create the new organism, and there are several accessory structures which assist in this process or take part in the subsequent development of the new individual.

The primary sexual organs, the testis in the male and the ovary in the female, each have a dual role: they produce the gametes and they secrete hormones which regulate the functions of the rest of the reproductive system. The secretion of these hormones is largely under the control of the pituitary gland.

1 - Male and female have different reproductive systems, both anatomically and functionally

2 - Testis

3 - Testis and ovary produce gametes

4 - Ovary

THE MALE SYSTEM

The reproductive system in the male consists of a primary gamete-forming sex organ — the testis — and a number of accessory structures which convey the gametes into the female genital tract.

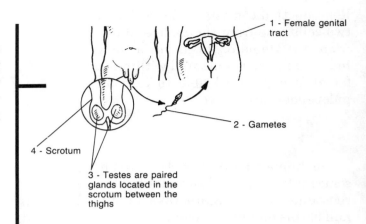

1 - Female genital tract

2 - Gametes

3 - Testes are paired glands located in the scrotum between the thighs

4 - Scrotum

The **testes** are paired glands located in the **scrotum** between the thighs; they are typically about 3 cm long and about 2 cm across, with a bean-like shape. Each testis is composed of a large number of **seminiferous tubules**, within the lumen of which the male gametes, the **spermatozoa**, are formed and develop. The tubules drain into a highly convoluted tubular structure, the **epididymis**, where the spermatozoa are stored and where they mature; this tube is about 7 m long in the human, and 86 m in the stallion. The epididymis leads into the muscular-walled **vas deferens** which runs in the spermatic cord (along with the testicular artery, veins and nerves), into the abdominal cavity, and then to the urethra at the base of the bladder. Each vas deferens is connected to a **seminal vesicle** lying just at the base of the bladder. The seminal vesicles, the vas deferens and the **prostate gland** all contribute components to the **seminal fluid** or semen, the fluid which the male donates to the female during sexual activity.

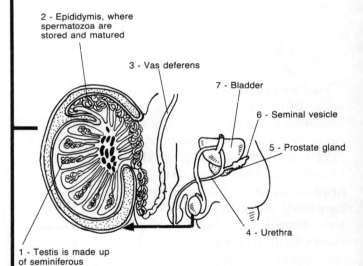

2 - Epididymis, where spermatozoa are stored and matured

3 - Vas deferens

7 - Bladder

6 - Seminal vesicle

5 - Prostate gland

4 - Urethra

1 - Testis is made up of seminiferous tubules in which the spermatozoa develop

After leaving the bladder the urethra runs in the **penis** or phallus, the main identifying male secondary sexual characteristic. At the base of the penis in the perineum the urethra passes through the muscular **bulbospongiosus**; the shaft of the penis consists of two **corpora cavernosa** and a **corpus spongiosus**, which contain erectile tissue. At the tip of the penis is the **glans penis**, a smooth area which is very richly endowed with sensory nerve endings, and which is covered (except in those who have been surgically circumcised) by a retractable sheath of skin, the **prepuce** or foreskin. The orifice of the urethra is at the tip of the penis, and serves for the exit both of urine and seminal fluid.

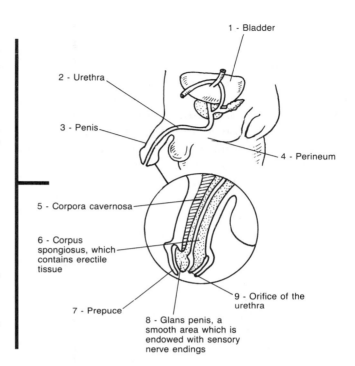

1 - Bladder

2 - Urethra

3 - Penis

4 - Perineum

5 - Corpora cavernosa

6 - Corpus spongiosus, which contains erectile tissue

7 - Prepuce

8 - Glans penis, a smooth area which is endowed with sensory nerve endings

9 - Orifice of the urethra

Gametogenesis

The male gametes are formed within the seminiferous tubules of the testis. In the walls of the tubules are primary **spermatogonia**, the stem cells which continuously divide to produce more spematogonia, and some of which divide to give rise to the gametes. The first product is the **primary spermatocytes** (still diploid), which undergo reduction division (meiosis) to form **secondary spermatocytes** (haploid). Each of these divides to form two **spermatids**, which develop into immature **spermatozoa**.

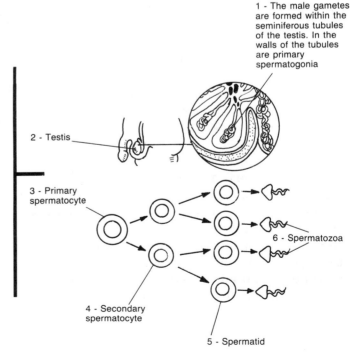

1 - The male gametes are formed within the seminiferous tubules of the testis. In the walls of the tubules are primary spermatogonia

2 - Testis

3 - Primary spermatocyte

4 - Secondary spermatocyte

5 - Spermatid

6 - Spermatozoa

The spermatids are still epithelioid in structure, but as they develop into spermatozoa they lose most of their cytoplasm, so that the spermatozoon consists of little more than a nucleus in its **head**, a small **body** containing mitochondria, and a long **tail** which exhibits flagellar activity and imparts motility to the sperm. Covering the head there is an **acrosome**, which may be analogous to the lysozome, containing enzymes which help the sperm to penetrate the egg.

The correct maturation and development of spermatozoa requires the conditions in the testis to be optimal. The temperature needs to be some degrees lower than that in the abdomen, and the testes are retained outside the abdominal cavity in the scrotum; they migrate there from the abdomen during fetal life, and failure to descend can lead to infertility. (It is interesting that the testes of the elephant remain within the abdominal cavity throughout life; elephants have little trouble with fertility, so presumably spermatogenesis can proceed at a higher temperature than in other mammals.)

The temperature of the testes is regulated by the function of the **dartos** muscle in the scrotum, and to a lesser extent by the **cremaster** in the spermatic cord. In a cold environment the muscles contract, bringing the testes closer to the abdomen, but on warm days the muscles relax and the testes hang at some distance from the heat of the abdomen.

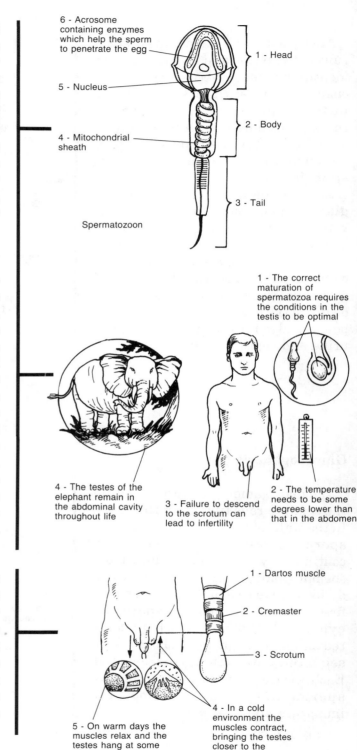

6 - Acrosome containing enzymes which help the sperm to penetrate the egg

1 - Head

5 - Nucleus

2 - Body

4 - Mitochondrial sheath

3 - Tail

Spermatozoon

1 - The correct maturation of spermatozoa requires the conditions in the testis to be optimal

4 - The testes of the elephant remain in the abdominal cavity throughout life

3 - Failure to descend to the scrotum can lead to infertility

2 - The temperature needs to be some degrees lower than that in the abdomen

1 - Dartos muscle

2 - Cremaster

3 - Scrotum

4 - In a cold environment the muscles contract, bringing the testes closer to the abdomen

5 - On warm days the muscles relax and the testes hang at some distance from the abdomen

In the seminiferous tubules there are also some supporting cells, the **Sertoli** cells, whose function is to provide nutrition and support to the developing and maturing sperms. These cells are much larger than the cells of the spermatogonia series.

The sperms found in the testes are not yet capable of fertilizing the egg, and in fact sperms from the seminiferous tubules are non-motile if they are introduced into the female genital tract. From the tubules the sperms pass into the epididymis, a long tube which they take some time (perhaps 25 days) to traverse. During this time the sperms undergo maturation, gradually acquiring the capacity to fertilize the ovum. The seminiferous tubules and epididymis secrete a watery fluid in which the spermatozoa are suspended.

The vas deferens conducts the seminal fluid to the base of the urethra, and in the seminal vesicles some citric acid and fructose are added for nutrition of the maturing sperms. The prostate gland contributes some other fluid components, including citric acid, calcium, phosphate and a clotting enzyme, as well as the prostaglandins, which are important in stimulating the female genital tract to receive the spermatozoa.

The **penis** is the main conduit for sperm into the female genital tract during sexual intercourse. It is normally a flaccid tube, but is capable of **erection**, a process in which it becomes longer, stiffer, and points upwards instead of hanging downwards between the legs; it is now ready to be inserted into the female's vagina for the act of coitus.

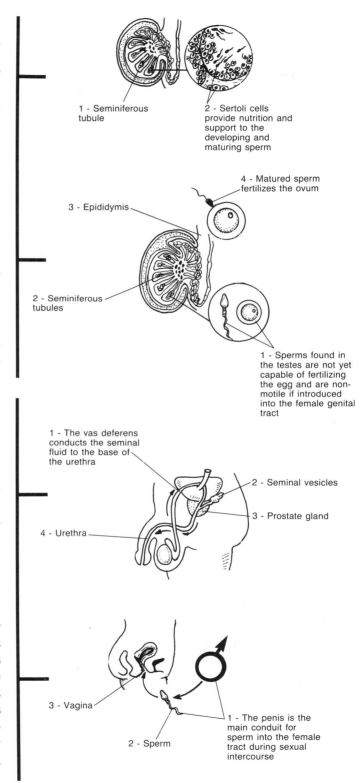

1 - Seminiferous tubule

2 - Sertoli cells provide nutrition and support to the developing and maturing sperm

3 - Epididymis

4 - Matured sperm fertilizes the ovum

2 - Seminiferous tubules

1 - Sperms found in the testes are not yet capable of fertilizing the egg and are non-motile if introduced into the female genital tract

1 - The vas deferens conducts the seminal fluid to the base of the urethra

2 - Seminal vesicles

3 - Prostate gland

4 - Urethra

3 - Vagina

2 - Sperm

1 - The penis is the main conduit for sperm into the female tract during sexual intercourse

Mechanism of erection

The corpus spongiosus and the corpora cavernosa have an extensive system of sinusoids, and these can become distended with blood by constriction of venules and dilatation of arterioles in the penis. This action is the result of parasympathetic impulses in the **nervi erigentes** (the pelvic visceral nerves) during sexual excitement. The transmitter is probably acetylcholine, and this is one of the few genuinely cholinergic vasodilator actions.

The mechanism requires the presence of an adequate blood supply to keep the flaccid arterioles open and the sinusoids distended; if the blood pressure is lowered, for example by antihypertensive drugs or alcohol, or sometimes even by standing up, the arterioles collapse and erection fails.

If the penis is inserted into the female vagina and moved in and out, or is stimulated in some other way, there is a bombardment of the central nervous system by sensory impulses causing an increasing excitement until **ejaculation** occurs.

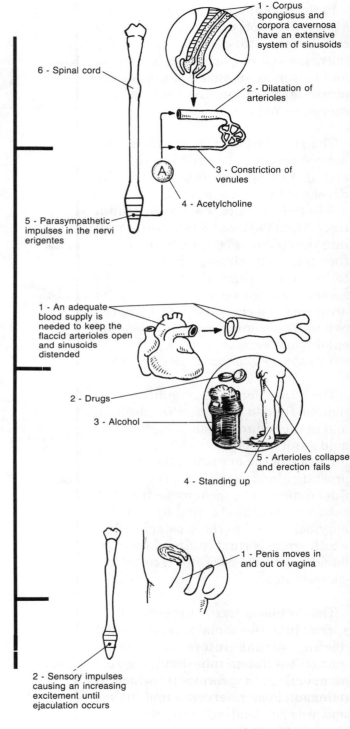

1 - Corpus spongiosus and corpora cavernosa have an extensive system of sinusoids

6 - Spinal cord

2 - Dilatation of arterioles

3 - Constriction of venules

4 - Acetylcholine

5 - Parasympathetic impulses in the nervi erigentes

1 - An adequate blood supply is needed to keep the flaccid arterioles open and sinusoids distended

2 - Drugs

3 - Alcohol

4 - Standing up

5 - Arterioles collapse and erection fails

1 - Penis moves in and out of vagina

2 - Sensory impulses causing an increasing excitement until ejaculation occurs

This is a reflex involving both autonomic and voluntary nervous systems, producing rhythmic contractions of the bulbospongiosus and contraction of the seminal vesicles, expelling seminal fluid out through the urethra and into the vault of the vagina.

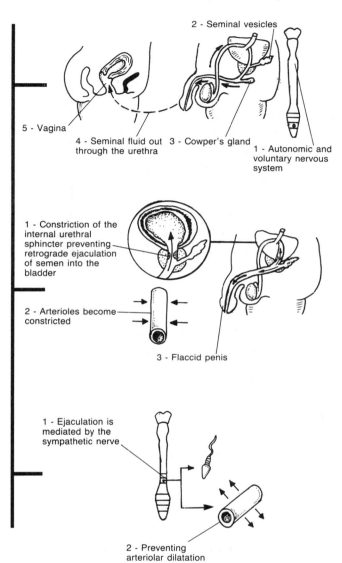

2 - Seminal vesicles

5 - Vagina

4 - Seminal fluid out through the urethra

3 - Cowper's gland

1 - Autonomic and voluntary nervous system

There is also constriction of the internal urethral sphincter, preventing retrograde ejaculation of semen into the bladder. The dilated arterioles become constricted, leading to flaccidity of the penis.

1 - Constriction of the internal urethral sphincter preventing retrograde ejaculation of semen into the bladder

2 - Arterioles become constricted

3 - Flaccid penis

The autonomic components of ejaculation are mediated by the sympathetic nerves, and sympathetic overactivity can inhibit erection (which is a parasympathetic activity) by preventing arteriolar dilatation, or may cause ejaculation to occur prematurely.

1 - Ejaculation is mediated by the sympathetic nerve

2 - Preventing arteriolar dilatation

Ejaculation is usually associated with a feeling of extreme pleasure and release of tension (known as **orgasm**), though the reflex can occur even in paraplegic patients, since it is a spinal reflex, and the intervention of higher centres is not entirely necessary.

Endocrine functions of the testis

Between the seminiferous tubules there are interstitial cells, the **Leydig cells**, which are responsible for secreting the testicular hormones. The main hormone is **testosterone**, a steroid androgen which is responsible for the male secondary sexual characteristics. These include the typical male pattern of musculoskeletal development and physique, the development of the external genitalia, the distribution of hair over the face and body (and also the male pattern of hair loss or baldness); they also include the deepening of the voice because of an increase in size of the larynx (voice-box), the onset of the male sexual drive, and perhaps the aggressive behaviour patterns which are supposed to be the characteristic of the male. Testosterone is also responsible for certain phases of sperm maturation.

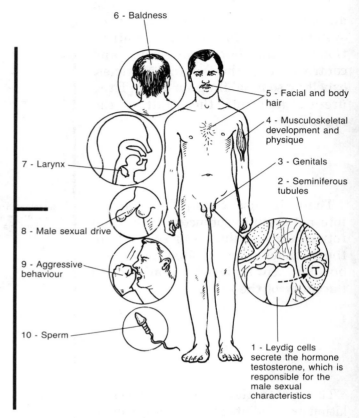

The secretion of testosterone by the Leydig cells (interstitial cells) is under the control of **luteinizing hormone (LH)**, one of the hormones of the anterior pituitary; it was formerly called interstitial cell-stimulating hormone (ICSH), until its true nature was recognized: it is identical to luteinizing hormone found in the female. The secretion of **LH** is controlled, in turn, by LH-releasing hormone (**LHRH**) produced in the hypothalamus and travelling in the portal capillaries to reach the pituitary.

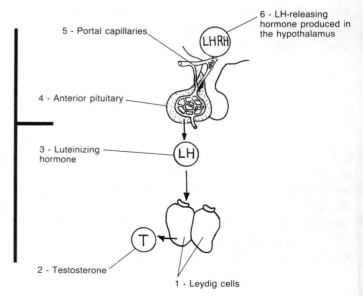

The other pituitary gonadotrophin is follicle-stimulating hormone (FSH), whose role in the female has long been well known; in the male it is responsible for stimulating the production of spermatozoa from spermatogonia.

Before puberty, when there is no **FSH**, the seminiferous tubules are scarcely discernible. At puberty (see below), the hypothalamus begins to secrete FSH-releasing factor and this stimulates the pituitary to produce FSH; once the testis is turned on by FSH the tubules develop and spermatogenesis begins.

The developing male (infant, child and immature adolescent) has very little testosterone activity. At **puberty**, which occurs between the ages of 13 and 16 years, the brain (via the hypothalamus) signals to the pituitary that LH secretion is to begin, and the Leydig cells are stimulated to begin production of testosterone. At this stage there is usually a spurt in growth, with development of a more muscular physique, enlargement of the external genitalia, the growth of hair over the body and particularly over the face and in the pubic region. The larynx enlarges, resulting in the voice becoming lower pitched. The boy usually begins to take a greater interest in members of the opposite sex, and experiences sexual urges; he may have vividly erotic dreams resulting in spontaneous ejaculation of semen while he sleeps ('wet dreams').

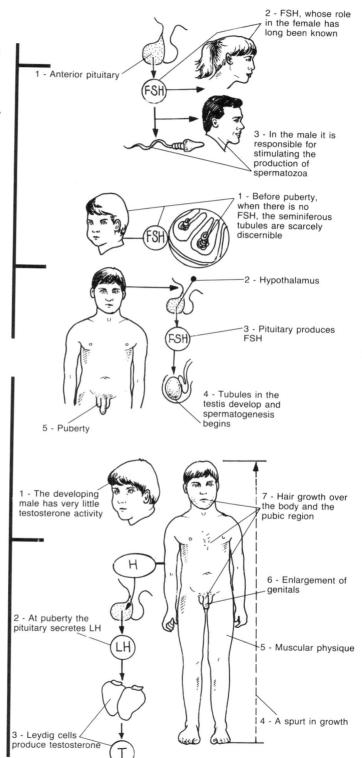

1 - Anterior pituitary

2 - FSH, whose role in the female has long been known

3 - In the male it is responsible for stimulating the production of spermatozoa

1 - Before puberty, when there is no FSH, the seminiferous tubules are scarcely discernible

2 - Hypothalamus

3 - Pituitary produces FSH

4 - Tubules in the testis develop and spermatogenesis begins

5 - Puberty

1 - The developing male has very little testosterone activity

2 - At puberty the pituitary secretes LH

3 - Leydig cells produce testosterone

7 - Hair growth over the body and the pubic region

6 - Enlargement of genitals

5 - Muscular physique

4 - A spurt in growth

THE FEMALE SYSTEM

The primary sexual organ in the female is the **ovary**, where the gametes (**ova** or eggs) are produced; the ovary also has important endocrine functions. The ovaries are situated within the abdomen, and release their ova into the peritoneal cavity. These are trapped by the open ends of the **Fallopian tubes**, which convey them to the **uterus** or womb; this is where the egg becomes implanted if it gets fertilized, and grows into a fetus, which is eventually born as a new individual. The uterine epithelium is highly vascular and very glandular for nutrition of the fetus; the walls consist of strong layers of smooth muscle which are essential for expelling the fetus during the process of birth.

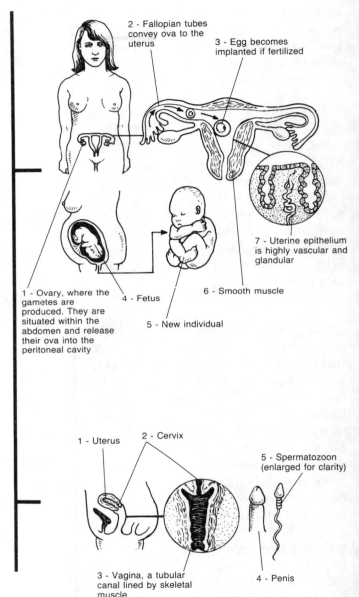

2 - Fallopian tubes convey ova to the uterus

3 - Egg becomes implanted if fertilized

7 - Uterine epithelium is highly vascular and glandular

1 - Ovary, where the gametes are produced. They are situated within the abdomen and release their ova into the peritoneal cavity

4 - Fetus

6 - Smooth muscle

5 - New individual

At the lower end of the uterus is an opening, the **cervix** or 'neck of the womb'. This leads into the **vagina** or sheath, a tubular canal lined by skeletal muscle, which accommodates the penis during coitus, and receives the spermatozoa.

1 - Uterus

2 - Cervix

5 - Spermatozoon (enlarged for clarity)

3 - Vagina, a tubular canal lined by skeletal muscle

4 - Penis

It subsequently acts as a conduit for the baby during the process of birth. The opening of the vagina in the perineum is known as the **vulva**, which has a pair of inner **labia minora** (minor lips) and a pair of outer **labia majora** (major lips). At the front of the vulva is the urethra, leading from the bladder, and above this is the **clitoris**, a small vestigial analogue of the male penis; at the rear is the orifice of the anus. This proximity of the genital tract to the openings from the gut and urinary tract has given rise to many of the misunderstandings and taboos about the process of reproduction ('love hath pitched his temple in the place of excrement' — William Blake).

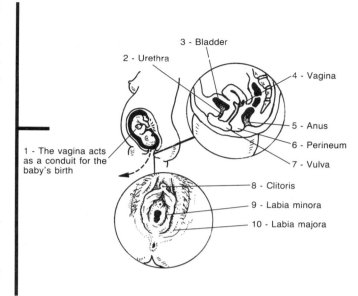

1 - The vagina acts as a conduit for the baby's birth
2 - Urethra
3 - Bladder
4 - Vagina
5 - Anus
6 - Perineum
7 - Vulva
8 - Clitoris
9 - Labia minora
10 - Labia majora

Gametogenesis (oogenesis)

The first stages of oogenesis take place while the female is still a fetus in her mother's uterus; the ovary is formed from a ridge in the coelomic lining. The epithelium forms a number of invaginations into the stroma of the gland, with small groups of cells surrounding the **oogonia** or primary sex cells.

1 - The first stages of oogenesis take place while the female is still a fetus in her mother's womb
2 - Ovary
3 - Epithelium
4 - Follicle
5 - Oogonia

These form the primordial ovarian follicles, each of which may potentially develop into a mature Graafian follicle with an egg capable of being fertilized.

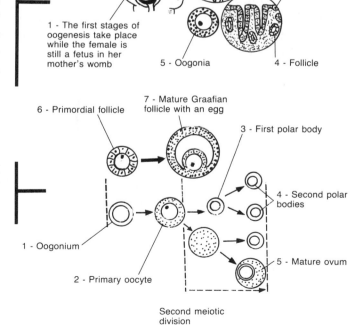

6 - Primordial follicle
7 - Mature Graafian follicle with an egg
3 - First polar body
4 - Second polar bodies
5 - Mature ovum
1 - Oogonium
2 - Primary oocyte

Second meiotic division

At this stage the reduction division (meiosis) from diploid to haploid cells has already taken place. By the time of birth the ovary already contains all of the eggs which the female will ever have: not all of the eggs will mature or be involved in the reproductive cycle, but no further eggs are formed during the woman's lifetime. This is in contrast to the situation in the male, who continuously produces new spermatozoa throughout his reproductive life.

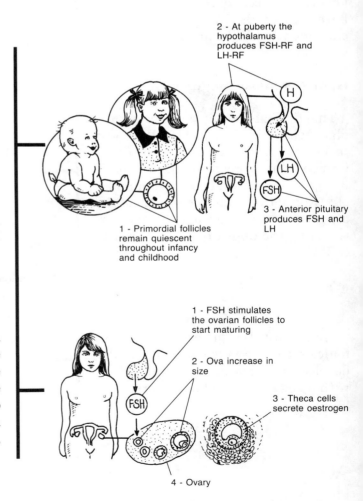

3 - In the male new spermatozoa are produced throughout his reproductive life

1 - By the time of birth the ovary already contains all the eggs which the female will ever have

2 - No further eggs are formed furing the woman's life

Puberty

The primordial follicles remain quiescent throughout infancy and childhood, and do not develop further until puberty, which is reached rather earlier in girls than in boys (about 11−15 years). At puberty, the hypothalamus starts to produce follicle-stimulating hormone-releasing factor (**FSH-RF**) and luteinizing hormone-releasing factor (**LH-RF**). The releasing factors trigger the production of the pituitary gonadotrophins FSH and LH.

2 - At puberty the hypothalamus produces FSH-RF and LH-RF

1 - Primordial follicles remain quiescent throughout infancy and childhood

3 - Anterior pituitary produces FSH and LH

Follicle-stimulating hormone is a small protein which stimulates the ovarian follicles to start maturing; the ova themselves increase in size and the surrounding **theca** cells begin to produce a fluid-filled cavity within each follicle, and start to secrete **oestrogen**, one of the main ovarian hormones.

1 - FSH stimulates the ovarian follicles to start maturing

2 - Ova increase in size

3 - Theca cells secrete oestrogen

4 - Ovary

The oestrogens stimulate maturation of many of the other organs and systems in the body: the **secondary sexual characteristics**. The uterus and the rest of the genital tract increase in size; the breasts begin to enlarge, partly by duct proliferation and partly by fat deposition. Fat is also deposited in other areas, particularly around the hips and thighs, to give the typical feminine body shape. The hair grows more thickly on the head, in the axillae and in the pubic region, while sparing the face. There is a spurt of growth in stature, just as in the male, and there is a widening of the pelvis; there is a growing sexual awareness, and most significantly the menstrual periods start.

The **menstrual cycle** is a sequence of cyclical changes in the ovary, uterus and pituitary gland, occurring at intervals of about 28 days. The most obvious manifestation is bleeding from the vagina: this is caused by sloughing of the uterine epithelium (**endometrium**) which has been preparing for a possible pregnancy that did not occur ('tears from a disappointed uterus').

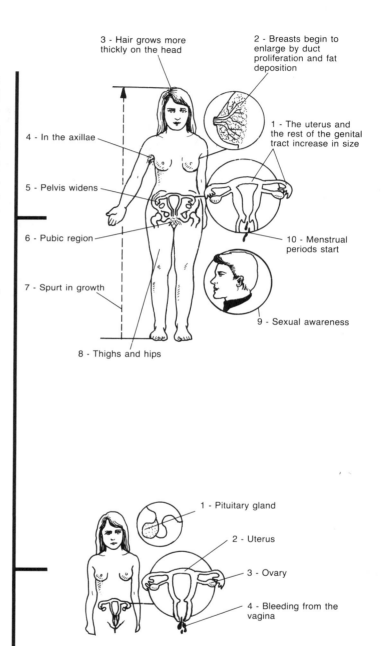

Menstrual cycle

At the start of the cycle (which is reckoned to begin on the first day of bleeding) there is an increase in FSH secretion, which causes a few follicles to start maturing. After a few days all but one of this group of follicles start to degenerate or become **atretic**, while one follicle begins to enlarge enormously, bulging out of the peritoneal surface of the ovary until it eventually bursts. The contents of the follicle, including the ovum, are released into the peritoneal cavity.

During the development of the follicle in the first two weeks of the menstrual cycle, there is an increasing secretion of oestrogen by the theca cells; this has a feedback effect on the pituitary, reducing the production of gonado-trophins. However, two weeks after the start of the cycle there is a sudden increase in the release of both FSH and LH, in a manner which cannot be explained by feedback control. This phenomenon requires initiation by a command from a higher centre, via the hypothalamic releasing factors. It is this surge in the concentrations of gonadotrophins which causes the rupture of the ovarian follicle.

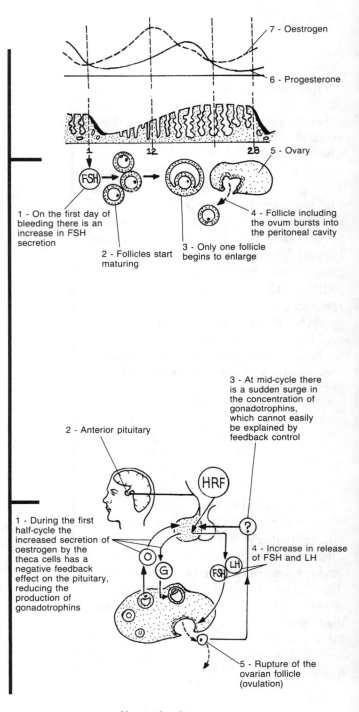

7 - Oestrogen

6 - Progesterone

5 - Ovary

1 - On the first day of bleeding there is an increase in FSH secretion

2 - Follicles start maturing

3 - Only one follicle begins to enlarge

4 - Follicle including the ovum bursts into the peritoneal cavity

3 - At mid-cycle there is a sudden surge in the concentration of gonadotrophins, which cannot easily be explained by feedback control

2 - Anterior pituitary

1 - During the first half-cycle the increased secretion of oestrogen by the theca cells has a negative feedback effect on the pituitary, reducing the production of gonadotrophins

4 - Increase in release of FSH and LH

5 - Rupture of the ovarian follicle (ovulation)

Menstrual cycle

The part of the follicle which remains in the ovary becomes filled with fibrin, and the cells of the lining continue to secrete hormones. The whole structure takes on a yellowish colour (**corpus luteum**) and the main hormone secreted is now **progesterone**, whose concentration rises during the second half of the mentrual cycle. The corpus luteum also secretes some oestrogen. The development of the corpus luteum and its hormone secretion are stimulated by **luteinizing hormone** from the pituitary gland. The concentration of LH quickly falls immediately after ovulation, but then rises again to maintain the secretory function of the corpus luteum.

The hormonal changes in the ovary cause changes in the uterine lining. After the period of bleeding, lasting from two to five days, the endometrium is considerably denuded and consists of the remnants of the bottoms of glands and some interstitial connective tissue. Under the influence of oestrogen the epithelial elements start to proliferate, producing a deep epithelium with numerous long thin flask-like glands. This early **proliferative phase** is followed (after ovulation, when the corpus luteum starts to secrete pro-gesterone) by the **secretory phase**, during which the glands become tortuous and are distended with gycogen and other nutritive material; this would help to support the develop-ing fetus if fertilization and implanta-tion were to occur.

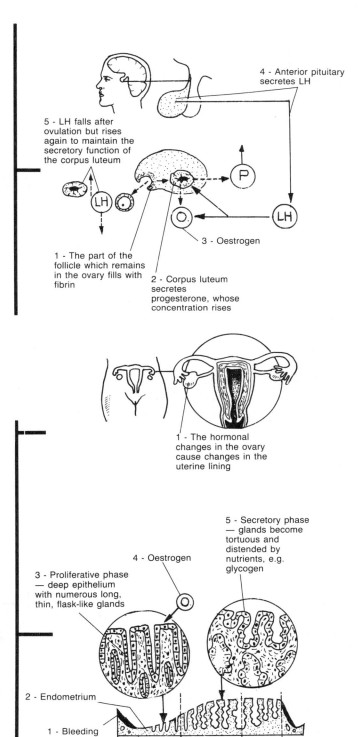

4 - Anterior pituitary secretes LH

5 - LH falls after ovulation but rises again to maintain the secretory function of the corpus luteum

3 - Oestrogen

1 - The part of the follicle which remains in the ovary fills with fibrin

2 - Corpus luteum secretes progesterone, whose concentration rises

1 - The hormonal changes in the ovary cause changes in the uterine lining

5 - Secretory phase — glands become tortuous and distended by nutrients, e.g. glycogen

4 - Oestrogen

3 - Proliferative phase — deep epithelium with numerous long, thin, flask-like glands

2 - Endometrium

1 - Bleeding

About 14 days after ovulation, if fertilization has failed to occur, and the ovary has not received its hormonal signal that conception has taken place, the production of progesterone suddenly ceases and the stimulation of the endometrium is suddenly withdrawn. This makes the spiral arteries in the endometrium go into spasm, causing ischaemic necrosis of the endometrial tissue and sloughing off of the dead epithelium, accompanied by a fair amount of blood.

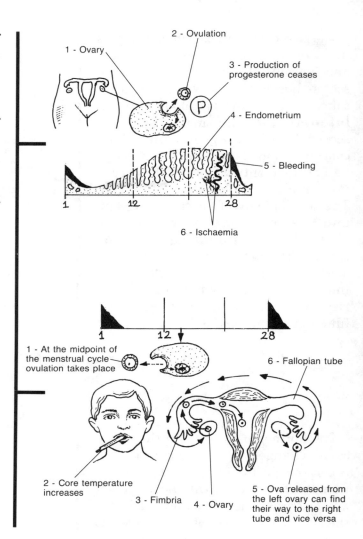

At the midpoint of the menstrual cycle ovulation takes place; the ovum is shed into the peritoneal cavity. At this point there is usually a sudden increase (about 0.5 °C) in the core temperature. The ovum is usually taken into the **fimbriated** end of one of the fallopian tubes; it is quite remarkable that ova released from the left ovary can find their way into the right tube and vice versa. It is not clear exactly how the ovum is caused to enter the tube, but the mechanism seems to be very efficient.

The contraction of the smooth muscle of the tubular walls and fimbriae, as well as the beating of cilia on the tubular epithelium, all help to get the ovum into the tube and to propel it towards the uterus. On its way down the tube, or in the uterine cavity, the ovum may encounter a spermatozoon, and fertilization may ensue; if it does not, the ovum simply degenerates and eventually is lost with the debris in the next menstruation.

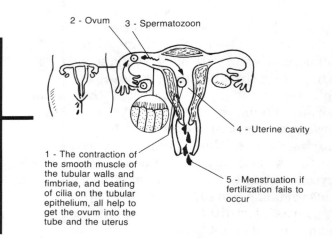

Fertilization

Coitus (copulation, sexual intercourse) is the act in which semen from the male is placed in the body of the female. It may result in fertilization of the ovum and the formation of a new individual, but humans, unlike most other species, regularly engage in the act for the sheer pleasure of it, without necessarily desiring to produce an infant. Fertilization can only occur if coitus takes place close to the time of ovulation.

The full penetration of the female by the male is usually preceded by a period of foreplay, during which the partners stimulate one another's **erogenous zones** (which include breasts, genitalia and perineal areas, in fact almost any part of the body, given appropriate circumstances). This produces a state of arousal. There is increasing emotional excitement, and the gradually accelerating stimulation causes erection of the penis in preparation for insertion into the vagina. Arousal of the female causes relaxation of the vaginal walls, oedema of the labia and secretion of lubricating fluid from the vaginal walls and the glands around the vulva; there is often erection of the clitoris, and sometimes erection of the nipples.

When both partners are aroused the penis is inserted into the vagina, and rhythmic movement in and out causes intense stimulation of the sensory nerves, particularly around the glans penis; this leads eventually to orgasm, with ejaculation of the semen into the vagina.

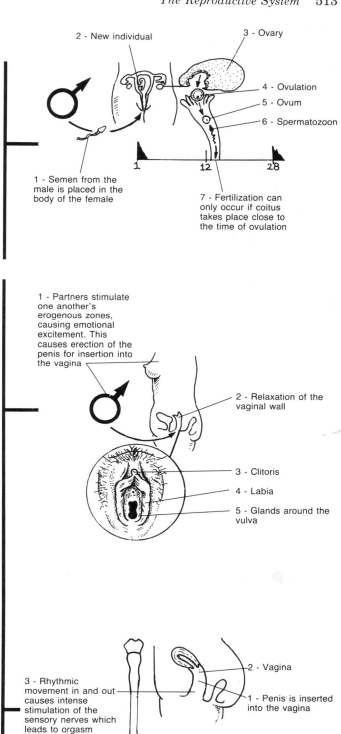

2 - New individual

3 - Ovary

4 - Ovulation

5 - Ovum

6 - Spermatozoon

1 - Semen from the male is placed in the body of the female

7 - Fertilization can only occur if coitus takes place close to the time of ovulation

1 - Partners stimulate one another's erogenous zones, causing emotional excitement. This causes erection of the penis for insertion into the vagina

2 - Relaxation of the vaginal wall

3 - Clitoris

4 - Labia

5 - Glands around the vulva

3 - Rhythmic movement in and out causes intense stimulation of the sensory nerves which leads to orgasm

2 - Vagina

1 - Penis is inserted into the vagina

4 - Spinal cord

In the female, orgasm is often more difficult to define or achieve, and it is not actually essential in order for fertilization to occur. However, it is probably a valuable accessory factor in ensuring efficient transport of sperm and successful union between sperm and ovum, and is certainly a desirable goal to achieve for successful and pleasurable sexual intercourse. Stimulation of the vaginal epithelium is often not enough to produce orgasm; stimulation of the clitoris, either by the shaft of the penis, or by the fingers or other parts before, during or after the insertion and ejaculation by the male, is often required to give the woman full satisfaction. If there is intense enough stimulation, the voluntary muscles around the clitoris undergo rhythmic contraction in a manner exactly analogous to the male orgasm, and the muscles of the vaginal vault may also contract rhythmically, adding to the pleasure of both the female and the male.

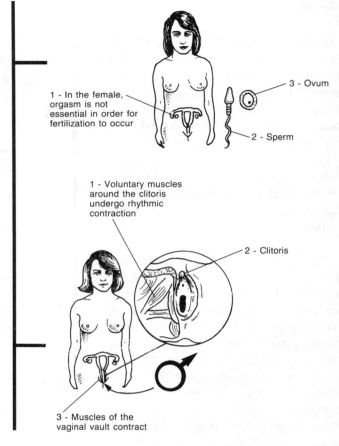

1 - In the female, orgasm is not essential in order for fertilization to occur

3 - Ovum

2 - Sperm

1 - Voluntary muscles around the clitoris undergo rhythmic contraction

2 - Clitoris

3 - Muscles of the vaginal vault contract

Contraction of the smooth muscles of the female genital tract is stimulated partly by sensory nervous activity, but also by the reflex release of oxytocin from the posterior pituitary, and by the **prostaglandins** secreted in the ejaculated fluid by the male.

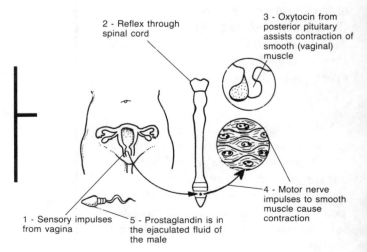

2 - Reflex through spinal cord

3 - Oxytocin from posterior pituitary assists contraction of smooth (vaginal) muscle

4 - Motor nerve impulses to smooth muscle cause contraction

1 - Sensory impulses from vagina

5 - Prostaglandin is in the ejaculated fluid of the male

Once they have been ejaculated, the spermatozoa have to find their way into the lumen of the uterus, and often as far as the fallopian tube, before they encounter the egg and can achieve fertilization. While spermatozoa have highly motile flagellar tails, these cannot generate the major propulsive power required to move them up to the site of fertilization; rather the function of sperm motility is to aid penetration of the egg once the correct site is reached.

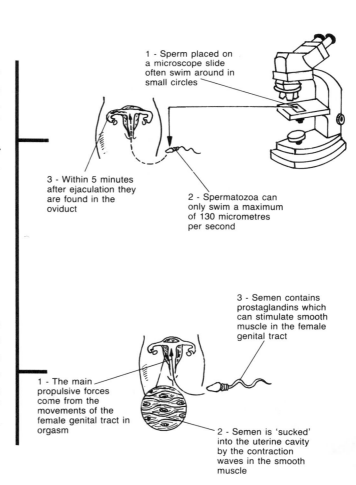

1 - Spermatozoa find their way into the uterus

5 - Fertilization

2 - Fallopian tube

3 - Egg

4 - Spermatozoa have highly motile flagellar tails, not for propulsion but to assist in penetration of ova

Sperm placed on a microscope slide often swim round in small circles; this is not a useful type of movement for a cell which has to migrate over distances of several centimetres. Spermatozoa can swim a maximum of 130 micrometres per second, yet they are found in the oviduct within 5 minutes after ejaculation.

1 - Sperm placed on a microscope slide often swim around in small circles

3 - Within 5 minutes after ejaculation they are found in the oviduct

2 - Spermatozoa can only swim a maximum of 130 micrometres per second

The main propulsive forces come from the movements of the female genital tract, either as a result of the reflexes in orgasm, or following the action of the prostaglandins in the male ejaculate. The semen is almost 'sucked' into the uterine cavity by the contraction waves in the smooth muscle.

3 - Semen contains prostaglandins which can stimulate smooth muscle in the female genital tract

1 - The main propulsive forces come from the movements of the female genital tract in orgasm

2 - Semen is 'sucked' into the uterine cavity by the contraction waves in the smooth muscle

If ovulation has recently occurred, there is a chance that fertilization might take place. At about this time the normally thick, sticky cervical mucus undergoes partial liquefaction under the influence of the ovarian hormones, and the sperm are transported through the cervix and the uterine cavity, to meet the ovum, which is usually found in the lumen of one of the fallopian tubes. Of the several million spermatozoa present in the ejaculate, several hundred may reach the site where the ovum is found. Only one of these sperms will fuse with the ovum.

6 - Only one sperm out of several million will fuse with the ovum

1 - Ovulation has occurred — there is a chance that fertilization might take place

5 - Ovum in the lumen of the fallopian tube

2 - Cervical mucus becomes less sticky

4 - Uterine cavity

3 - Sperm

In order for a sperm to penetrate the ovum, a process of **capacitation** must occur; this requires several hours in the female genital tract, and involves loss of the membrane covering the acrosome, presumably making the lysosomal enzymes more effective at penetrating the coverings of the ovum.

3 - The membrane covering the acrosome is lost

1 - For the sperm to penetrate the ovum capacitation must occur

2 - This requires several hours in the female genital tract

If one sperm penetrates the ovum, it appears to secrete some substance which prevents other spermatozoa from penetrating the membrane.

1 - When one sperm penetrates the ovum it secretes a substance which prevents other sperm penetrating the ovum

The head of the successful spermatozoon swells, forming the male pronucleus, which migrates towards the female pronucleus. The two haploid pronuclei fuse to form a single diploid nucleus, the basis of a new, unique human being.

Shortly after this the cell begins repeatedly to undergo ordinary mitotic division, and the single fertilized cell soon becomes a multicellular ball, the **blastocyst**.

Implantation

The fertilized embryo is propelled into the uterine cavity, and becomes lodged in the endometrium, which by now has completed its proliferative phase and is very glandular.

The embryo secretes enzymes which enable it to erode its way deep into the endometrial wall, and obtain nourishment from the blood vessels of the uterine epithelium.

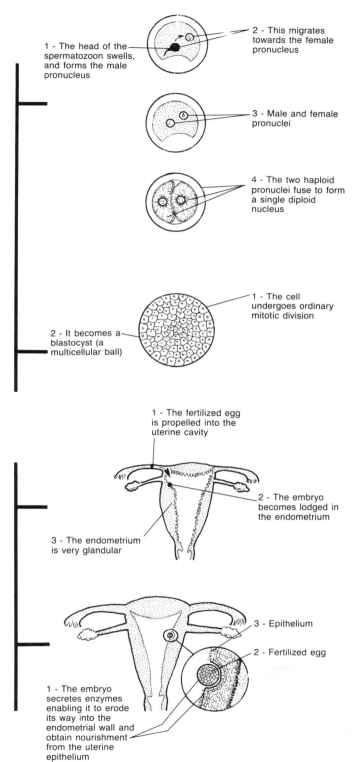

Within a few days the embryo becomes organized into two main parts: one part develops into the body and organs of the eventual baby, and the other part develops into the organs for support and nutrition of the fetus.

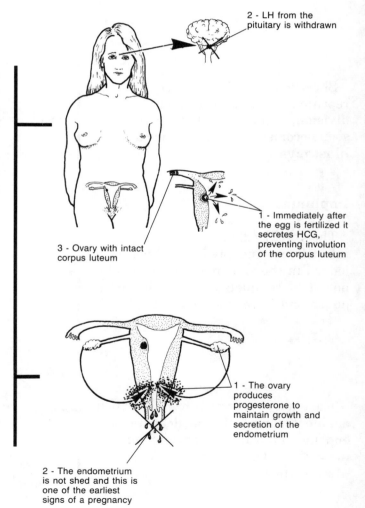

2 - The body and organs of the fetus

3 - Organs for support and nutrition (placenta)

1 - Within a few days the embryo becomes organized into two main parts

Almost immediately after the egg is fertilized, the embryo begins to secrete **human chorionic gonadotrophin (HCG)**, a hormone which stimulates the corpus luteum in the ovary, prevents its involution and enables it to survive even when the LH from the pituitary would normally be withdrawn.

2 - LH from the pituitary is withdrawn

1 - Immediately after the egg is fertilized it secretes HCG, preventing involution of the corpus luteum

3 - Ovary with intact corpus luteum

This enables the ovary to continue producing progesterone and maintains the growth and secretions of the endometrium which is now not shed: the menstrual period is missed, and this is one of the earliest signs of pregnancy.

1 - The ovary produces progesterone to maintain growth and secretion of the endometrium

2 - The endometrium is not shed and this is one of the earliest signs of a pregnancy

PREGNANCY

The placenta

The part of the embryo concerned with obtaining nutrition from the mother is the **trophoblast**. From this develops the **placenta**, which is the organ of interface between the fetus and its mother, and the fetal membranes (**amnion** and **chorion**) which eventually surround the developing baby and contain the amniotic fluid which protects it.

As the fetus grows and develops a circulatory system, the placenta develops in complexity, being attached to the developing fetus by the umbilical cord, which contains two arteries and a vein. The trophoblast throws out large numbers of finger-like processes, the **villi**, which erode into the maternal tissue and lie within the mother's blood vessels. The core of each villus contains the blood vessels of the fetus, and these are surrounded by the trophoblastic epithelium, which comes into direct contact with the mother's blood.

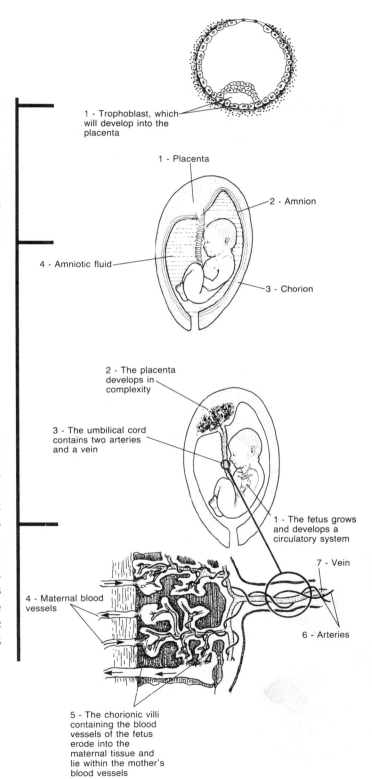

1 - Trophoblast, which will develop into the placenta

1 - Placenta
2 - Amnion
4 - Amniotic fluid
3 - Chorion

2 - The placenta develops in complexity
3 - The umbilical cord contains two arteries and a vein
1 - The fetus grows and develops a circulatory system
7 - Vein
4 - Maternal blood vessels
6 - Arteries
5 - The chorionic villi containing the blood vessels of the fetus erode into the maternal tissue and lie within the mother's blood vessels

It is very easy for nutrients and waste products (including oxygen and carbon dioxide) to be exchanged between the mother and fetus. All of the substances exchanged across the placenta are subject to passive diffusion; there is no active transport of substances between the mother and baby.

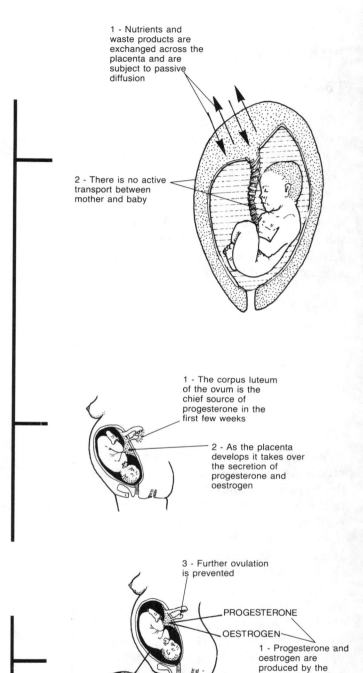

1 - Nutrients and waste products are exchanged across the placenta and are subject to passive diffusion

2 - There is no active transport between mother and baby

As well as exchanging nutrients, the placenta has an important endocrine function. The corpus luteum of the ovary is the chief source of progesterone in the first few weeks of pregnancy, but as the placenta develops it begins to secrete progesterone and oestrogen, and after the first few weeks it becomes the main supplier of these hormones and the role of the ovary becomes less and less.

1 - The corpus luteum of the ovum is the chief source of progesterone in the first few weeks

2 - As the placenta develops it takes over the secretion of progesterone and oestrogen

Both oestrogen and progesterone are required for the full maintenance of the pregnancy: for the continued growth of the uterus (both muscle layer and endometrium), prevention of further ovulation during the pregnancy, and the growth of the placenta itself.

3 - Further ovulation is prevented

PROGESTERONE

OESTROGEN

1 - Progesterone and oestrogen are produced by the placenta

2 - This encourages the growth of the uterus and placenta

The placenta also secretes **human chorionic somatomammotrophin** (placental lactogen), a hormone which causes many of the systemic changes of pregnancy in the mother, including various circulatory changes and the development of the mammary glands.

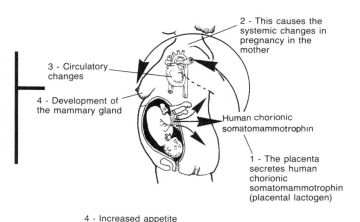

2 - This causes the systemic changes in pregnancy in the mother

3 - Circulatory changes

4 - Development of the mammary gland

Human chorionic somatomammotrophin

1 - The placenta secretes human chorionic somatomammotrophin (placental lactogen)

Maternal changes

During pregnancy there is a general increase in maternal body weight. Not all of this is due simply to the weight of the fetus; at term the fetus may weight 3−4 kg, the placenta may weigh about 500 g, the amniotic fluid may contribute up to 1 kg, and the increase in uterine size may contribute another 500 g. There is also an increase in the size of the breasts (see discussion of lactation, below). The increased appetite (see below) may cause a generalized increase in weight by deposition of fat.

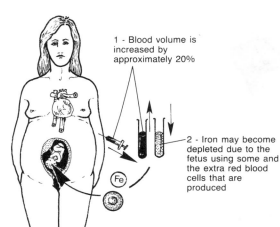

4 - Increased appetite may cause an increased deposition of fat

3 - There is an increase in breast size

2 - At full term the fetus may weigh 3 kg, the placenta 500 g, and the anmiotic fluid 1 kg

1 - Increase in body weight

There are several cardiovascular adjustments to the increased work of being pregnant. The blood volume increases by about 20%, and there is an increase in haemopoiesis, although this may not keep pace with the increase in plasma volume, so that there is a relative anaemia. The mother's stores of iron may become depleted, as the fetus uses up some of the maternal iron and some goes into the extra red cells made during the pregnancy.

1 - Blood volume is increased by approximately 20%

2 - Iron may become depleted due to the fetus using some and the extra red blood cells that are produced

With the extra maternal tissue to perfuse and the additional requirements of the fetus, the cardiac output increases by up to 20%; some of this increase is required by the extra cardiac and respiratory work of perfusing the other tissues.

As a consequence of the generalized inhibitory effect of progesterone on smooth muscle (see below), the walls of the veins become flaccid, causing distended varicose veins and piles (haemorrhoids). These venous problems are compounded by the mechanical obstruction due to the presence of the fetus in the pelvis.

During pregnancy the corpus luteum produces 'relaxin', a hormone which loosens the ligaments around the body, and especially those of the symphysis pubis; this effect is also caused by oestrogen and progesterone. The various joints become much more mobile, and this will eventually be important during the process of parturition. In the meantime, various joints become unstable, particularly those of the pelvis and spine, and backache becomes a prominent and annoying symptom just before term.

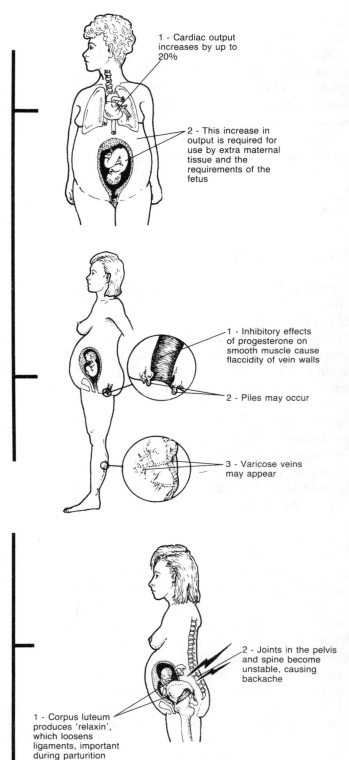

1 - Cardiac output increases by up to 20%

2 - This increase in output is required for use by extra maternal tissue and the requirements of the fetus

1 - Inhibitory effects of progesterone on smooth muscle cause flaccidity of vein walls

2 - Piles may occur

3 - Varicose veins may appear

2 - Joints in the pelvis and spine become unstable, causing backache

1 - Corpus luteum produces 'relaxin', which loosens ligaments, important during parturition

The respiratory system responds to pregnancy by increasing ventilation by about 40%, though oxygen uptake increases by only 20%. Respiratory movements become increasingly difficult in the later stages of pregnancy as the developing fetus occupies more and more of the abdominal cavity.

In the digestive system, the changes include an increased appetite to supply the fetus and extra tissues with nourishment. However, in the early weeks of pregnancy there is often troublesome nausea and vomiting ('morning sickness'), whose hormonal basis is poorly understood.

The mother also frequently suffers constipation, or dyspepsia due to slowed gastric emptying; this results partly from the inhibitory effects of progesterone on smooth muscle motility in general (see below), but is also due to the enlargement of the fetus and uterus within the abdomen.

The maternal kidney is called upon to eliminate the wastes from the fetus as well as the mother; there is often a tendency to retain fluid during pregnancy, though oedema, proteinuria and hypertension are pathological findings. The renal threshold for glucose is often raised, and mild harmless glycosuria is often detected.

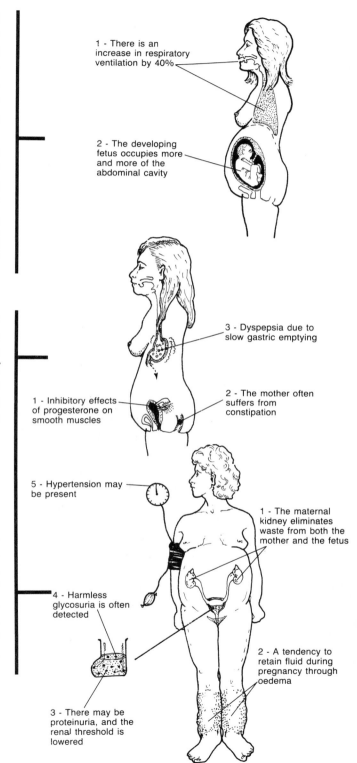

1 - There is an increase in respiratory ventilation by 40%

2 - The developing fetus occupies more and more of the abdominal cavity

3 - Dyspepsia due to slow gastric emptying

1 - Inhibitory effects of progesterone on smooth muscles

2 - The mother often suffers from constipation

5 - Hypertension may be present

1 - The maternal kidney eliminates waste from both the mother and the fetus

4 - Harmless glycosuria is often detected

2 - A tendency to retain fluid during pregnancy through oedema

3 - There may be proteinuria, and the renal threshold is lowered

Development of the fetus

Gestation or pregnancy in the human lasts on average nine months, or 40 weeks from the beginning of the menstrual period just before conception (i.e. about 38 weeks from the time of conception).

The first three months are largely occupied by differentiation of the fetal tissues to form primitive organs and organ systems; the second three months are occupied by an increase in complexity and maturity of all of the organ systems, and the third three months are largely spent in getting bigger and more able to lead an independent existence. The detailed changes during development are the province of the embryologist or anatomist.

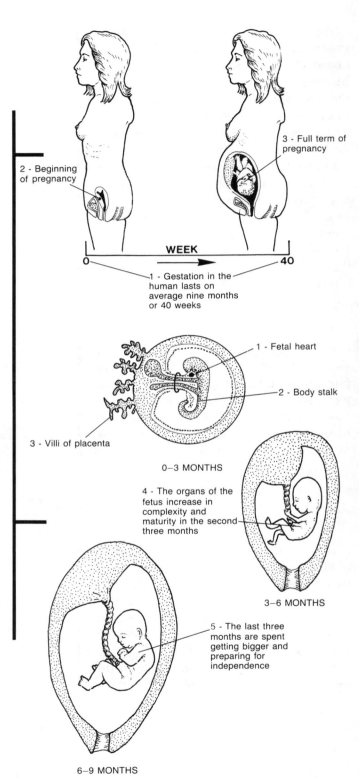

2 - Beginning of pregnancy

3 - Full term of pregnancy

WEEK

0   40

1 - Gestation in the human lasts on average nine months or 40 weeks

1 - Fetal heart

2 - Body stalk

3 - Villi of placenta

0–3 MONTHS

4 - The organs of the fetus increase in complexity and maturity in the second three months

3–6 MONTHS

5 - The last three months are spent getting bigger and preparing for independence

6–9 MONTHS

The fetal circulation develops at an early stage, and as well as pumping blood around the baby's own tissues the heart has to perfuse the placenta through the umbilical vessels to allow exchange of nutrients and wastes with the mother. The haemoglobin in fetal blood has a higher affinity for oxygen than maternal blood (the oxygen dissociation curve is shifted to the left), so the fetus is able to extract oxygen from the mother even at low oxygen tensions.

The fetal lungs develop, but since they are filled with fluid, not air, they have no very obvious function before birth; the main respiratory organ is the placenta.

Nevertheless, the fetus *in utero* has been observed to perform rhythmic thoracic movements very like breathing, and there is some evidence that this intra-uterine 'respiration' is essential for the maturation of the lungs and particularly for the production of alveolar surfactant.

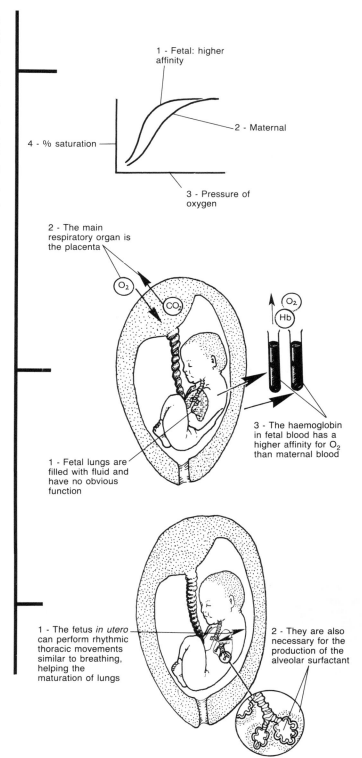

1 - Fetal: higher affinity

2 - Maternal

4 - % saturation

3 - Pressure of oxygen

2 - The main respiratory organ is the placenta

3 - The haemoglobin in fetal blood has a higher affinity for O_2 than maternal blood

1 - Fetal lungs are filled with fluid and have no obvious function

1 - The fetus *in utero* can perform rhythmic thoracic movements similar to breathing, helping the maturation of lungs

2 - They are also necessary for the production of the alveolar surfactant

The fetal kidneys produce urine which is shed into the amniotic cavity and contributes to the volume of amniotic fluid, but this is not an excretory function; the main excretory organ is the placenta, which transfers the fetal wastes to the mother.

The fetus drinks the amniotic fluid, and there is some passage of materials through the gut, although it is unusual for defaecation to occur *in utero* unless the fetus is distressed during labour.

The fetal nervous system increases in complexity during gestation, and there is often considerable motor activity, with much movement of limbs. The fetus is able to respond to noises, to pressures and even to light while it is in the uterus.

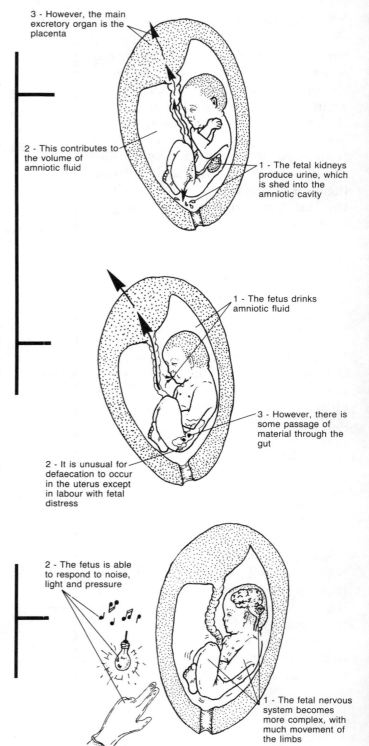

3 - However, the main excretory organ is the placenta

2 - This contributes to the volume of amniotic fluid

1 - The fetal kidneys produce urine, which is shed into the amniotic cavity

1 - The fetus drinks amniotic fluid

3 - However, there is some passage of material through the gut

2 - It is unusual for defaecation to occur in the uterus except in labour with fetal distress

2 - The fetus is able to respond to noise, light and pressure

1 - The fetal nervous system becomes more complex, with much movement of the limbs

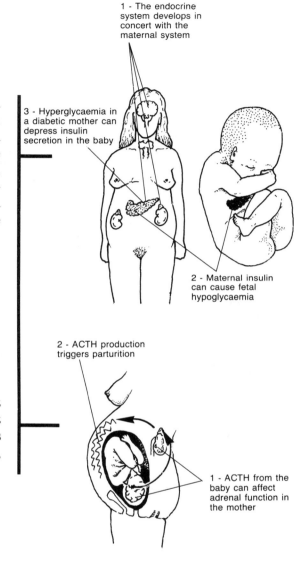

The endocrine system develops in concert with the maternal system; many of the maternal hormones can cross the placenta and influence the fetus, and vice versa. For instance, maternal insulin can cause fetal hypoglycaemia, and hyperglycaemia in a diabetic mother can depress the secretion of insulin by the baby.

1 - The endocrine system develops in concert with the maternal system

3 - Hyperglycaemia in a diabetic mother can depress insulin secretion in the baby

2 - Maternal insulin can cause fetal hypoglycaemia

ACTH from the baby can affect adrenal function in the mother, and it may be that a surge of fetal ACTH is the event that triggers parturition, signalling the end of pregnancy.

2 - ACTH production triggers parturition

1 - ACTH from the baby can affect adrenal function in the mother

Parturition

After nine months the fetus is expelled from the uterus. We are still uncertain as to the nature of the trigger for this event, but fetal secretion of ACTH, prostaglandins or hormones which have not yet been identified have all been suggested.

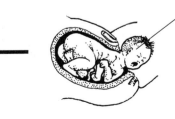

1 - After nine months the fetus is expelled from the uterus, possibly due to ACTH, prostaglandins or other hormones

The virgin or non-pregnant uterus has not much intrinsic spontaneous contractile activity, as the membrane of the smooth muscle cells is rather depolarized. Oestrogen hyperpolarizes the membrane slightly, bringing the potential into the range where spontaneous activity can occur; progesterone further hyperpolarizes the membrane so that the potential is too high for spontaneous activity to take place, and also reduces the efficacy of cell-to-cell conduction of excitation. The net result is that during most of pregnancy the motility of the uterus is suppressed. This depression of smooth muscle activity is also seen in other systems: the effects on the gut and veins have already been described.

At the end of pregnancy the block caused by progesterone is removed, making depolarization of the uterine smooth muscle possible.

The secretion of oxytocin by the pituitary and the release of prostaglandins stimulates the uterine muscle to undergo rhythmic waves of depolarization with action potentials and associated contractile activity, and labour begins.

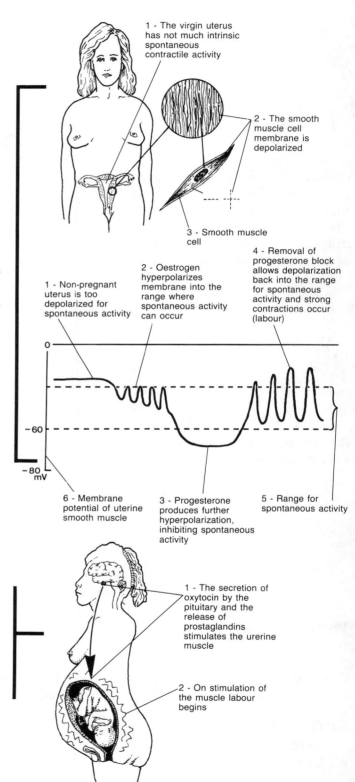

1 - The virgin uterus has not much intrinsic spontaneous contractile activity

2 - The smooth muscle cell membrane is depolarized

3 - Smooth muscle cell

1 - Non-pregnant uterus is too depolarized for spontaneous activity

2 - Oestrogen hyperpolarizes membrane into the range where spontaneous activity can occur

4 - Removal of progesterone block allows depolarization back into the range for spontaneous activity and strong contractions occur (labour)

6 - Membrane potential of uterine smooth muscle

3 - Progesterone produces further hyperpolarization, inhibiting spontaneous activity

5 - Range for spontaneous activity

1 - The secretion of oxytocin by the pituitary and the release of prostaglandins stimulates the urerine muscle

2 - On stimulation of the muscle labour begins

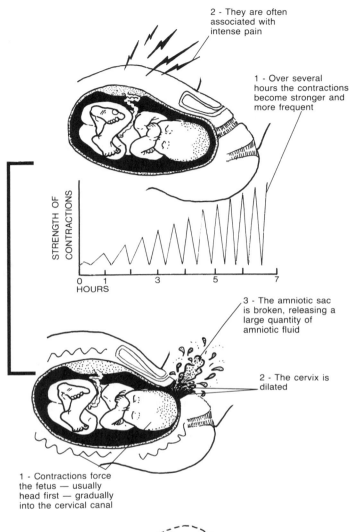

2 - They are often associated with intense pain

1 - Over several hours the contractions become stronger and more frequent

There is a series of rhythmic contractions and relaxations; at first they are weak and infrequent, but over several hours they become stronger, more frequent and more efficient. They are often associated with intense pain. Their first effect is to force the fetal presenting part (usually the head) gradually into the cervical canal, dilating the cervix and moving into the maternal pelvis. The amniotic sac is usually broken and considerable quantities of amniotic fluid are shed.

STRENGTH OF CONTRACTIONS

0 1   3   5   7
HOURS

3 - The amniotic sac is broken, releasing a large quantity of amniotic fluid

2 - The cervix is dilated

1 - Contractions force the fetus — usually head first — gradually into the cervical canal

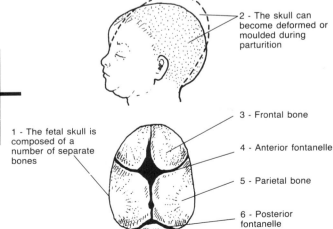

2 - The skull can become deformed or moulded during parturition

The fetal skull is composed of a number of separate bones which can move relative to one another, and the head can become considerably deformed or 'moulded' during this process.

1 - The fetal skull is composed of a number of separate bones

3 - Frontal bone

4 - Anterior fontanelle

5 - Parietal bone

6 - Posterior fontanelle

When the cervix has become fully dilated by the plunger-like action of the fetal head, the presenting part begins to move through the pelvic canal, considerably distorting the maternal anatomy in the process.

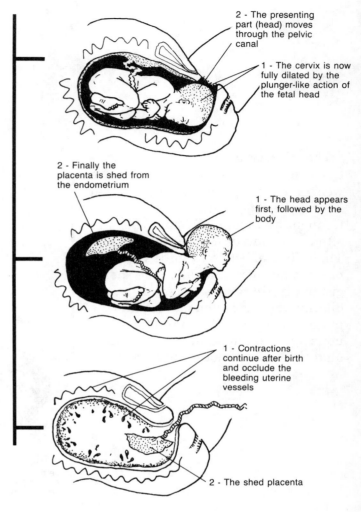

2 - The presenting part (head) moves through the pelvic canal

1 - The cervix is now fully dilated by the plunger-like action of the fetal head

2 - Finally the placenta is shed from the endometrium

1 - The head appears first, followed by the body

First the head and then all the rest of the body emerges into the outside world, and finally the placenta is shed from the endometrium.

1 - Contractions continue after birth and occlude the bleeding uterine vessels

Usually the contractions of the uterus continue and occlude the bleeding uterine vessels, forming 'muscular ligatures'.

2 - The shed placenta

Neonatal changes

Once it has been born, the infant has to change rapidly from being totally dependent upon the mother to coping with the outside world by itself.

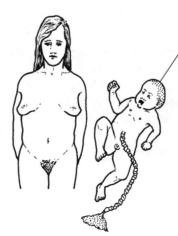

1 - Once the baby is born it must change to cope with the outside world itself

As soon as the umbilical link with the mother is interrupted, the baby must breathe for itself, derive its nutrition from its gut and excrete wastes through its own kidneys. It also has to regulate its own body temperature against environmental stresses, and its nervous system is exposed to a barrage of new stimuli by sight, sound, smell and feeling.

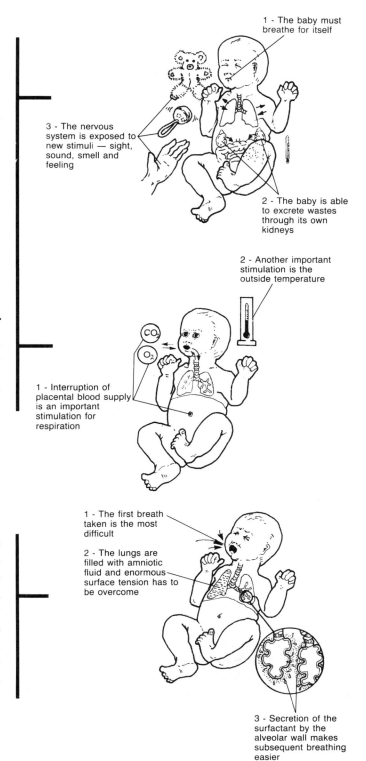

1 - The baby must breathe for itself

3 - The nervous system is exposed to new stimuli — sight, sound, smell and feeling

2 - The baby is able to excrete wastes through its own kidneys

The hypoxia due to interruption of the placental blood supply is an important stimulus to respiration, but cold and the general sensory stimulation of the outside world are other contributory factors.

2 - Another important stimulation is the outside temperature

1 - Interruption of placental blood supply is an important stimulation for respiration

The first breath the baby takes is probably the most difficult in its whole life, as it has to inflate fluid-filled lungs with air, and enormous surface tension forces have to be overcome. Normally the presence of pulmonary surfactant makes subsequent breathing easier, but premature babies lacking surfactant have continuing problems with respiration.

1 - The first breath taken is the most difficult

2 - The lungs are filled with amniotic fluid and enormous surface tension has to be overcome

3 - Secretion of the surfactant by the alveolar wall makes subsequent breathing easier

Hypoxia is also the stimulus for several changes in the cardiovascular system. The fetal circulation differs from that of the neonate and adult in having a number of shunts between the right and left sides of the heart, and in having the umbilical vessels. Blood returning from the fetal tissues to the right atrium is mixed with blood from the umbilical vein.

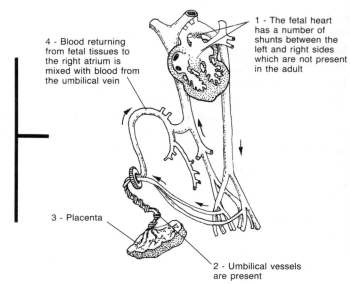

4 - Blood returning from fetal tissues to the right atrium is mixed with blood from the umbilical vein

1 - The fetal heart has a number of shunts between the left and right sides which are not present in the adult

3 - Placenta

2 - Umbilical vessels are present

Since there is no air in the lungs, there is little point in perfusing the lungs and most of the blood in the right atrium passes through the **foramen ovale** into the left atrium for pumping to the rest of the body.

2 - Left atrium

3 - Right atrium

4 - Superior vena cava

1 - The foramen ovale, through which most of the blood from the right atrium to the left atrium passes

5 - Inferior vena cava

The blood passing from the right atrium into the right ventricle is similarly diverted away from the lungs and into the systemic circulation through the **ductus arteriosus**, an arterial connection between the pulmonary artery and the aorta.

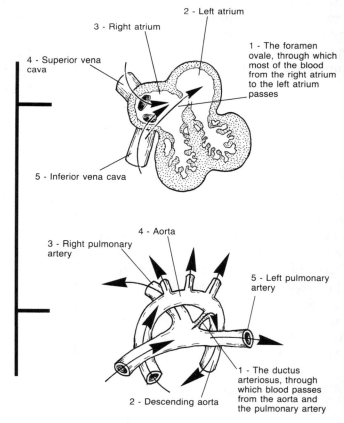

4 - Aorta

3 - Right pulmonary artery

5 - Left pulmonary artery

1 - The ductus arteriosus, through which blood passes from the aorta and the pulmonary artery

2 - Descending aorta

Following birth the placental vessels are removed from the circulation. The removal of a major parallel pathway increases systemic vascular resistance and raises systemic arterial pressure, causing the pressure in the left atrium to rise and tending to close the foramen ovale. At the same time the inflation of the lungs reduces right-sided vascular resistance and causes a lower pressure in the right atrium, helping to close the foramen ovale.

3 - Inflation of the lungs reduces right-sided vascular resistance

4 - This causes a lower pressure in the right atrium which helps to close the foramen ovale

1 - Following birth the placental vessels are removed from the circulation

2 - Systemic arterial pressure and vascular resistance increase

An increase in oxygen tension affects the smooth muscle of the ductus arteriosus, causing it to go into spasm and thus closing off the other major right-to-left shunt, and within a few minutes or hours after birth the circulation is transformed into a full dual system like that of the adult.

1 - Increase in O$_2$ tension causes the smooth muscle of the ductus to go into spasm

2 - Within a few hours (or minutes) after birth the circulation is transformed into a dual system

The newborn infant has to perform thermoregulation as soon as it is separated from its mother; this is often inefficient for several hours or days, particularly if the infant is premature. The smaller the infant, the greater is the ratio of surface area to volume and therefore the greater is the potential problem of heat loss.

1 - The newborn baby has to perform thermoregulation as soon as it is separated from its mother

2 - This is often inefficient for several hours or days

3 - The smaller the infant the greater is the ratio of surface area to volume

4 - The potential problem of heat loss is greater

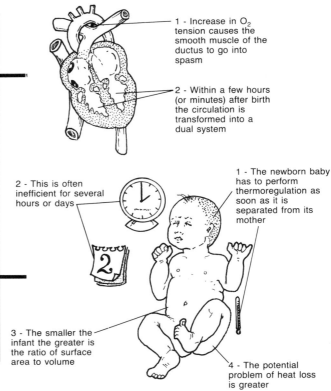

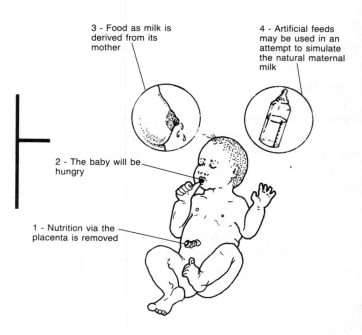

Soon after its removal from direct nutrition via the placenta, the baby will be hungry and will require to feed. It either derives its food as milk from its mother (see below) or it has to be given artificial feeds which attempt to simulate the natural maternal milk.

Lactation

Milk is secreted by the mother's breasts or **mammary glands**, situated on the anterior thoracic wall. The breasts are modified sweat glands, capable of intense secretory activity.

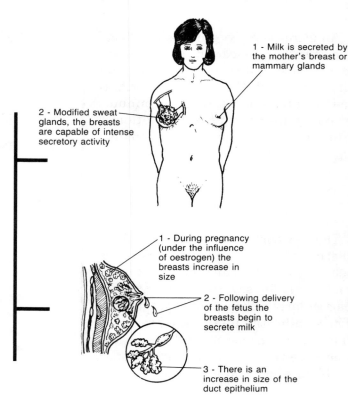

For most of a woman's life they are quiescent, but during pregnancy under the influence of oestrogens they increase in size, with proliferation of duct epithelium, and following delivery of the fetus they begin to secrete milk.

Their development and the secretion of milk are under the control of the anterior pituitary hormone **prolactin** (which is, in turn, regulated by the hypothalamic **prolactin inhibitory factor**).

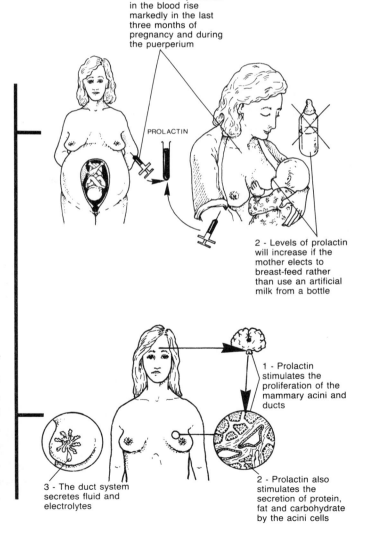

1 - Breast development and the secretion of milk are under the control of the anterior pituitary hormone prolactin

2 - Prolactin secretion is regulated by the hypothalamic prolactin inhibitory factor

1 - Levels of prolactin in the blood rise markedly in the last three months of pregnancy and during the puerperium

The levels of prolactin in the blood rise markedly in the last three months of pregnancy and during the puerperium, particularly if the mother elects to breast-feed her infant rather than feeding with artificial milk from a bottle.

PROLACTIN

2 - Levels of prolactin will increase if the mother elects to breast-feed rather than use an artificial milk from a bottle

Prolactin stimulates proliferation of mammary acini and ducts; it also stimulates the secretion of protein, fat and carbohydrate by the acinar cells and the secretion of fluid and electrolytes by the duct system. An increase in prolactin secretion is caused by a decrease in secretion of prolactin inhibitory factor by the hypothalamus.

1 - Prolactin stimulates the proliferation of the mammary acini and ducts

3 - The duct system secretes fluid and electrolytes

2 - Prolactin also stimulates the secretion of protein, fat and carbohydrate by the acini cells

The mechanism of protein synthesis and secretion in the breast is identical to that in the pancreas (see chapter on the digestive system). Ribosomes at the basal end of the acinar cells assemble the amino acid chains; these are gathered together into clumps and packaged by the Golgi apparatus into granules, which are subsequently released at the apices of the acinar cells by a process of exocytosis.

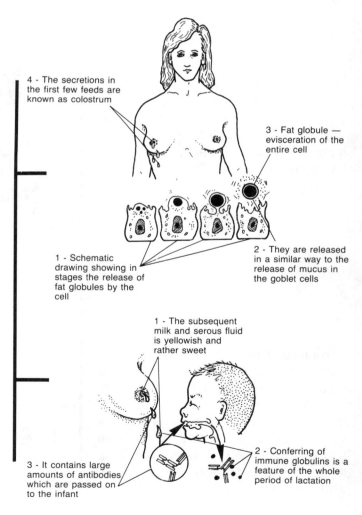

4 - Acinar cells

3 - Ribosome

2 - Ribosomes at the basal end of the acinar cells assemble the amino acid chain together into granules, which are released at the apices of the cells by a process of exocytosis

1 - The mechanism of protein synthesis and secretion in the breast is identical to that in the pancreas

Fats are synthesized by other cells into large globules which are released in a manner rather similar to the way in which the mucus of goblet cells is released: essentially the evisceration of the entire cell.

The secretions in the first few feeds after birth are different from the normal milk, and are known as **colostrum**.

4 - The secretions in the first few feeds are known as colostrum

3 - Fat globule — evisceration of the entire cell

2 - They are released in a similar way to the release of mucus in the goblet cells

1 - Schematic drawing showing in stages the release of fat globules by the cell

There is much less protein or fat than in the subsequent milk, and the yellowish serous fluid is rather sweet. It contains large amounts of antibodies, conferring passive immunity on the infant; the secretion of immune globulins is a feature of the whole period of lactation.

1 - The subsequent milk and serous fluid is yellowish and rather sweet

2 - Conferring of immune globulins is a feature of the whole period of lactation

3 - It contains large amounts of antibodies which are passed on to the infant

Between the infant's feeds a considerable quantity of milk accumulates within the duct system, and when the infant begins to suckle the sensory nerve endings around the nipple are stimulated, relaying an intense sensory volley to the central nervous system. Signals reaching the hypothalamus make the posterior pituitary gland secrete oxytocin, which travels in the blood to reach the mammary gland and causes contraction of the **myo-epithelial cells** lining the walls of the mammary ducts. The contraction ejects the stored milk from the nipple — the so-called 'let-down' reflex.

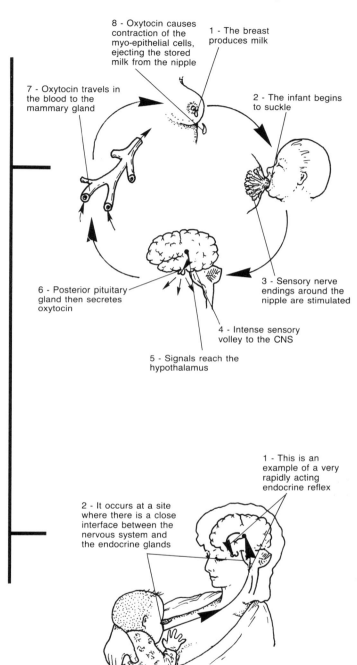

8 - Oxytocin causes contraction of the myo-epithelial cells, ejecting the stored milk from the nipple

1 - The breast produces milk

7 - Oxytocin travels in the blood to the mammary gland

2 - The infant begins to suckle

6 - Posterior pituitary gland then secretes oxytocin

3 - Sensory nerve endings around the nipple are stimulated

4 - Intense sensory volley to the CNS

5 - Signals reach the hypothalamus

This is an instance of a very rapidly acting endocrine reflex, occurring at a site where there is a close interface between the nervous system and the endocrine glands.

1 - This is an example of a very rapidly acting endocrine reflex

2 - It occurs at a site where there is a close interface between the nervous system and the endocrine glands

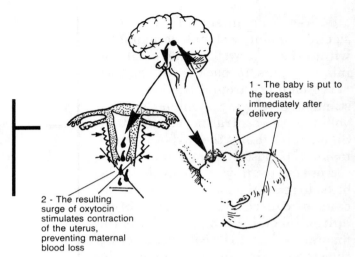

If a baby is put to the breast immediately after delivery, the reflexly secreted surge of oxytocin is very beneficial in stimulating contraction of the uterus and preventing maternal blood loss.

1 - The baby is put to the breast immediately after delivery

2 - The resulting surge of oxytocin stimulates contraction of the uterus, preventing maternal blood loss

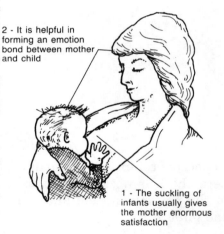

The suckling of infants usually gives the mother enormous satisfaction, and is very helpful in forming an emotional bond between mother and child.

2 - It is helpful in forming an emotion bond between mother and child

1 - The suckling of infants usually gives the mother enormous satisfaction

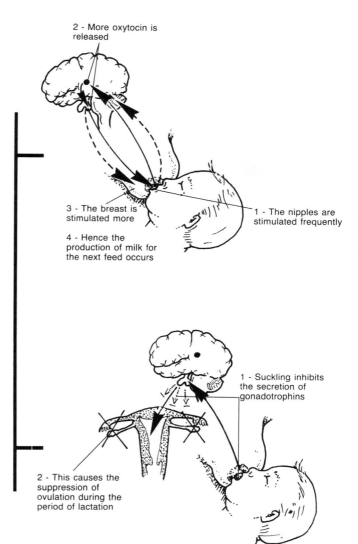

2 - More oxytocin is released

3 - The breast is stimulated more

4 - Hence the production of milk for the next feed occurs

1 - The nipples are stimulated frequently

The more the nipples are subsequently stimulated by suckling, the more oxytocin is released and the more the breast is stimulated; suckling also promotes the secretion of prolactin and hence the production of milk for the next feed.

1 - Suckling inhibits the secretion of gonadotrophins

2 - This causes the suppression of ovulation during the period of lactation

It also inhibits the secretion of gonadotrophins and hence suppresses ovulation during the period of lactation, though this is by no means reliable as a method of contraception.

Index

Index compiled by John Gibson